the
newborn baby

fifth edition

the
newborn baby

fifth edition

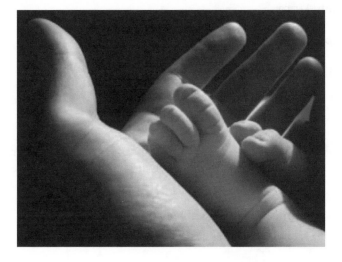

VC HARRISON
MMed (UCT), MD (UCT), DCH (RCP & S)
Emeritus Associate Professor
School of Child and Adolescent Health, University of Cape Town

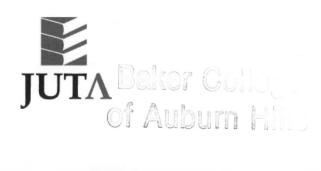

JUTA

The Newborn Baby: Fifth edition

First published 1978
Third edition 1996
Second impression 1999
Fourth edition 2002
Reprinted 2004
Fifth edition 2008
Reprinted 2008

Juta & Company Ltd
Mercury Crescent
Wetton, 7780
Cape Town, South Africa

© **2008** Juta & Company Ltd

ISBN 978 0 702 17708 8

Disclaimer
The author and publisher have exerted every effort to ensure that drug selections and dosages set forth in this text are in accord with current recommendations and practice at the time of publication. However, readers are urged to check the package insert for each drug for any change in indications of dosage and for added warnings and precautions. The information in this book is provided in good faith. The author and publisher cannot be held responsible for errors, individual responses to drugs and other consequences.

Typeset in 10/12 Palatino Regular

Project Manager: Sarah O'Neill
Editor: Danya Ristić
Illustrator: Bronwen Lusted
Typesetter: Mckore Graphics, Parow, Cape Town
Cover designer: Pumphaus Design Studio
Printed in South Africa by Mills Litho, Cape Town.

Contents

Preface

Most newborn babies are normal. But what is normal? Does this include a non-retractable foreskin, enlarged breasts or vaginal bleeding in the first week? These features are of concern to parents and throughout this book the acceptable variations of structure and function are stressed. 'Do no harm' is a primary consideration in Medicine so it is essential to master the range of normal. Only then will the abnormal become obvious.

Common problems such as colic, constipation and feeding difficulties are rarely addressed by the experts who care for sick infants; they have neither the time nor the inclination. But these complaints comprise a significant proportion of a health professional's consultations, particularly in primary care units, and are therefore covered in the relevant sections of this book.

Even a healthy newborn baby is susceptible to noxious factors such as hypothermia, hypoxaemia, hypoglycaemia, hyperbilirubinaemia and infection. Prevention is essential and the risks and treatment of these complications are discussed in detail.

Most students, nurses and doctors have little or no contact with very ill babies in intensive care units and consequently this matter is not fully addressed. This textbook therefore is not suited to those who wish to specialise in Neonatology.

Lastly, a mother knows best. She has an intimate knowledge of her infant and can sense deviations from normal before they are obvious. Never ignore her concerns. You will regret it!

Vincent Harrison

About the author

Vincent Harrison graduated in Medicine at the University of Cape Town and obtained his degree in Paediatrics from the same institution. Following a three year fellowship in Neonatology at Groote Schuur and Vanderbilt University (USA) hospitals he was appointed to the first dedicated neonatal post in South Africa at Mowbray Maternity Hospital. During his tenure from 1968 to 1999 he pursued interests in fetal physiology and in respiratory and gastrointestinal function. His work in these fields has been published in a variety of peer-reviewed journals and books. He was privileged to experience the great advances in Neonatology during the 1960's and 1970's that have now realised the best care that babies have ever received. However, significant problems remain unsolved, prematurity and hypoxic brain damage being most pressing. He believes that these can only be addressed in association with Obstetric colleagues and anticipates a fruitful combination of skills in the future.

CHAPTER 1

Perinatal Terminology

The care of newborn babies received a tremendous boost in the 1960s with the introduction of intensive care, remarkable discoveries, technical innovations and a better understanding of physiology. Within several decades the infant mortality and morbidity rates (*mortalis* = fatal; *morbidus* = sick) had declined significantly in industrialised countries, but these factors complemented the excellent standards of housing, income, nutrition and antenatal care that already existed. The benefits of recent advances can be experienced only once the basic structures for adequate health of mother and baby have been established. Currently, South Africa is still in a transitional stage.

Half of the deaths in early life, for example birth asphyxia, occur within hours or days of delivery, and most of the predisposing factors are present before birth.

This has prompted a detailed study of fetal well-being, and has led to the development of perinatology (*peri* = around), a specialised field in which obstetric and paediatric care are closely associated. The following definitions are pertinent to this phase of life.

PERIODS

Pregnancy

This is timed from the first day of a mother's last menstrual period and its duration is expressed in completed weeks. Pregnancy is divided into three stages:

1. *First trimester*, which includes the first 13 weeks.
2. *Second trimester*, which extends from 14 to 26 weeks.
3. *Third trimester*, which dates from 27 weeks to birth.

Perinatal period

This extends from the 24th week of pregnancy, which is the approximate time of infant viability, to the end of the first week of life.

Neonatal period

This starts at birth and ends after a month (28 days). It is divided into the:

- *early neonatal period*, which extends from birth to seven completed days
- *late neonatal period*, which begins on the 8th day and ends on the 28th day.

BIRTHS AND DEATHS

Standard definitions based on birthweight are used by the World Health

Organisation (WHO) so that perinatal statistics may be meaningful throughout the world. Weight is often the only measurement recorded on infants in underdeveloped regions. A baby with a birthweight of 500 grams (g) is approximately 24 weeks' gestation and is considered to be viable, while one of 1 000 g is about 28 weeks' gestation.

In South African law, viability extends from six months, and those under 1 000 g who die do not require a death certificate. However, for international comparisons, statistics should include all infants of 500 g or more.

Live birth
This is a baby over 500 g in weight, irrespective of gestation, who shows signs of life after delivery, that is, heartbeats, respirations or muscle movements.

Stillbirth
An infant over 500 g in weight, irrespective of gestation, who shows no signs of life after delivery is considered to be stillborn.

Abortion
This refers to a fetus of less than 500 g in weight who may or may not show evidence of life after delivery.

It also refers to the expulsion or extraction of the placenta or membranes without an identifiable fetus.

Neonatal death
Infants who die within 28 days of birth are classified as neonatal deaths. A further division includes:
- *early neonatal death*, which refers to the death of an infant within the first week

- *late neonatal death*, which includes the death of an infant between 8 and 28 days.

Perinatal death
Stillborn infants and babies who die within the first week (early neonatal death) are included in this category.

MORTALITY RATES
Neonatal mortality rate
This is expressed as the number of neonatal deaths per 1 000 liveborn infants.

Perinatal mortality rate
This includes stillbirths and early neonatal deaths and is expressed per 1 000 total births.

It is a sensitive index of the health of the mother and baby and reflects the quality of ante- and postnatal care.

A steady decline has occurred in industrialised countries and the major causes of death worldwide include prematurity, asphyxia, infection and congenital abnormalities.

LOW BIRTHWEIGHT RATE
Infants who weigh less than 2 500 g at birth are considered to be of low birthweight. Many are born prematurely (p. 60) and some, though born at term, have suffered impaired growth *in utero* (p. 76).

The rate of low birthweight babies is a manifestation of the health of a community. The rate is calculated by multiplying the number of infants of less than 2 500 g by 100 and dividing the result by the total number of births. In underdeveloped regions, the rate can be as high as 15% – twice that of industrialised countries.

CHAPTER 2

Intrauterine Growth and Gestational Age

INTRAUTERINE GROWTH

Human development and growth are customarily divided into pre- and post-natal stages.

Prenatal period

The remarkable transformation of a single cell into a complex individual begins at fertilisation, when an oocyte and a sperm combine to form the zygote. The zygote divides into a multicellular morula and then into a blastocyst, which is implanted in the uterus to form an embryo (Fig. 2.1).

The embryonic period is concerned with the formation of major organs and extends from the second to the ninth week.

The developing human is now a fetus until birth.

Fetal growth

The overall rate of growth accelerates in a linear fashion in the fetus and body

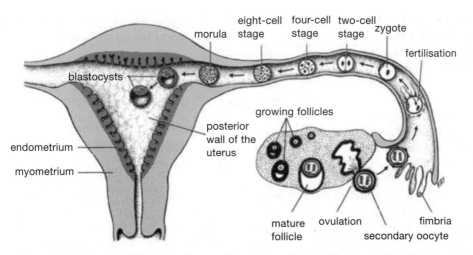

Fig. 2.1 *The early stages of human development (From Moore, K. 1977.* The Developing Human. *2 ed. Philadelphia: WB Saunders)*

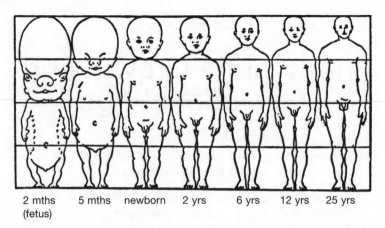

| 2 mths (fetus) | 5 mths | newborn | 2 yrs | 6 yrs | 12 yrs | 25 yrs |

Fig. 2.2 *Stages of growth: Relative proportions of head, trunk and limbs for various ages (From Robbins, WJ et al. 1928.* Growth. *New Haven: Yale University Press)*

proportions alter significantly. The head and brain, for example, are relatively larger than at any other stage of life (Fig. 2.2).

Growth curves for weight, length and surface area are shown in Fig. 2.3. The maximum velocity in linear growth occurs at about 20 weeks' and in weight gain at approximately 34 weeks' gestation.

Fetal growth is influenced by important factors such as:
- chromosomes
- energy and food substrates
- hormones
- uteroplacental blood supply.

Chromosomes: While fetal genes determine ultimate size after birth, they hardly influence intrauterine growth, which depends on maternal rather than paternal size. A small woman produces small babies, presumably because of a small uterus and placenta.

Abnormal chromosomes impair fetal growth, as seen in Down's syndrome (p. 117) and trisomy 18 (p. 119).

Energy and food: Glucose is the main source of energy for the fetus and is obtained continuously from the mother. It is essential for normal fetal growth and metabolism, and the blood level is about two-thirds that of the mother.

Amino acids also cross the placenta and significantly influence fetal growth, which is impaired if the mother is depleted of proteins.

Other substrates include lipids, ketones and acetate.

Hormones: Insulin is an important growth hormone. It does not cross the placenta, and is produced by the fetal pancreas. It promotes the cellular uptake of amino acids which are then converted into protein, particularly in the liver, skeletal muscle and heart.

Blood supply: An adequate blood supply to the intervillus space ensures that sufficient oxygen and nutrients can reach the fetus. The blood supply increases during pregnancy, but its mode of regulation is as yet unknown. Oestrogen may play a role in enhancing placental blood flow.

Fetal maturation
The last weeks of pregnancy probably constitute a stage of fetal 'ripening' and are associated with major changes in maternal hormones. Plasma oestrogen rises, while the progesterone level falls, and this coincides with increased formation of liver glycogen in the fetus, the deposition of additional subcutaneous

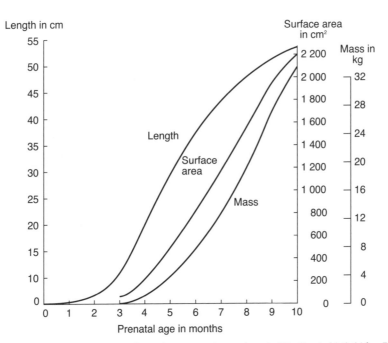

Fig. 2.3 *Graphs of prenatal growth: Length, surface area and mass from fertilisation to birth (After Boyd, E. In: Anson, BJ. 1966. Morris Human Anatomy. 12 ed. New York: McGraw Hill)*

fat, and the maturation of organs such as the lungs, liver and gut.

This process is usually completed by the beginning of the 38th week. Most (80%) normal babies are born between 38 and 42 weeks' gestation and are referred to as 'term' infants. At this stage, their chance of survival and normal development is optimal.

Infants who are born before the 38th week are considered to be 'preterm' or premature, as most have not experienced these changes and have immature organs.

Organ maturation accelerates when intrauterine growth is impaired, probably in anticipation of early birth, and the lungs of a growth-retarded fetus usually mature before the 38th week.

Birth before the 38th week or after the 42nd week is associated with increased morbidity and mortality rates.

Postnatal period

The quality of intrauterine growth is reflected in the weight, length and head circumference of a newborn baby. These are plotted on percentile charts that indicate the normal range for a particular gestational age.

Weight
Method
See p. 12.

Normal weight
The weights of most babies fall between the 10th and 90th percentile on a growth chart (Fig. 2.4). This range is termed 'appropriate for gestational age'.

Normal variations in weight may be related to the following:
Sex – female babies tend to be lighter than males.

Parity – first-born babies are often lighter than subsequent ones.

Maternal weight gain – large gains in weight during pregnancy are associated with heavy babies.

Parental size – small parents tend to have small babies.

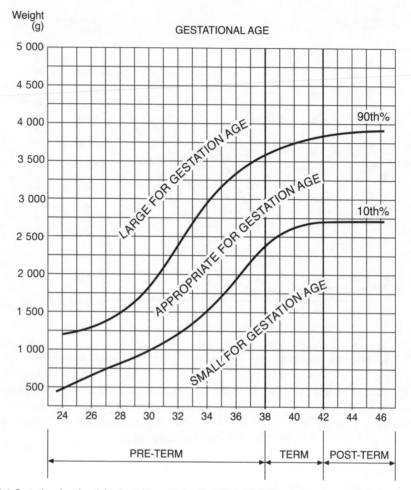

Fig. 2.4 *Gestational and weight chart (From Battaglia, FC and Lubchenco, LO. 1967. J Pediatr 71: 159–63)*

Social group – differences occur in various social groups, for example babies from high socioeconomic groups weigh more than those from less affluent groups. These variations are probably related to socioeconomic factors.

Height above sea level – babies born at sea level tend to weigh more than those born at high altitudes. The chart for weight in Fig. 2.4 was drawn up for babies born at a high altitude in Colorado and the 10th percentile is equivalent to the 3rd percentile at sea level.

Multiple pregnancy – on average, twins are smaller than singletons.

Abnormal weight
The pattern of growth is considered to be abnormal if an infant's weight falls outside the 10th or 90th percentile for a specific gestational age.

Birthweight below 10th percentile: An infant with a weight below the 10th percentile is underweight or 'small for gestational age'. The various factors that may impair intrauterine growth are discussed on p. 76.

Birthweight above 90th percentile: An infant in this category is considered to be over-weight or 'large for gestational age'. Factors associated with excessive growth are discussed on p. 80.

Length

Method
See p. 12.

Normal length (Fig. 2.5)
Variations in length can be related to the following:
Sex – males tend to be longer than females.
Altitude – infants born at high altitudes tend to be shorter at birth than those born at sea level.

Abnormal length
Abnormally long babies are seen in cases of fetal hypothyroidism (p. 276).

Abnormally short babies may be seen in dwarfism, such as achondroplasia (p. 282), and type I intrauterine growth retardation (p. 77).

Head circumference

This is an important measurement at birth as it indirectly reflects fetal brain growth.

Method
See p. 12.
Growth curves are illustrated in Fig. 2.6.

Normal variations
Sex – males tend to have larger heads than females at birth.
Altitude – infants born at high altitudes tend to have smaller heads than those born at sea level.

Abnormal measurements
A head circumference below the normal range may be associated with:
- microcephaly (p. 138)
- small-for-gestation infant (p. 76).

Head measurements above the normal range may be owing to:
- hydrocephalus (p. 136)
- intracranial bleeding or cerebral oedema (p. 141)
- megalencephaly (p. 138).

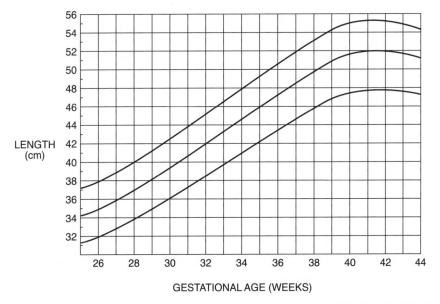

Fig. 2.5 *Percentile chart for length (From Usher, R and McLean, F. 1969. J Pediatr **74**: 901–10)*

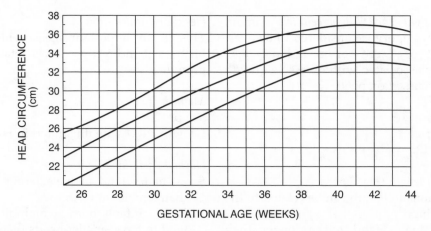

Fig. 2.6 *Percentile chart for head circumference (From Usher, R and McLean, F. 1969.* J Pediatr **74**: 901–10)

Body proportions (Fig. 2.2)

Proportions of the neonate vary considerably from those of the child or adult. For example, at birth the head forms 25% of the total body length, compared with 11% in adulthood.

The umbilicus of the newborn is situated about 2,5 cm below the middle of the body, and lower limbs are shorter than the trunk.

TABLE 2.1

Other body measurements at birth	
Measurement	*cm*
Sitting height	33,5
Arm length	20,0
Leg length	19,0
Foot length	8,3
Hand length	7,2
Thorax circumference (in nipple line)	32,2

The ratio of crown to symphysis pubis and symphysis pubis to soles of feet measurement is 1,7:1 at birth. This diminishes progressively to reach 1:1 at 10 years of age. In other words, when the child is 10 years old, the symphysis pubis forms the mid-point of the body.

The cranial vault, that is, the portion that contains the brain, is relatively large in the newborn in comparison with the face. Facial bones grow rapidly so that by adulthood the face forms the larger portion of the head as a whole.

ESTIMATION OF GESTATIONAL AGE
Before birth

During pregnancy, gestational age can be estimated from the following:

Menstrual history: The period of amenorrhoea is probably the most reliable single sign for estimating the duration of pregnancy. It is measured from the first day of the last menstrual period.

Physical signs and symptoms: Fundal height, fetal size and the onset of movement offer a clinical guide to gestational age.

Special investigations:
Human chorionic gonadotropin: When the fertilised ovum is implanted in the uterus, this hormone, produced by the embryo, gains access to the maternal circulation. It can be detected in urine between 23 and 28 days (menstrual).

Ultrasound: This detects the embryo between 32 and 35 days and determines gestational age most accurately before 20 weeks.

Measurements: Serial skull measurements (bipariatal diameter) may be made after 11 weeks. Other measurements include crown–rump length (before 13 weeks) and femur length (after 11 weeks).

After birth

Infants are divided into the following categories depending on their age (Fig. 2.4):
- Preterm – less than 37 completed weeks, or 259 days.
- Term, or full-term – 38 to 42 weeks.
- Post-term – more than 42 weeks.

The accuracy of estimating gestational age can be enhanced through the use of various scoring systems that evaluate physical or neurological characteristics.

The Farr system

This system is based on physical signs only. It is easy to perform and sufficiently accurate for the majority of infants.

To ensure accuracy:
- assess an infant within five days of birth
- keep the baby warm during the examination
- determine skin colour before the baby cries.

Method

Eleven external features are assessed (Table 2.3). Each is assigned a score, for example 0, 1, 2, 3, etc. A half-score is recorded when the assessment falls between two definitions. Low scores imply immature signs, whereas high scores indicate mature features.

The total score is read off a chart to give gestational age (Table 2.2).

An approximation of gestation

Formal gestation scoring is rarely done in busy primary care units. Nevertheless a distinction should be made between term and preterm. This can be done rapidly and fairly accurately by noting the birthweight and the presence or absence of breast nodules, which appear under the areola at 36 weeks of gestation and can be felt between a forefinger and thumb. An infant under 2 500 g with palpable breast tissue is likely to be mature and close to term. One without breast nodules and weighing less than 2 500 g is probably under 36 weeks of gestation and thus is preterm.

Posture of the limbs offers a further subdivision for the preterm infant: good flexion implies a gestation over 32 weeks.

TABLE 2.2

Conversion of total maturity score to predicted gestational age					
Score	Gestational age (wks)	Score	Gestational age (wks)	Score	Gestational age (wks)
5	28,1	15	35,9	25	40,3
6	29,0	16	36,5	26	40,6
7	29,9	17	37,1	27	40,8
8	30,8	18	37,6	28	41,0
9	31,6	19	38,1	29	41,1
10	32,4	20	38,5	30	41,2
11	33,2	21	39,0	31	41,3
12	33,9	22	39,4	32	41,4
13	34,6	23	39,7	33	41,4
14	35,3	24	40,0	34	41,4

*(From Farr, V; Kerrigde, DF; Mitchell, RG. 1966. **Develop Med Child Neurol** 8: 657–80)*

TABLE 2.3

External (superficial) criteria						
External sign	0	1	2	3	4	Assessment of external features
Oedema	Obvious oedema of hands and feet, pitting over tibia	No obvious oedema of hands and feet, pitting over tibia	No oedema			Skin over the lower tibia is depressed with a finger for five seconds
Skin texture	Very thin, gelatinous	Thin and smooth	Smooth, medium thickness. Rash or superficial peeling	Slight thickening. Superficial cracking and peeling, especially hands and feet	Thick and parchment-like, superficial or deep cracking	Assessed by inspection and picking up a fold of abdominal skin
Skin colour	Dark red	Uniformly pink	Pale pink variable over body	Pale. Only pink over ears, lips, palms or soles		This sign is noted while baby is quiet or sleeping, as crying alters the colour
Skin opacity	Numerous veins and venules clearly seen, especially over abdomen	Veins and tributaries seen	A few large vessels clearly seen over abdomen	A few large vessels seen indistinctly over abdomen	No blood vessels seen	Veins over the abdomen are inspected in a good light
Lanugo	No lanugo	Abundant: long and thick over whole back	Hair thinning, especially over lower back	Small amount of lanugo and bald areas	At least half of back devoid of lanugo	Infant is held up to a good light and hair on back is inspected
Plantar creases	No skin creases	Faint red marks over anterior half of sole	Definite red marks over more than anterior half; indentations over less than anterior third	Indentations over more than anterior third	Definite deep indentations over more than anterior third	Creases on the sole of the foot are assessed with toes extended
Nipple formation	Nipple barely visible; no areola	Nipple well defined; areola not raised	Areola edge raised			Areola and nipple are observed in a good light
Breast size	No breast tissue palpable	Breast tissue on one or both sides < 0,5 cm	Breast tissue both sides; one or both 0,5–1,0 cm	Breast tissue both sides; one or both > 1 cm		Size and amount of tissue are determined by palpation between finger and thumb
Ear form	Pinna flat and shapeless, little or no incurving of edge	Incurving of part of edge of pinna	Partial incurving whole of upper pinna	Well-defined incurving whole of upper pinna		The upper portion of the ear is inspected above external meatus
Ear firmness	Pinna soft, easily folded, no recoil	Pinna soft, easily folded, slow recoil	Cartilage to edge of pinna, soft in places, ready recoil	Pinna firm, cartilage to edge, instant recoil		Edge of the upper pinna is rolled between finger and thumb to feel cartilage
Genitalia: Male	Neither testis in scrotum	At least one testis high in scrotum	At least one testis right down			Testes are palpated with a finger, starting at the inguinal canal and working towards scrotum to detect a retractile testis
Genitalia: Female	Labia majora widely separated, labia minora protruding	Labia majora almost cover labia minora	Labia majora completely cover labia minora			Legs are abducted to inspect labia

(From Farr V, Kerrigde DF, Mitchell RG. 1966. *Develop Med Child Neurol* 8: 657–80)

CHAPTER 3

The Physical Examination

PERINATAL INFORMATION

The health of a baby is significantly influenced by that of the mother and by factors that may have occurred during pregnancy, labour and birth. The relevant information is obtained from obstetric and anaesthetic records, and can be summarised on an Infant Card (Figs. 3.1 and 3.2) by staff in the labour ward. Study the following details before examining the baby.

Mother
Name
Age
Marital status
Socioeconomic status
Blood group and VDRL
Illnesses, for example diabetes, anaemia, heart disease

Fetus
Lie and presentation
Growth and movements *in utero*
Heart-rate pattern before and during labour

Pregnancy
Expected date of delivery
Complications, for example pregnancy-induced hypertension, urinary tract infection, vaginal bleeding
Drugs, for example smoking, alcohol, sedatives, diuretics, antibiotics, contraceptives, anticonvulsants, antipyretics
Infections, for example HIV, syphilis, herpes, cytomegalo virus, toxoplasmosis, rubella

Labour
Onset – spontaneous or induced
Drugs – sedatives, analgesics, anaesthetics

Induction agents, for example prosta-glandin, oxytocin
Duration of first and second stages
Duration of rupture of membranes
Amount and colour of liquor
Maternal pyrexia
Signs of chorioaminonitis

Birth
Time and date
Mode – vertex, breech, section
Instruments – vacuum, forceps
Apgar rating
Resuscitation
Meconium-staining

Placenta
Weight
Cord
Maternal surface
Fetal surface

Also obtain information regarding previous pregnancies and the birthweights and health of other children.

After birth
Record the following details of the baby:
- Vitamin K_1 injection.
- Identification.
- Blood group.
- Gestational age.
- BCG and polio immunisation at discharge.

Measurements
Weight
Length
Head circumference

These are usually determined soon after birth.

Weight
Place the unclothed infant in a weighing pan lined with a clean strip of paper towelling, and read the weight on the scale.
A suitable weighing scale should:

- have a pan large enough to accommodate a newborn baby
- be unaffected by movement of the infant
- measure to the nearest 10 g
- be mobile and rest on a flat surface.

The accuracy of the instrument ought to be checked against known weights several times a year.

At birth, most full-term babies weigh between 2 700 and 3 800 g (Fig. 2.4, p. 6).

Length
Crown–heel length is measured in a calibrated crib (Fig. 3.3).

Place the baby supine with the head touching the upper end and knees pressed to the surface to keep the legs straight.

Bring the movable board up to the feet, which are held at right angles to the surface.

The length of a full-term baby averages 51 cm, with a range of 48 to 54 cm (Fig. 2.5, p. 7).

If a calibrated crib is not available, don't use a tape measure, as this gives a highly inaccurate reading. It is better to omit the measurement altogether.

Head circumference
This important measurement is an indirect reflection of brain growth.

Place a clean measuring tape around the head to cover the most prominent points on the forehead and occiput.

The head circumference averages 35 cm in the full-term baby, with a range of 33 to 37 cm (Fig. 2.6, p. 8).

METHOD OF EXAMINATION
Examine a baby on the following occasions:
- *At birth:* Ensure there are no major congenital abnormalities or gross disease.

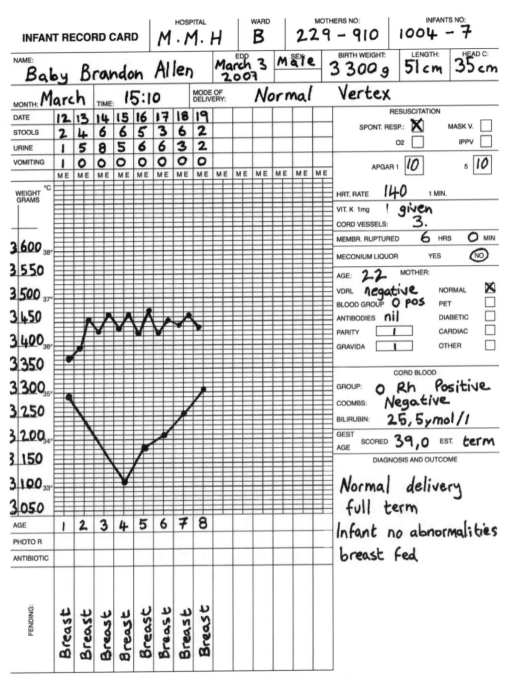

INFANT RECORD CARD	HOSPITAL	WARD	MOTHERS NO:	INFANTS NO:
	M . M . H	B	229 – 910	1004 – 7

NAME:	EDD	SEX	BIRTH WEIGHT:	LENGTH:	HEAD C:
Baby Brandon Allen	March 3 2007	Male	3 300 g	51 cm	35 cm

| MONTH: March | TIME: 15:10 | MODE OF DELIVERY: | Normal | Vertex |

DATE	12	13	14	15	16	17	18	19						
STOOLS	2	4	6	6	5	3	6	2						
URINE	1	5	8	5	6	6	3	2						
VOMITING	1	0	0	0	0	0	0	0						
	M E	M E	M E	M E	M E	M E	M E	M E	M E	M E	M E	M E	M E	M E

RESUSCITATION

SPONT. RESP.: ☒   MASK V. ☐

O2 ☐   IPPV ☐

APGAR 1 10   5 10

HRT. RATE 140   1 MIN.

VIT. K 1mg   1 given

CORD VESSELS: 3.

MEMBR. RUPTURED   6 HRS   0 MIN

MECONIUM LIQUOR   YES   (NO)

AGE: 22   MOTHER:

VDRL negative	NORMAL ☒
BLOOD GROUP O pos	PET ☐
ANTIBODIES nil	DIABETIC ☐
PARITY 1	CARDIAC ☐
GRAVIDA 1	OTHER ☐

CORD BLOOD

GROUP: O Rh Positive

COOMBS: Negative

BILIRUBIN: 25,5 ymol/l

GEST AGE SCORED 39,0 EST. term

DIAGNOSIS AND OUTCOME

Normal delivery
full term
Infant no abnormalities
breast fed

WEIGHT GRAMS °C

3 600	38°
3 550	
3 500	37°
3 450	
3 400	36°
3 350	
3 300	35°
3 250	
3 200	34°
3 150	
3 100	33°
3 050	

AGE	1	2	3	4	5	6	7	8				
PHOTO R												
ANTIBIOTIC												

FENDING:

| Breast | Breast | Breast | Breast | Breast | Breast | Breast | Breast | | | | |

Fig. 3.1 *The outer cover of an infant record chart*

- *Within 24 hours of birth:* Perform a full physical and neurological examination.
- *Within the first week:* A deviation from the normal pattern of growth or behaviour would prompt a repeat examination.
- *On discharge:* Repeat the physical and neurological assessment.

PREVIOUS PREGNANCIES:

1
2
3
4   Primip.
5
6
7
8

HISTORY OF PREGNANCY:

BOOKED [✗ AMA] PMH | GSH | MOU | OTHER | EMERG. | UNBOOKED

AMNIOCENTESIS   [YES]   [NO]

HISTORY OF LABOUR:

1st Stage : Spontaneous onset
no complications
no drugs

2nd Stage:

EXAMINATION

AGE: 13/3/2007   SIGNITURE:

HEAD: Moulding

FONTANELLES: Normal

SUTURES: Mobile

MORO: Normal   GRASP: Present

EYES: Light reflex present

EARS: Shape and position normal

NOSE: Patent nostrils

MOUTH: Normal

PALATE: Intact

HEART: Normal sounds

CHEST: Normal

ABDOMEN: No masses

CORD: 3 vessels

HIPS: Stable not dislocatable

GENITALIA: Testes down   URINE: Passed

ANUS: Patent   MECONIUM: Passed

FEMORALS: Palpable   RADIALS: Normal

SPINE: no abnormality

SKIN: Normal

HANDS: Normal   FEET: Normal

DRUGS GIVEN TO MOTHER:

Antenatal

During Labour Pethidine 100mg IMI
at 11h00

ABNORMALITIES NOTED AT BIRTH:

Nil detected

PLACENTA

WEIGHT: 562g

UMBILICAL CORD: Central insertion. 3 vessels

MEMBRANES: clear

GENERAL: No abnormalities

MAT. SURFACE: minimal calcification

FOETAL SURFACE: Few subchorionic thrombi

IDENTIFICATION

NAME: J. Harvard   SIGNATURE: J.Harvard.

WITNESSED BY: Fiona Nujent
NAME: Rm Rm   SIGNATURE: Fiona Nujent Rm Rm

I HAVE CHECKED THE IDENTITY AND AM SATISFIED THAT THIS IS MY INFANT.

LABOUR WARD   WARD

MOTHER'S SIGNATURE   MOTHER'S SIGNATURE
LGAllen

Fig. 3.2 *The inner cover of an infant record chart*

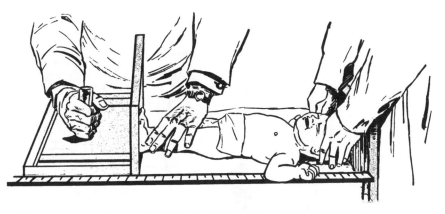

Fig. 3.3 *The measurement of the length of the infant (Adapted from Jelliffe, DB. 1966. The Assessment of the Nutritional Status of the Community.* **WHO Monograph Series** *54)*

Requirements
Obtain a stethoscope, a diagnostic set and a measuring tape.

Ensure that your hands are washed and that the baby is protected from cold. Before examining the baby in the presence of the mother, ask her if she is concerned about any features. This will avoid embarrassment if you overlook minor defects, such as syndactyly, which she is sure to have noticed.

Observation is the essence of the examination.

General appearance
Obtain an overall impression by noting size, facial appearance, colour of

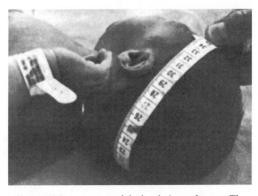

Fig. 3.4 *Measurement of the head circumference. The tape is placed around the most prominent points on the occiput and the forehead*

mucosae, posture, limb proportions and movements.

Do not undress or disturb a quiet baby; examine the following at this stage:
■ Eyes (p. 19).
■ Breathing pattern (p. 20).
■ Patency of nostrils (p. 19).
■ Heart position and sounds (p. 20).
■ Palpation of abdomen (p. 21).

Once undressed, the baby usually cries. This affords the opportunity to inspect the buccal cavity (p. 19).

Now examine the baby from head to toe.

Head
Size (p. 7)
Shape
Sutures
Fontanelles
Swellings
Hair
Scalp lesions

Shape
This is influenced by gestational age and by the moulding that occurs during pregnancy and birth.

Vertex delivery: The head is lengthened in the mentovertical axis. It differs from the rounded one of an infant born by

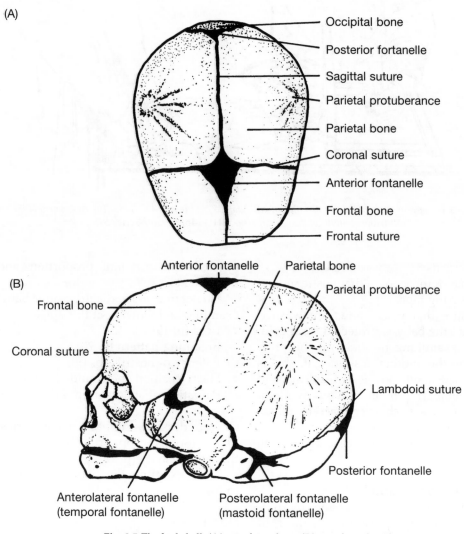

(A)

Occipital bone

Posterior fortanelle

Sagittal suture

Parietal protuberance

Parietal bone

Coronal suture

Anterior fontanelle

Frontal bone

Frontal suture

(B)

Anterior fontanelle   Parietal bone

Frontal bone

Parietal protuberance

Coronal suture

Lambdoid suture

Posterior fontanelle

Anterolateral fontanelle
(temporal fontanelle)

Posterolateral fontanelle
(mastoid fontanelle)

Fig. 3.5 *The fetal skull:* (**A**) *seen from above;* (**B**) *seen from the side*

Caesarean section before the head has engaged in the pelvis.

Breech delivery: The head is lengthened in the fronto-occipital plane with a rounded forehead and a narrow occiput that has a prominent protuberance.

An abnormally shaped skull is usually the result of premature closure of sutures (or synostosis p. 280).

Sutures (Fig. 3.5)

The skull bones are separated from one another by membranous sutures which permit expansion of the skull and growth of the brain.

The skull bones include:

- one *frontal* suture between frontal bones
- one *sagittal* suture between parietal bones
- two *coronal* sutures, one on each side between parietal and frontal bones

- two *lambdoid* sutures, one on each side between parietal and occipital bones.

The size of the sutures depends on the degree of moulding, and they may not be palpable if the bones overlap, or they may be up to 0,5 cm wide when the bones are separated.

Determine mobility of sutures by gently depressing the adjacent bones with your thumbs (Fig. 3.6). Movement excludes synostosis.

Fontanelles (Fig. 3.5)
The skull has six membranous fontanelles, two of which are palpable. They are the anterior and posterior fontanelles, which are situated at either end of the sagittal suture.

Posterior fontanelle: This small depression is usually the size of a fingertip or less.

Anterior fontanelle: This diamond-shaped area has an average length and width of 2,1 cm, with a range of 0,5 to 3,5 cm.

Place your extended fingers over the area so that they rest on the surrounding bones. Do this with the baby lying supine. The fontanelle is slightly depressed.

A bulging fontanelle signifies raised intracranial pressure. A markedly depressed one indicates underhydration.

Craniotabes: These are areas of the skull that often indent on palpation. The parchment-like regions are usually present in parietal and temporal bones adjacent to the sutures, but they can occur anywhere in the cranium.

The phenomenon is due to faulty ossification and is found in 2 to 3% of full-term babies and in many preterm babies. It is usually of no significance and is corrected within weeks or months.

Swellings
The scalp is frequently discoloured

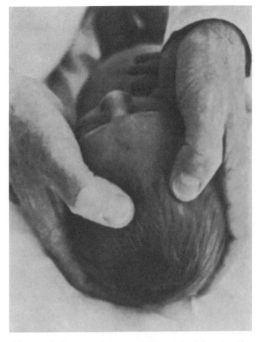

Fig. 3.6 *Palpation of the cranial bones to determine the mobility of sutures*

and swollen. This is known as a 'caput succedaneum' (p. 257).

Subperiosteal bleeding can result in a cephalhaematoma (p. 258), which is usually situated over a parietal bone. It enlarges over 24 hours and subsides within four to eight weeks. A subaponeurotic haemorrhage (p. 259) causes the whole head to enlarge and may result in anaemia.

Midline swellings are frequently caused by congenital defects, for example encephalocele (p. 135).

Hair
The full-term infant usually has a good growth of scalp hair. Individual strands do not adhere together, as they do in the preterm infant. In lighter-skinned babies, the colour of the hair is not a guide to its future shade.

Scalp lesions
The techniques used to monitor the fetus

and to rupture membranes during labour have led to an increase in the incidence of scalp trauma. Lesions may be missed at birth when the head is covered with blood and vernix.

Inspect the scalp carefully, once the hair has been washed and dried, to detect lesions such as scalp electrode cuts (p. 259).

Midline abnormalities, for example punched-out ulcers over the occiput, are usually congenital in origin (p. 251).

Face

Features vary in different races and it is advisable for you to know the facial characteristics of the parents before considering a baby's appearance to be abnormal.

Note the shape of the face.

Fetal posture may produce facial asymmetry, particularly when the jaw has been compressed against a shoulder. The lips are asymmetrical and the jaw appears to be angulated. The nose may be deviated to one or other side. This straightens with growth.

Observe the facial movements during crying to exclude a seventh-nerve palsy (p. 148).

Minor blemishes are common and include milia (p. 248) and 'stork bites' or 'salmon patches' (p. 255).

Bruising and petechiae

A difficult labour may be associated with facial bruising. This characteristically occurs over the mouth and nose.

Petechiae may be noted, but seldom extend below the level of the shoulders, when associated with trauma (Fig. 3.7).

Ears

Position

A horizontal line through the inner canthi of both eyes would pass through and not above the ear. Excessively low ears occur in renal agenesis (p. 238).

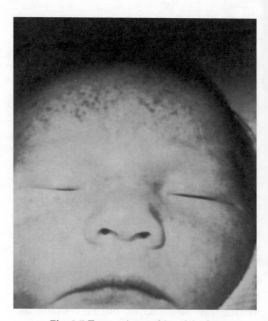

Fig. 3.7 *Traumatic petechiae of the face*

Shape

The normal structure of the external ear is shown in Fig. 3.8.

Incomplete folding of the helix is not unusual, but gross deformities may be associated with abnormalities elsewhere, for example certain heart defects and numerous genetic syndromes.

Nose

At birth the nose may be somewhat saddle-shaped, with upturned nares.

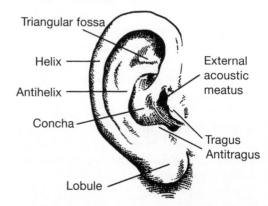

Fig. 3.8 *Normal structure of the external ear*

To determine airway patency, listen over each nostril with a stethoscope while occluding the other with your finger. The newborn is an obligate nose breather and air is heard to rush out during expiration.

A blocked nostril may be due to dried secretions and rarely to choanal atresia (p. 157).

Eyes

Note the shape, size and position.

The distance between the inner canthi ranges from 1,5 to 2,5 cm in the full-term infant.

Epicanthic folds or slanting of the palpebral fissures can occur as a variation of normal, particularly if seen in other members of the family. Down's syndrome (p. 117) is the most common abnormality associated with this feature.

Look for persistent tearing. This is abnormal and may indicate a blocked lachrymal duct (p. 154). If the lids are closed, gently open them and inspect the eyeball using a torch. Subconjunctival haemorrhages may be seen, particularly if delivery was difficult.

Note
Various congenital defects (p. 153) can be missed if the eyes are not inspected properly.

Focus an ophthalmoscope (set on 0) into each eye to elicit a light reflex. This presents a yellowish-red circle devoid of central black opacities caused by cataracts.

Buccal cavity

Inspect the lips for clefts or asymmetry. Thickened patches, termed 'sucking blisters' (Fig. 3.9), are sometimes seen on the lips.

Inspect the gums. Teeth are uncommon (p. 208). Retention cysts may be seen on the gum margins.

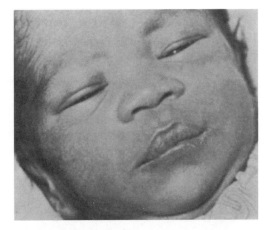

Fig. 3.9 *'Sucking blisters' on the upper lip*

Note the colour, size and mobility of the tongue. This structure is normally pink and relatively large at birth. An excessively large tongue, which usually cannot be contained in the mouth, is associated with hypothyroidism (p. 207), Down's syndrome (p. 117), Beckwith syndrome (p. 207) and glycogen storage disease (p. 273). Microglossia occurs in Pierre Robin syndrome (p. 207).

In so-called 'tongue tie', the frenum linguae from the floor of the mouth is inserted into the anterior portion of the tongue. It is a variation of normal and usually does not impair sucking or interfere with speech in later life (p. 207).

Inspect the palate to exclude a cleft (p. 206).

Small, grey-white papules are often noted in the midline of the posterior portion of the palate. They are termed 'epithelial pearls' (Fig. 3.10).

Neck

This is examined by extending or rotating the head. Inspect for webbing, clefts or swellings (p. 210). A sternomastoid 'tumour' may be seen in the muscle. This painless swelling is not obvious at birth and appears only after several weeks

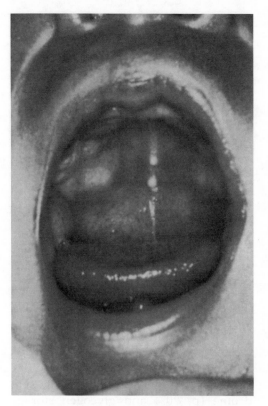

Fig. 3.10 *'Epithelial pearls' of palate*

(p. 288). A thyroid goitre is an unusual swelling (p. 277).

Palpate the clavicles to exclude crepitus or tenderness caused by a fractured bone (p. 289).

Chest
The distal end of the xiphisternum is often prominent.

The nipples are situated in the midclavicular line. Their areolae are well developed and breast nodules are palpable. Accessory nipples may be seen along the nipple line.

One or both breasts may enlarge and fill with milky secretions. These swellings can occur in male and female babies and may be uni- or bilateral. They persist for weeks to months and must not be squeezed, as this can lead to infection (Colour plate XII).

Respiration
Observe breathing while the baby is quiet. The abdomen rises in inspiration and there is very little movement of the chest cage. The rate averages 30 to 45 breaths per minute.

Air entry should be heard equally on both sides of the chest. Rib recession and tachypnoea, which is indicated by a rate persistently over 60, is abnormal and reveals respiratory distress (p. 172).

Cardiovascular system
Heart
The apex beat is difficult to palpate, but may be located in the third or fourth left intercostal space in the nipple line.

Listen to both sides of the chest and locate the area of maximum intensity of the heart sounds. This is usually confined to the centre or to the left side. In dextrocardia, the sounds are heard best on the right side.

Heart sounds are of equal intensity and a systolic murmur may be audible for the first few days of life. This is often an ejection murmur over the pulmonary area and along the left sternal border. In some cases it is localised to the pulmonary area. It may be caused by the increased flow of blood across the pulmonary valve or by a patent ductus arteriosus (p. 194).

Pulses
The radial artery is easy to locate. A femoral pulse may be palpated with the hip abducted. It is felt about a fingerbreadth medial to the anterior superior iliac spine. This pulse is not easily detected in every infant and an experienced person may need to confirm its presence. An absent femoral pulse is indicative of coarctation of the aorta (p. 194).

Pulse rate (p. 189).

Blood pressure (p. 189).

Abdomen

The abdomen is moderately protuberant. The liver can be palpated in the epigastrium and its edge extends about 1,5 cm below the costal margin. The kidneys and tip of spleen can be felt in thin infants. The bladder is an abdominal organ and when full is felt as a globular mass above the pelvis. It should not be palpable after micturition.

In a male baby a distended bladder associated with persistent dribbling of urine indicates posterior urethral valve obstruction (p. 239).

Umbilical cord

Count the vessels if the cord has not dried out.

The cord normally contains two arteries and one vein. In 0,2 to 1,0% of births, a single artery may be present. This can occur as a variation of normal, but should alert you to the possibility of other congenital abnormalities.

Genitalia

Male

The scrotum is well developed and covered with transverse skin folds.

Testes should be palpable in the sac.

A retractile testis can be pushed along the inguinal canal into the sac (p. 244).

A truly undescended testis cannot be sited in the scrotum, which appears underdeveloped and lacks skin folds on the affected side (p. 243).

A hydrocele is frequently present (p. 244); it usually disappears within days.

Inspect the penis and identify the meatus. The prepuce normally adheres to the glans and cannot be fully retracted. If urine is passed, the stream should be strong and not a constant dribble.

Female

Separate the legs to inspect the labial region.

The labia minora and clitoris are prominent. A hymenal skin tag (Colour plate X) may protrude from the vagina; it regresses after a few weeks. A white discharge or bleeding may be observed in the first week (p. 245), which is normal.

Anus

Inspect the anus to determine patency. Do this by retracting the buttocks to expose a puckered mucous membrane surface.

Anal skin tags are occasionally seen and they shrink within a few weeks.

Limbs

Note the size and shape. The lower legs may be bowed as a variation of normal (p. 283).

Inspect the hands and feet. A single palmar crease is seen in the hand in about 4% of normal infants and is also found in various chromosome anomalies, for example Down's syndrome (Fig. 3.11). Count the fingers and toes. Partial syndactyly of second and third toes is common.

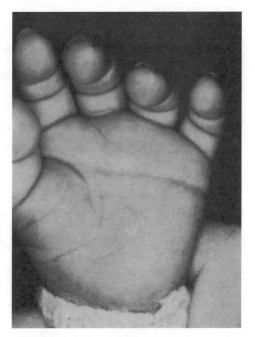

Fig. 3.11 *A single palmar crease*

Back

Turn the infant over to inspect the back for midline abnormalities, for example meningocele (p. 135), or sinuses.

A sacral dimple is often present. An underlying sinus can be excluded by retracting the skin margins and at the same time inspecting the base of the dimple through an auroscope.

Hips

Developmental dysplasia, or congenital dislocation, of the hip joint should be excluded by the following tests.

Ortolani test (Figs. 3.12 and 3.13)

Place the infant supine and grip each thigh between a thumb and forefinger so that both hips are flexed to 90° and the knees are fully bent. Abduct the hips as fully as possible. The thighs should reach the underlying surface.

Limitation of abduction is an important sign of congenital dislocation of a hip (p. 286).

Barlow test (Fig. 3.14)

Grip a thigh between the thumb and forefinger and hold it in mid-abduction

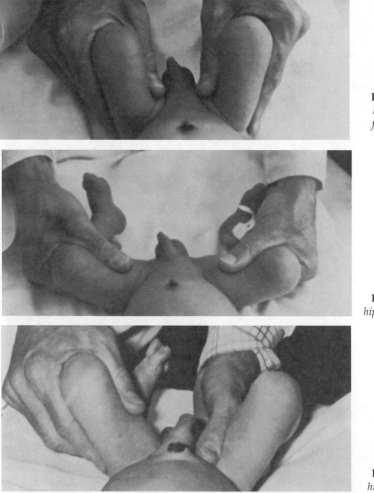

Fig. 3.12 *Examination of the hips. The hips and knees are flexed and the upper legs are gripped as illustrated*

Fig. 3.13 *Examination of the hips. The Ortolani test (see text)*

Fig. 3.14 *Examination of the hips. The Barlow test (see text)*

with the hip and knee flexed. Rock the head of the femur between the thumb and forefinger while exerting downward pressure along the shaft of the femur. The opposite pelvis is steadied during this procedure.

The hip joint should remain steady. A dislocated hip springs forward into the socket with an audible 'clunk'. Note that many hips, while being stable, can also produce a clicking sound during these tests. They are considered to be normal, but should be re-tested within two weeks.

Some hips are unstable, as the head of the femur can jump out of the socket, but is readily relocated. The instability usually subsides within three months, but the hips should be re-examined until this has been established.

Skin

Various blemishes or rashes may be present at birth or may appear within a few days (p. 249). Most are of no concern, but the mother usually needs reassurance.

Conclude the physical examination by relating weight, length and head circumference to gestational age.

Neurological examination

See p. 125.

EXAMINATION OF THE PLACENTA

Membranes
Cord
Fetal surface
Maternal surface
Weight

The organ should be examined immediately after birth, but can be refrigerated overnight in a plastic bag. Wear rubber gloves while handling the placenta.

Membranes

Place the placenta on a flat surface and spread out the membranes to reconstruct the fetal sac. The chorion, or outer layer, is shiny and adherent to the amnion. Identify the site of rupture and note whether any portion is missing. If so, note which portion it may be.

Cord

The attachment to the placenta may be central or lateral. Occasionally, the cord is inserted into the membranes (vellamentous) and the vessels lacking support may have ruptured.

Cut off the cord at its point of insertion and then transect it in the middle to study the vessels. There are two small thick-walled arteries and a thin-walled vein. A single umbilical artery may be associated with congenital abnormalities in the infant.

Fetal surface

This is glistening and blue-grey. It may be dull in amniotic infection or yellow in meconium-staining.

White plaques, or subchorionic thrombi, are frequently seen under the chorion. They consist of fibrin and are of no functional significance.

Maternal surface

Wash off the thin layer of freshly clotted blood that is present, and inspect the cotyledons. Note any missing portions. Superficial white specks of calcium are often seen. These gritty deposits are of no physiological significance.

Weight

The placenta and membranes are now weighed. The normal placenta to infant weight ratio at term is 1:5.

A disproportionately large placenta may be associated with congenital syphilis (p. 157) or Rh incompatibility (p. 101).

Slice the placenta at narrow intervals to study the underlying tissues. Ensure that firm portions are cut for inspection.

The villous tissue is usually dark red or pink, but may be pale in cases of blood loss, such as erythroblastosis and transfusion syndrome (p. 82). Infarcts are usually white and triangular, with the apex extending to the fetal surface. They are of no consequence when situated at the periphery.

If the placenta appears to be abnormal, send it for histological examination in a carton of preservative, like Bouin solution. Enclose details of the mother and infant.

Nursery Care

ROUTINE CARE
At birth

Fluid oozes from an infant's nostrils and mouth as the face emerges through the vagina. Crying commences as soon as the chest has been extruded and within half a minute the bluish mucosae become pink. The initial vigorous crying is followed by regular and shallow breathing. This process clears lung fluid (p. 160) from the nostrils and pharynx and there is no need to suction the upper airways, which could damage mucosal surfaces, thereby allowing bacteria to enter the body, or could produce reflex apnoea. Suction is indicated only when breathing is impaired and the airway needs to be cleared of fluid, blood or meconium (p. 168).

Clamping the umbilical cord

An infant's blood volume is related to the time of cord clamping after birth (p. 223). In normal full-term babies, it is probably advantageous to clamp the cord between 30 and 60 seconds. This permits a significant volume of placental blood to enter the infant during initial crying.

Apply two Spencer Wells forceps at approximately 5 and 6 cm from the umbilicus and sever the cord between them with a sterile pair of scissors. Rest the lower point of the scissor blade in the palm of your hand to avoid nicking the infant's skin. Later, attach a disposable sterile clamp about 1 cm above the umbilicus. This plastic device is closed by finger pressure and the cord above is cut off (Fig. 4.1).

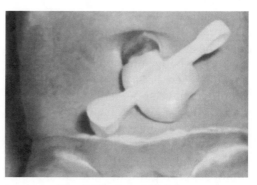

Fig. 4.1 *Plastic umbilical clamp*

Prevention of hypothermia

The environmental temperature of a delivery suite should be maintained above 23 °C and the room must be free of draughts.

Dry the wet infant with a sterile surgical drape. Discard all moist coverings and wrap the baby in a clean dry towel that covers the head and body. Avoid any exposure to cold.

Place the baby on the mother's chest to be fondled and suckled. Skin-to-skin contact is recommended. This ensures that the maternal body heat will maintain the baby's temperature within a normal range, and it also promotes colonisation with the mother's innocuous skin organisms. See page 62 for care of a preterm baby.

Delivery by Caesarean section

Carry the baby in a sterile drape to a warm resuscitation table. Dry, then briefly examine and rewrap the infant in a clean towel. Show the identified baby to the father and ensure that routine procedures such as weighing, eye prophylaxis and vitamin K_1 injection have been completed before the baby leaves the delivery suite.

If delivery was done under general anaesthesia, keep the infant in a nursery until the mother is fully conscious. Reunite the two as soon as possible.

Suckling

The bond of love between a mother and her infant commences during pregnancy. It can be enhanced by encouraging her to suckle the baby soon after delivery, and she may even assist in the birth after the shoulders have appeared.

This early union has many physiological advantages. It enables the baby to establish a pattern of sucking and also promotes the flow of colostrum. The infant's sterile gut and skin can be colonised by the mother's harmless bacteria rather than by pathogens from hospital staff.

Oxytocin is released from the maternal pituitary during sucking and contracts the uterus. This aids expulsion of the placenta and reduces the possibility of postpartum haemorrhage.

Identification (Fig. 4.3, p. 32)

Place a plastic bracelet around the baby's wrist and another around an ankle. This states the infant's name and sex.

Physical examination

The parents' first concern – "Is our baby normal?" – needs to be addressed as soon as possible. Expose the baby on the warmed surface of a resuscitation table and examine briefly to exclude obvious abnormalities such as congenital defects, respiratory distress (p. 172), pallor (p. 223) and birth trauma (p. 146).

Measurement

After a period of suckling, take the baby from the mother to a warm area or room designated for immediate care. Here eye prophylaxis, a vitamin K_1 injection and measurements may be completed.

Measure and record weight, head circumference and length (p. 12).

Prevent hypothermia during these procedures.

Vitamin K_1

Inject vitamin K_1 1 mg into the anterolateral thigh muscle (p. 305) to prevent haemorrhagic disease.

Note

Never do this in the labour ward as injections intended for the mother may inadvertently be given to the baby.

Gonococcal ophthalmia prophylaxis

Prophylaxis against gonococcal or chlamydial eye infection is recommended in regions where antenatal attendance or care is inadequate and where unbooked pregnancies abound.

Open an eye by separating the lids between the forefinger and thumb and instil half the contents of a chloramphenicol applicap. Do the same to the other eye.

Erythromycin ointment, if available, is preferable, for it destroys both types of organisms.

Cord blood collection

This is a routine in many hospitals to screen for hypothyroidism. It is also done to determine blood groups and is essential when:

- the mother is Rh negative, or the Rh state is unknown
- the mother's VDRL is positive or unknown.

Transference to ward

Place the baby in the mother's arms and accompany both to the ward. Ensure that relevant information is recorded in the infant chart.

After birth – immediate care

Wherever possible, do not separate the baby and mother. Keep the baby in a crib at the bedside and ensure adequate warmth.

In the case of an abnormal delivery, for example Caesarean section, the period of separation should be as brief as possible, providing the baby is normal.

Nursing staff should complete the following procedures:

Cord

Check the clamp and swab the cord with spirits (methylated or surgical). Keep it exposed to promote drying.

Bathing (p. 33)

Clotted blood and meconium may be removed after birth, while opinion about the necessity to bath an infant varies from one institution to another. Vernix is considered to have antibacterial properties and there is no need to wash it off.

Dress

Clothe the baby in a cotton vest and a short gown which ties at the back. Fit a disposable napkin and wrap the infant in two woollen blankets.

Arrange these so that movement is not impeded.

Temperature

Maintain the environmental temperature in a ward between 23 and 25 °C.

Record the baby's axillary temperature on a mercury thermometer. It should be in the range of 36,5 to 37 °C. Use a low-reading thermometer if the temperature is below normal.

The infant who cannot maintain a normal temperature needs incubation (p. 64) or kangaroo care (p. 65).

Respiration

Count and record the breathing rate half-hourly for the first two hours. In normal full-term infants it averages 44 (breaths per minute, or bpm), peaking at 48 bpm by three hours and gradually declining to the lower 40s thereafter.

The following signs are abnormal:

- A sustained rate of over 60 per minute.
- Rib or sternal recession.
- Grunting.
- Cyanosis of lips and tongue.

These indicate respiratory distress, which needs urgent investigation and treatment in a special care unit.

Neurological function

Assess movement and behaviour half-hourly for two hours. The following factors are abnormal:

- Excessive drowsiness.
- Irregular breathing or apnoea.

- A tense fontanelle.
- Seizures (p. 145).
- Inadequate suck reflex.

These features may be indicative of oversedation (p. 301), intracranial bleeding (p. 142) or neonatal encephalopathy (p. 139). The infant requires urgent treatment in a special care unit.

Birth injuries
The following signs are indicative of birth trauma:
- The infant cries excessively when moved or picked up, for example fracture of clavicle (p. 289).
- Facial asymmetry on crying, for example facial nerve palsy (p. 148).
- Flaccid limb, for example nerve palsy (p. 147).

Congenital abnormalities
Obvious abnormalities should be detected at the first examination.

Occult abnormalities may be suspected in the presence of certain features, such as the following:
- Constant drooling – may be a sign of oesophageal atresia (p. 209).
- Inability to suck – may be associated with a cleft palate (p. 206).
- Persistent vomiting – may be a sign of a high intestinal obstruction, like duodenal atresia (p. 214).

The period of observation depends on the state of the mother and infant. It usually does not exceed one to two hours. The time will have to be extended if the mother is unable to receive her baby, for example after Caesarean section.

Blood glucose monitoring (p. 262)
This is necessary in the first six hours for babies who are too large (> 4 000 g) or too small (< 2 500 g). These groups are prone to hypoglycaemia.

Feeding
A normal baby and mother remain together, and demand-feeding is encouraged. Ensure that an infant who has been separated from the mother receives a feed within an hour of birth. Expressed colostrum may be used if the mother is incapable of putting the baby to the breast.

After birth – continuing care
A baby ought to be examined fully on the first day, and gestational age (p. 8) may be assessed within five days.

The following checks are completed daily by a nurse, who should record and report any features of concern:

Skin
Inspect the baby's body for:

Rashes
Erythema toxicum (p. 249), heat rash (p. 249) and phototherapy rashes (p. 107) are harmless. Report any other types.

Pustules
These indicate a staphylococcal infection and require treatment immediately (p. 260).

Scratches
Abrasions on the cheeks are usually caused by the baby's fingernails. Trim these horizontally with a pair of small, blunt-nose scissors or use an emery board. Do not use a nail clipper as this can cut off a fingertip.

Perineal redness
Wash the buttocks with soap and water and apply Vaseline to the anal region. Discard soiled nappies as soon as possible to prevent skin contact. If this is not successful consider a candida infection (p. 251).

Peeling
Superficial skin may peel off the hands, feet and trunk. This frequently occurs in post-term, growth-retarded or meconium-stained babies, but it may also be a feature of congenital syphilis (p. 157).

Peripheral cyanosis
The hands and feet may remain blue for hours or days after birth. This is normal, provided that the baby is warm and the lips and tongue are pink.

Jaundice
This commonly occurs after 48 hours. It starts on the face and can spread to the trunk and limbs. The distribution is related to the level of serum bilirubin.
Face only: bilirubin is less than 150 μmol/l
Face and trunk: bilirubin is less than 200 μmol/l
Whole body: bilirubin is more than 200 μmol/l

Jaundice is abnormal when it:
- appears within 24 hours of age
- involves more than the face
- persists beyond 10 days of age
- is associated with hepatosplenomegaly.

If any of these apply, obtain a specimen of heel-blood for bilirubin measurement (p. 232) and refer the infant for assessment.

Temperature
Check and record the axillary temperature twice a day (p. 33), and ensure that the environmental temperature is satisfactory.

Weight
A baby loses 3–5% of birthweight over the first three days. This physiological event is thought to be owing to the small intake of fluid, the loss of meconium and lung fluid, insensible water loss and the utilisation of glycogen stores in the liver.
The following patterns are abnormal:
- Excessive weight loss, that is, 10% or more of birthweight.
- Failure to gain weight after the fourth day, or persistent weight loss.
- Excessive weight gain, that is, more than 200 g/d, which may indicate fluid retention (oedema).

Cord
Swab the umbilicus three times a day with spirits (p. 33).

Report
- Redness or oedema.
- Bleeding or discharge.
- Offensive smell.

Eyes
Remove crusted material from the nasal margins with a moist swab.

Report
- A discharge from the eyes.

Nose
Cautiously remove crusted secretions from the nostrils with moist cotton wool buds.

Report
- A nasal discharge.

Note
A blocked nose is common and is often associated with sneezing. This does not imply flu or a cold; it is a normal event.

Mouth
Inspect the mucosa of the lips and cheeks for thrush (p. 220).

Stools
Note the colour and consistency of each stool (p. 201), and record the number passed daily.

Report
- A delay in passing meconium, that is, more than 24 hours.
- Diarrhoea.
- Blood in the stool.

Urine
Check the daily output by counting the number of wet nappies (p. 234).

Report
- A delay in micturition, that is, more than 36 hours.
- Constant dribbling (p. 239).

Feeding
Breast-feeding poses difficulty for many mothers and a considerable portion of a nurse's time is spent in explaining or treating various problems.

Common difficulties are a delay in milk production, sore nipples, engorged breasts, uncertainty as to the amount of milk taken at each feed, an excessively drowsy baby and refusal to suck at the breast.

The following problems need immediate attention:
- Inadequate sucking reflex.
- Persistent vomiting.

Mother–baby relationship
Inadequate bonding in early life has been implicated in baby battering, behaviour problems, abnormal parental concern and failure to thrive.

Staff must provide an environment in which the bond between mother and baby is not threatened.

Keep the two together throughout their stay in a maternity hospital. Ensure rooming-in facilities; quietness, especially at night; and relatively unrestricted visiting for family members. Answer queries with sympathy and respect, and assist the mother to master the art of breast-feeding. It is her best investment for the baby's future health.

Visitors
Many maternity institutions have unrestricted visiting. Children in the family are allowed to be with their mother and new sibling. This makes the acceptance of a baby easier and does not increase the chances of cross-infection. However, do not permit persons with colds or other infectious illnesses to visit or touch a newborn baby.

Discharge
The following checks and arrangements are important:
- Establish that the baby is feeding and thriving adequately.
- Conduct a full physical examination.
- Confirm the name on identification bracelets.
- Ensure that the mother knows how to breast-feed and is able to bath her baby and clean the cord.
- Check that BCG and polio immunisations (p. 34) have been given.
- Issue a Health Card, which will be used to record milestones, immunisations and other aspects of growth in the preschool stage.

Follow-up
Well babies should be examined at least once after discharge. This can be done at six weeks of age when the mother is checked at a postnatal clinic.

Babies should attend their local infant welfare clinic for routine weighing, milestone assessment and immunisations. These details are entered in the Health Card. Remind the mother to bring this card to the clinic or hospital.

Breast-feeding clinic
The mother who breast-feeds her infant needs constant encouragement and advice after discharge from hospital. This is best provided at a feeding clinic run by a nursing sister and staff who are experienced in the art of breast-feeding.

Accommodation and equipment

Rooming-in is recommended for normal babies. This implies keeping the mother and baby together at all times. Nursing staff are responsible for the immediate care of an infant after birth. Thereafter, the mother takes over this role and the baby sleeps at her bedside in a crib.

A nurse is charged with the important task of teaching babycraft so that a mother should be capable of:
- cleaning the umbilical cord
- bathing her baby
- breast-feeding with confidence.

Space
Suitable wards should accommodate up to six mothers. Decor is as attractive as possible and curtains are needed to screen off beds. Each mother and baby should be allocated a minimum area of 7,5 sq. m.

Single wards are needed for those who require isolation for infectious diseases like maternal chickenpox (p. 96).

Temperature
The environmental temperature of 23–24 °C is comfortable for adults and enables full-term babies to maintain adequate warmth when clothed and covered by two woollen blankets. The room must be free of draughts.

Wash basins
Foot-, elbow- or automatic-controlled units should be situated in each ward. They must provide warm running water and be stocked with paper towels and liquid soap.

Bins
Foot-controlled bins fitted with plastic bags are placed in each ward. Separate bins are required for dirty linen and refuse. Closed bags are placed outside the ward for collection. On no account should any article be removed from the bags in the ward.

Bassinets
Cots made of unbreakable plastic are designed to serve as a bath and as a bed (Fig. 4.2). They rest on a rust-proof mobile frame and must be easy to clean. Compartments are built onto the frame for storage of clothing, linen, swabs, soap, Vaseline and a thermometer.

Identification particulars of the infant must be clearly displayed. Sufficient bassinets must be available so that several can be out of service for cleaning and repair without disrupting the running of the ward.

Nursery techniques
All members of staff must be instructed in the approved techniques. They will be held responsible for the correct implementation of these procedures.

Hand-washing
Hands must be cleaned immediately before touching a baby; they are otherwise regarded as contaminated.

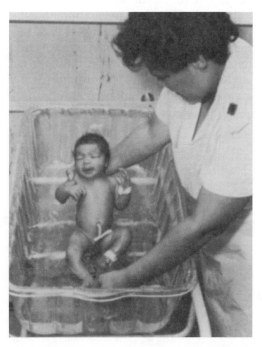

Fig. 4.2 *Plastic bassinet: This serves as a cot and a bath*

Use an antiseptic soap, for example Hibiscrub, to wash hands, wrists and forearms.

- Rinse thoroughly under running water.
- Use only elbow-, foot- or automatic-controlled taps.
- Dry on disposable paper towels.
- Keep fingernails short and clean.

Repeated hand-washing is impracticable when non-infected babies are constantly handled, for example in a nursery or an intensive care unit. After an initial scrub, spray your palms with an antiseptic solution (chlorhexidine gluconate in alcohol) before touching a baby.

Identification (Fig. 4.3)
A baby is identified:
- in the labour ward
- in the postnatal ward or nursery
- on discharge.

In the labour ward
Prepare two identification bracelets to indicate the baby's name, sex and hospital number. Ensure that the mother confirms the information and then attach one band to the baby's wrist and the other to an ankle. The mother is shown and ideally given her identified infant.

Identification information is then entered on the baby's chart. The mother signs the baby's chart to indicate she has witnessed the identification procedure.

In cases of delivery under anaesthesia, two members of the nursing staff should witness the identification of the infant and sign the record chart to this effect.

In some institutions the mother's fingerprints and the baby's footprint are recorded and filed in the record chart.

In the ward
Show the infant to the mother and confirm identification when she is admitted to a ward from the delivery room.

Under no circumstances must identification bands be removed. An infant is discharged with these in place.

In the nursery
Confirm identification and compare it with the particulars on the chart.

Label the bassinet or incubator with the infant's name, number, date of birth and weight.

On discharge
Confirm the infant's name on the bracelet with the mother and have her sign that she has received her infant. Identification bracelets remain on and can be removed at home.

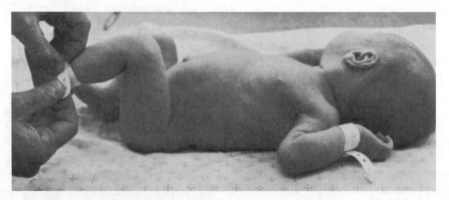

Fig. 4.3 *Identification bands are attached to an ankle immediately after birth and left in place until the baby has been discharged*

Umbilical cord care

The cord is cleaned three times a day: after the daily bath, in the early afternoon and in the early evening.

It is cleaned three-hourly if moist or when the baby is in an incubator.

Requirements

- A packet of clean swabs.
- A clipper in a container of methylated spirits.
- A spray bottle of spirits (methylated or surgical).
- A chlorhexidine gluconate/alcohol spray for cleaning your hands.
- A container for dirty items.

All equipment is placed on a clean trolley, which is wheeled from one baby to the next.

Method

Spray your hands with the antiseptic solution. Place the baby on the mother's bed on a plastic sheet, securing hands and feet.

Spray two clean swabs with spirits. Hold the top of the cord with one swab. Clean around the base and up the sides with the other swab. Discard swabs.

Use the clipper to remove the cord clamp 24 hours post delivery. If the cord is still on at the time of discharge, instruct the mother to continue drying out the base with methylated or surgical spirits.

After separation of the cord, the area is washed daily with soap and water. Avoid spirits as it can cause bleeding at this stage.

Axillary temperature

A mercury thermometer must be available for each infant. It is washed in cold water each day and kept in a small test tube that is autoclaved daily.

Method

Spray your hands with an antiseptic solution. Wipe the thermometer with a clean swab and shake it so that the mercury settles below the lowest reading.

Hold the thermometer in the axilla for two minutes with infant's upper arm pressed against thorax. Record the temperature. Normal range is from 36,5 to 37 °C.

Wipe the thermometer with a swab and replace it in the container.

Bathing

This is optional and probably unnecessary unless an infant is covered in meconium, blood or contaminated liquor. Various procedures are used, depending on the degree of contamination. This method describes a full bath. Ensure that it is done in a warm room and that the baby is exposed as briefly as possible.

Requirements

- Bland soap (neutrogena).
- Baby clothes.
- Disposable napkin.
- Packet of clean swabs.
- Jar of Vaseline.
- Two clean bath towels.
- Savlon® 1:200, or detergent spray.

Method

Assemble towels and clothes and position a cord trolley nearby. Spray your hands with chlorhexidine gluconate/alcohol before touching the baby. Verify the infant's name and sex and record the axillary temperature. Bathing is commenced when this is above 36 °C.

Lift the baby out of the bassinet and wrap in a clean towel. Hold the infant securely in your left arm while wiping the table-top, mattress and bassinet with Savlon® or detergent.

Place the mattress on the table and lay the baby (wrapped in towel) on it.

Undress the baby and examine for obvious abnormalities. The buttocks may be cleaned with a moist swab if meconium has been passed.

Vernix
Remove vernix from the head, axillae and groin with soap-impregnated swabs. Rewrap the infant to immobilise arms and legs.

Eyelids, face, ears
Wipe eyelids from nasal to temporal side with moist swabs. The face and ears are also cleaned and dried with swabs.

Bath water
Run warm water (38 °C) into the bassinet. Your elbow should feel comfortably warm when immersed in the water.

Hair
Hold the baby over the bassinet supported in your left arm, with the head and neck cradled in your left hand. Soap and rinse hair twice and then dry it when the baby is back on the mattress. Bath water may need to be changed if excessively dirty.

Body and limbs
Unwrap the baby and soap the body and limbs, omitting the hands. Slide your left hand under the baby's shoulders to grip the opposite arm, then slip your right hand under the buttocks and grip the left thigh. Immerse the baby in the water, rinse off soap and wash the infant's hands while maintaining support with your left hand.

Dry the baby with a clean towel, paying attention to skin folds in the neck, axillae and groins.

Dress
Clothe the baby in a vest and nightgown and fold them so that the cord can be cleaned (p. 33). Rub the buttocks with Vaseline and put on a nappy. Wrap the infant securely in a blanket.

Completion
Empty the bassinet and hold the baby in the left arm while bassinet, mattress and table-top are wiped with Savlon or detergent and then dried.

Replace the mattress in the bassinet and cover it with a sheet. Lay the infant in the cot and cover with two blankets.

Kangaroo care or incubation (pp. 64, 65) may be needed if the axillary temperature is less than 36 °C.

Tidy up and record details of examination, any abnormalities, passage of meconium and urine.

Immunisations
Babies are immunised against tuberculosis and polio within five days of birth.

Tuberculosis
BCG vaccination: this is essential in regions with a high incidence of tuberculosis.
  Contraindications: Infants who are ill and those with symptomatic Aids.

Intradermal method
A live attenuated strain of *Mycobacterium bovis* injected into the skin affords a 60–80% protection against disseminated tuberculosis.
Dose: 0,05 ml of reconstituted powder drawn up in a special syringe.
Site: Inject this into the skin at the base of the right deltoid muscle to raise a bleb. Natural responses at the site of injection are as follows:
- Three weeks – redness.
- Six weeks – a papule.
- Ten weeks – a shallow ulcer.
- Fourteen weeks – a dry healing ulcer.
- Three to six months – a scar.

Neither cover the area nor apply any antiseptic. A few small axillary glands (< 1 mm) may be palpable.

Polio
Trivalent oral vaccine.

Method

Squeeze two drops of vaccine from the plastic container into the infant's mouth. To ensure sterility, do not let the dropper touch the oral cavity.

Keep the vaccine refrigerated after use.

Each container has approximately 30 doses of vaccine.

Cleaning of nurseries and equipment

Floors are mopped daily with a solution of chlorine, for example Biocide D®. The mopping may be preceded by vacuum cleaning, provided an approved cleaner is used. This must be fitted with a suitable bacterial filter and a disposable paper bag.

Mops should have detachable heads and these can be autoclaved daily, together with the metal buckets used for cleaning.

Walls

The periodic washing of walls is desirable on grounds of cleanliness, but is not necessary for the control of cross-infection.

Table surfaces

All surfaces are cleaned daily with a detergent solution, and then wiped with methylated spirits.

Disposable cloths are used for this purpose.

Equipment

Items such as incubators, chairs, bassinets and infusion pumps are cleaned in a similar manner to table surfaces. Instruments that can withstand heat treatment are autoclaved.

Sinks

These sites are a potential hazard for the growth of bacteria such as *Pseudomonas*. The plughole area must be cleaned daily by particulate matter being removed and then the hot-water taps being allowed to run at maximum heat for two minutes. If this is not feasible (in the case of an automatic tap, for instance) then boiling water from a kettle should be poured down the plughole each day.

Ideally, bacteriological cultures should be obtained from various sites each week.

PRIMARY CARE

This is of fundamental importance for mothers and infants in underdeveloped regions.

Midwife Obstetric Unit

A successful perinatal model has been developed in the Cape Peninsula, South Africa, called the Midwife Obstetric Unit (MOU). As the name implies, the midwife is central to its function and is responsible for the overall care of low-risk mothers and their offspring. There are no resident medical staff, and rigorous clinical criteria ensure timely transference to hospital of women who develop complications before or during labour.

MOUs are best sited in densely populated urban regions, located within easy distance from home, and readily accessible to regional and tertiary hospitals.

An MOU ensures a reduction in maternal and perinatal mortality and morbidity rates, as well as an improvement in the general health of women and infants, if the following are provided:

- Sufficient well-trained staff.
- Continual education for staff and patients.
- Relevant equipment and drugs.
- Apt criteria for referral to hospital.
- Suitable channels of communication with designated hospitals.
- Adequate transport facilities.
- Regular perinatal audits.

- Community acceptance and partici-
  pation.

Continual perinatal education is paramount. This includes orientation courses
for new midwifery staff, monthly perinatal mortality and morbidity discussions, case presentations, the outcome
and relevance of hospital referrals, and
a review of current practices and procedures. These are attended and presented
by visiting obstetricians, neonatologists
and senior midwives.

Patient education is provided
by midwives at each antenatal clinic.
It includes formal lectures, practical
demonstrations, informal discussions,
poster presentations and audiovisual
programmes.

The objective is to impart information
and skills that encourage women to
monitor their own health efficiently
during pregnancy.

MOU care of the newborn

Nursing staff manage all routine newborn care after birth and are expected to:
- give prophylactic eye treatment
  (p. 27)
- give vitamin K_1 (p. 26)
- examine the infant after birth (p. 12)
- ensure that breast-feeding is established (p. 48)
- carry out and record appropriate
  observations after birth (p. 13)
- instruct the mother on the cleaning of
  the cord (p. 33) and being attentive to
  possible problems
- give BCG vaccination (p. 34), and the
  first dose of polio drops (p. 34)
- supervise baby care in the first
  week (p. 30) and do appropriate
  investigations, for example bilirubin
  level.

The nurse is expected to be familiar with
emergency treatment, in particular the
resuscitation of an asphyxiated infant
at birth (p. 168), the initial care of a low
birthweight infant (p. 63) and treatment
of one who has respiratory distress (p.
172).

Following stabilisation of blood sugar,
temperature and oxygen saturation, the
appropriate details are entered on the
infant chart and the nurse communicates
with the base hospital to arrange transference of the infant.

A nurse also deals with the formalities
of a stillbirth. This includes certification,
advice about burial, counselling of parents, and if necessary consultation with
the doctor in charge.

Role of a visiting doctor

Teaching is of paramount importance
and the knowledge and skills needed
for newborn care must be continually
imparted to resident nursing staff.

A follow-up service is provided for
referrals from MOU staff and for high-
risk babies after discharge from hospital.
This includes developmental screening.

Neonatal data is collected for audit
and presentation at monthly perinatal
meetings.

Availability is essential at all times,
be it on a telephone or at the MOU. This
ensures a close liaison with nursing staff
should problems arise.

Contact is also maintained with the
staff of the base hospital to ensure conti-
nuity and compatibility of care.

Equipment

Most infants leave the MOU with their
mothers within six hours of birth.

Standard items are needed for those
who require resuscitation, oxygen,
phototherapy or incubation. These
include face-mask ventilators and relevant
equipment (p. 171), piped oxygen or gas
cylinders, several closed incubators and
phototherapy units.

Infants who require care after birth are kept in a warm nursery until discharge or transference to hospital.

SPECIAL CARE

This is an integral part of the neonatal health services of many countries. The evolution of such care stems from two concepts:

1. Newborn babies are vulnerable to factors which cause irreversible physical or mental damage.
2. The physical and physiological characteristics of the newborn differ significantly from those of older infants.

Hazardous factors

The following can be harmful:

- Hypoxaemia.
- Hypoglycaemia.
- Hyperbilirubinaemia.
- Hypothermia.
- Infection.

A high-risk baby may be defined as one who is likely to develop permanent disabilities as a result of exposure to one or more of these complications.

Hazardous therapy

In unskilled hands, various forms of treatment, like oxygen therapy, can be as harmful as the underlying disease itself.

Aims

Intensive care aims to prevent complications by identifying the infant at risk even before birth and providing the appropriate treatment immediately after birth.

The skills and knowledge necessary for optimum care of ill babies are best acquired and applied in an intensive care unit. Such a unit can indirectly improve the care of newborns in a whole area or province.

Trained medical and nursing personnel should visit outlying hospitals and primary care units to instruct their staff in proper techniques of care, and the staff should then spend a period of study in a special care unit.

Location

An intensive care unit is best situated in a maternity hospital that handles high-risk obstetric cases. It should be accessible by road to surrounding primary care units.

Treatment can be instituted immediately and close co-operation can be promoted between obstetric and paediatric staff.

The smallest hospital that is viable from the point of view of intensive care should have no less than 2 500 deliveries a year. Such a hospital would also have to cater for infants born elsewhere.

Approximately 10–20% of liveborn babies require special care for their first few days of life.

Criteria for admission

A vulnerable infant should be identified and immediately transferred for observation and care. The majority are preterm and suffer from respiratory distress.

Indications for admission are listed in Table 4.1.

TABLE 4.1

Important indications for special care
Low birthweight (less than 2 000 g)
Perinatal asphyxia
Respiratory distress or apnoea
Hypoglycaemia
Rhesus disease
Severe infection, e.g. septicaemia
A diabetic mother
Convulsions or failure to suck
Cyanotic heart disease
Treatable congenital abnormalities, e.g. oesophageal atresia

Transference

An infant born in an outlying hospital or primary care unit and who needs special care (Table 4.1) must be transported under optimal conditions.

A nursing sister, paramedic or doctor trained in intensive care travels to the point of collection in an air or land ambulance. The vehicle must be equipped with a portable incubator, oxygen supply, a ventilator, a constant infusion pump, a telethermometer and various items that may be needed for resuscitation (p. 171) or for intravenous therapy.

Stabilise the baby before transfer. This implies that hypoxaemia, hypoglycaemia and hypothermia are corrected or prevented before the journey.

In most cases, the primary care staff would have established adequate warmth, set up a peripheral or umbilical vein drip of 10% dextrose water, and supplied extra oxygen through a perspex™ head-box. In severe respiratory distress, endotracheal intubation and artificial ventilation may be needed before the baby is transferred to the ambulance.

If radiological facilities are available, obtain an X-ray of the chest to determine the cause of distress. A tension pneumothorax will require immediate treatment (p. 180).

Obtain a detailed history of the pregnancy, labour and birth. This includes drugs used to treat the mother at various stages.

Take clotted and unclotted specimens of blood from the mother and from the placenta, if available. These may be needed later for investigations, for example blood grouping, antibodies, IgM levels.

Record the name, address and telephone number of the parents and of the referring doctor.

Show the mother her identified infant and ensure that vitamin K_1 has been given.

A parent, usually the mother, accompanies the infant to the main hospital. If this is not possible, obtain written consent for investigations that may be necessary, such as cardiac catheterisation.

During the journey, which may last several hours, maintain the infant in an optimal state. Pay particular attention to temperature control (p. 63) and oxygen saturation (p. 163).

Benefits
Immediate
The introduction of special care has resulted in a 50% decrease in neonatal mortality rates for low-birthweight babies.

Long-term
The efficiency of intensive care becomes apparent only over a number of years.

An overall improvement has occurred in the neurological and intellectual functions of infants weighing between 1 000 and 1 500 g. The incidence of such abnormalities has declined from 70% to below 10% since the introduction of intensive care.

Babies weighing under 1 000 g still have significant morbidity and mortality rates.

Follow-up studies
Infants who have received special care need careful assessment in the early years of life. Use this period to detect any deviation from normal in the physical and/or mental development. An early assessment of senses, such as hearing and eyesight, can be made, but formal IQ and DQ testing is practicable only at four to five years of age.

The early school period should be covered in order for learning difficulties, such as an inability to read, to be detected.

Future planning
The pattern of perinatal disease indicates that most problems are of antenatal origin,

and future care lies in the prevention of such disorders, for example premature onset of labour. Present-day planning must be flexible enough to adapt to this fact. As far as possible, the transportation of an infant should be *in utero* and every attempt must be made to detect and correct factors that are associated with the onset of preterm labour (p. 62).

Further details are beyond the scope of this book, and you are referred to the many excellent texts on special care.

Breast-feeding

SIGNIFICANCE

Breast milk is the specific food of the human infant. Its qualities have been perfected through evolutionary development and the natural way for a baby to obtain nourishment is to nurse at the breast. This may well be a law of nature.

Babies who receive only human milk have unique advantages.

Nutritional benefits
Protein
Lactalbumin predominates and is highly nutritious and easily digested. The protein is non-allergenic.

Carbohydrates
Lactose is converted to glucose for energy and to galactose for lipid synthesis in the nervous system. An undigested portion of lactose promotes the growth of lactobacilli in the large bowel.

Fat
Most of breast milk fat is easily absorbed (95%) and contains essential fatty acids such as gamma linolenic acid, which is needed for prostaglandin synthesis. Fatty acids are also used for brain and retinal growth. The milk fat globule contains readily available fatty acids and cholesterol for micellar absorption, as well as growth factors and vitamins.

Minerals and electrolytes
Calcium and iron are readily absorbed, and zinc, selenium and magnesium are transported through the bowel by various milk enzymes.

Growth inducers
Several factors are important for the growth and development of the gut after birth. They include epithelial growth factor (EGF), nerve growth factor (NGF), somatomedin, prolactin and insulin.

Protection against infection
Breast milk contains elements that reduce the risk of both enteral and parenteral infections. Some known constituents are as follows:

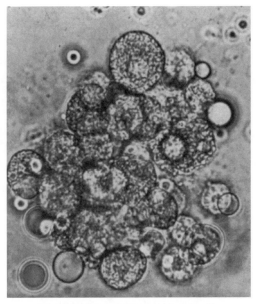

Fig. 5.1 *The macrophages in breast milk*

Immunoglobulins
Colostrum and milk contain significant amounts of IgG, IgA and IgM antibodies. These are absorbed into the infant's circulation and the secretory portion of IgA remains in the gut. It is protected from stomach acids and reaches the small bowel intact. The immunoglobulins can destroy various viruses, like poliovirus, and bacteria, such as *E. coli.*

Cells
Macrophages account for 90% of the cellular content of mature milk (Fig. 5.1) and are thought to phagocytose bacteria, whereas lymphocytes are considered to synthesise IgA immunoglobulin.

Lysozyme
This is abundant and remains stable in the acid environment of the stomach. It destroys the cell walls of bacteria.

Complement
The C3 and C4 fractions can lyse bacteria.

Lactoferrin
This iron-binding protein is capable of inhibiting the growth of staphylococci and *E. coli* organisms.

Lactoperoxidase
This is believed to aid in the destruction of streptococci.

Other agents
Milk lipids damage viruses while mucins adhere to bacteria and viruses and help to eliminate them.
    Interferon and fibronectin have antiviral properties.

Bowel flora regulants
Bifidobacterium (*Lactobacillus bifidus*) constitutes 99% of the stool flora in the wholly breast-fed baby. Colonisation is promoted by specific factors as well as by the pH, lactose, low-protein and low-phosphate content of the milk. This organism adheres to the wall of the large bowel, prevents the implantation of pathogenic bacteria and enhances the infant's immune system.

Protection against allergy
Allergies such as asthma and eczema occur more frequently in infants who are fed cow milk than in those who are wholly breast-fed.
    Secretory IgA in human milk is considered to react with various food allergens and to prevent their absorption through the relatively porous gut wall. This state lasts for the duration of breast-feeding.

Economy
Breast-feeding saves on food and doctors' bills. A built-in milk supply is available at all times and does not entail extra work for the mother.

Other advantages
Iron deficiency and rickets are rarely encountered.

Hyperosmolar dehydration is unlikely to occur.

Convulsions due to hypomagnesaemia and hypocalcaemia are not seen.

Constipation does not occur.

The interval between pregnancies is extended in a breast-feeding woman. This contraceptive effect depends on frequent suckling.

PROMOTION

The implementation of successful breast-feeding requires a 'baby friendly' environment. This can be achieved by implementing the steps of the Baby Friendly Hospital Initiative. They are as follows:

- Assure a written breast-feeding policy.
- Provide appropriate training for staff to carry out the policy.
- Ensure that pregnant women are aware of the benefits and proper technique of breast-feeding.
- Assist mothers to breast-feed within 30 minutes of delivery.
- Keep mother and baby together throughout the day and night.
- Show mothers how to breast-feed and to maintain lactation even when separated from the baby.
- Breast-feed babies on demand.
- Maintain exclusive breast-feeding for six months.
- Avoid artificial teats and dummies.
- Encourage breast-feeding support groups.

An institution's breast-feeding policy must be prominently displayed and conveyed to all members of staff, who should receive at least 18 hours of training in the anatomy of the breast, and in the theory and practical aspects of breast-feeding. They must be taught to communicate effectively with mothers and to impart valid information.

Formula milk may be required for specific infants, but leaflets or posters should not be sponsored by the manufacturers of such products.

STRUCTURE AND FUNCTION OF THE BREAST

The breasts originate from skin as specialised ectodermal structures. Each is made up of 15 to 20 lobes supported by connective tissue and fat cells. The lobes are subdivided into lobules containing clusters of alveoli, which open into collection ductules. These in turn drain into a lactiferous duct (one from each lobe) that broadens into a sinus where milk can be temporarily stored. From each sinus a duct leads on to the surface of the nipple through a skin pore. Sinuses cannot be detected on ultrasound studies and there is now some doubt as to their presence. The pigmented areola that encircles the base of the nipple contains small nodules, Montgomery follicles, which secrete an oily lubricant for the nipple (Fig. 5.2).

Various physiological changes take place in the breasts during pregnancy under the influence of oestrogen and progesterone hormones.

First trimester

There is branching and extension of the duct system.

Second trimester

New alveoli are formed and secretions appear in their luminae. The breasts are now capable of making milk, but are prevented from doing so by the high levels of progesterone and oestrogen.

Third trimester

The vascularity of the lobules increases and these structures occupy much of the space previously filled by the fat and connective tissue.

The diameter of the areola and nipple

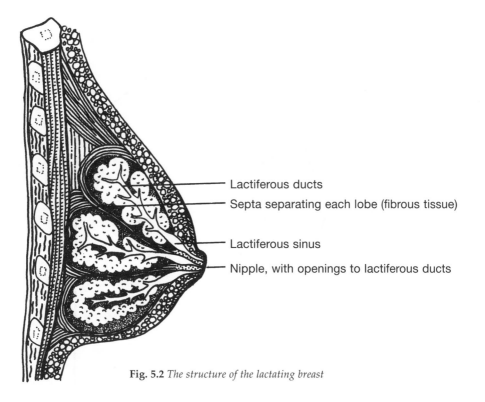

Fig. 5.2 *The structure of the lactating breast*

— Lactiferous ducts
— Septa separating each lobe (fibrous tissue)
— Lactiferous sinus
— Nipple, with openings to lactiferous ducts

increases throughout pregnancy. The nipple also becomes mobile and protractile, making it easy for the infant to grasp.

LACTATION

This is initiated by the hormones prolactin and oxytocin, which stimulate the breasts to secrete and drain milk.

Milk synthesis (Fig. 5.3)

Milk is synthesised by the alveolar cells of the breast under control of prolactin, a hormone secreted by the anterior pituitary gland. The levels of progesterone and oestrogen decrease rapidly after birth and prolactin promptly stimulates the alveolar cells to manufacture large amounts of fat, protein and milk sugar.

Fat

Fat globules are formed in the basal region of an alveolar cell and move towards the apex where they bulge through the cell wall. These globules, enveloped by a layer of plasma membrane, continue to protrude until the base is nipped off from the epithelial cell and they are released into the lumen (Fig. 5.3A).

Protein

Milk proteins appear as fine granular material in the Golgi apparatus of the alveolar cell and these granules are extruded into the lumen.

Sugar

The milk sugar, lactose, is formed in the alveolar cell from glucose and galactose in the presence of synthetases.

Prolactin secretion

The baby provides a major stimulus for prolactin secretion. When the breast is suckled, a series of nerve impulses is transmitted from the mother's nipple to her spinal cord and hypothalamus, which stimulates the anterior portion of the pituitary gland to release prolactin.

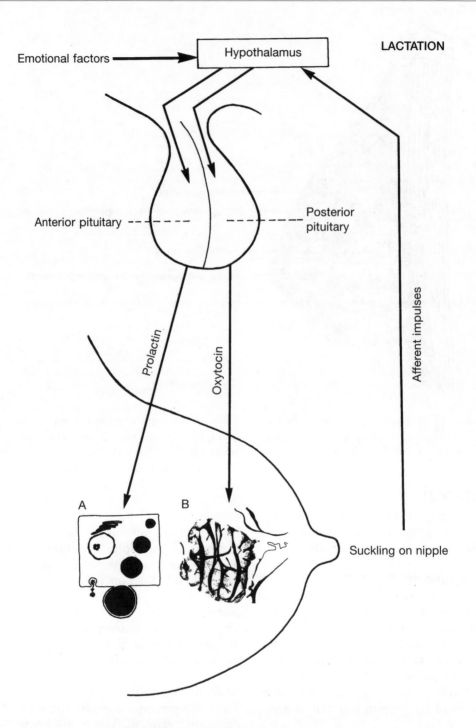

Fig. 5.3 *Lactation: Diagrammatic representation (see text)*
A. *The formation of milk in an alveolar cell. The dark circles represent a fat globule that forms at the base of the cell,*
then rises to bulge through the cell membrane and is finally extruded into the alveolar lumen
B. *An alveolus surrounded by the contractile myoepithelial fibres*
(Adapted from Richardson, KE. 1949. Proceedings of the Royal Society **136**: 30–45)

Large quantities of the hormone appear in the blood during nursing and for several hours thereafter.

Colostrum

The initial secretion from the breast is a thick yellow fluid, colostrum. Small amounts are actually produced during the last trimester of pregnancy and the quantity increases to about 50 ml a day after birth. There is a gradual change to mature milk after the second day post-partum, and this transition is usually completed within a week.

A comparison between colostrum and milk is tabulated as follows:

	Colostrum	Breast milk
Colour	Lemon-yellow	White
Specific gravity	1 040–1 060	1 030
Protein	8,6%	1,1–1,5%
Carbohydrate	3,2%	7,0%
Fat	2,3%	4,0%
Mineral salts	0,3%	0.2%
Water	85,6%	87,3%

Milk drainage (Fig. 5.3)

Nipple stimulation by sucking also causes the hormone oxytocin to be released from the posterior pituitary gland. This substance is found in the blood within three minutes of nursing, and it constricts myoepithelial cells. The bundle-like cells surround and compress each alveolus (Fig. 5.3B) to release a large quantity of fat-enriched 'hindmilk' into the ducts and sinuses. This strong ejection, the 'draught' or 'let down' reflex, depends on an adequate production of oxytocin. Milk secreted between feeds accumulates in the ducts as 'formilk'

Characteristics of 'foremilk'

This is the initial portion of milk that is ingested. It constitutes a third of the total output. The fat (2%) and protein content are low and the milk appears watery and blue.

A faulty let down reflex will result in the infant receiving 'foremilk' only and remaining hungry owing to the ingestion of too little fat.

Maintenance of lactation

The delicate balance between milk secretion and milk drainage must be maintained to ensure successful breast-feeding.

This depends on a number of factors:
- Hormones.
- Suitable nipples.
- Sucking reflex.
- Physical and emotional state of the mother.
- Attitude of the father, and of the medical and nursing staff.
- Fluid intake and diet.
- The technique of feeding.
- Adequate emptying of the breasts.

Hormones

The optimum production of milk depends on adequate quantities of prolactin and oxytocin. These hormones act best when oestrogen and progesterone are either absent or present in small quantities.

Contraceptive tablets containing oestrogen can impair milk secretion. Ergot preparations, as well as oestrogenic compounds, like stilboestrol, can decrease the output of prolactin.

Suitable nipples

In order to appreciate the role of the nipple, it is important to understand the method whereby an infant obtains milk from the breast.

The nipple is sucked far back into the baby's mouth (Fig. 5.4), to be cushioned between the cheeks, palate and dorsum of the tongue with the nipple-tip resting against the hard palate.

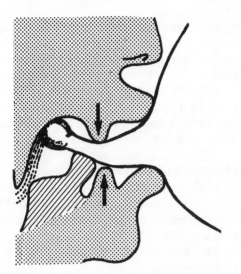

Fig. 5.4 *Sucking movements of the tongue and cheeks create a negative pressure at the back of the throat. At the same time the areola is compressed by the gums and milk flows against hard palate (From Appelbaum, RM. 1970. The modern management of successful breast-feeding. Pediatric Clinics of N America **17**: 203–25)*

Here it is protected from the force of suction created by the tongue and cheeks. This position of the nipple also enables the lips and jaws to come well up onto the periphery of the areola. The gums compress the underlying sinuses and milk is injected into the mouth.

Unsuitable nipples

An infant may be unable to grasp a nipple which is too large, too small or retractile. In such cases, the nipple lies at the front of the mouth with the areola out of reach of the baby's gums. Milk cannot be squeezed out effectively and the nipple surface bears the brunt of the suction. This results in a painful or cracked nipple, as well as improper drainage of milk from the breast. A vicious circle may follow as the nipple becomes oedematous and more difficult to grasp when it is buried in an over-distended breast.

Inverted nipples

When the areola margin is gently squeezed between a thumb and forefinger, the nipple usually protrudes. In some cases it will retract and thus be unsuitable for breast-feeding (Fig. 5.5). This difficulty can be overcome by specific treatment given in the last few months of pregnancy (Fig. 5.6).

Treatment

Place the tips of each thumb at the base of the nipple and stretch the skin towards the areolar margin (Fig. 5.6). If this movement is done several times a day, in both the horizontal and vertical planes, it often results in the nipple becoming protractile by the time the infant is born.

Another method of treatment is to fit a small plastic cup, the 'Woolwich shell', over the nipple during the last four to eight weeks of pregnancy. The rim of the cup presses against the areola when this device is worn under a tight bra, and causes the nipple to protrude into the cup.

Sucking reflex

Vigorous sucking is the single most important requirement for adequate lactation. Failure to empty the breast properly leads to milk stasis, venous and lymphatic engorgement, and finally to

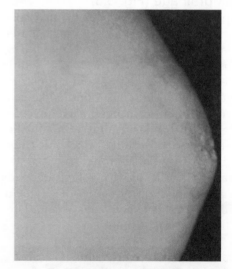

Fig. 5.5 *A retracted nipple*

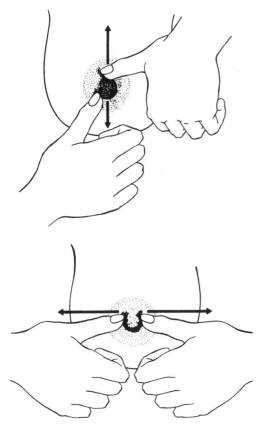

Fig. 5.6 *Antenatal treatment for an inverted nipple. The base of the nipple is stretched to break down adhesions (Adapted from Hoffmann, J. 1953.* American Journal of Obstetrics and Gynecology **66**: 346)

pressure atrophy of myoepithelial and alveolar cells, when no further milk will be produced.

Sucking can be impaired by:
- prematurity
- mechanical difficulties, such as
  - cleft palate
  - blocked nose
  - facial palsy
  - thrush
- oversedation
- illness, like respiratory distress
- mental retardation
- cerebral birth injury, or hypoxia.

The physical and emotional state of the mother

Fatigue caused by lack of sleep, ill health or the too-early resumption of work may impair lactation. Significantly, a third of the total output of prolactin is secreted during the hours of peaceful sleep. The smooth operation of the let down reflex is favoured by a tranquil mind. It can be hindered by the tensions, grief and fears that so commonly occur during the postpartum period. Such anxiety can often be dispelled by treating the mother with sympathy and giving her a full explanation of her particular problem.

Breast-feeding is often abandoned because a mother is considered to be "too nervous", or it is "too much strain for her". But will she as a consequence be free from nervous tension? Such anxiety is often best relieved by doing something successfully, and in this respect breast-feeding can be the finest tranquilliser.

The attitude of the father and the staff

A mother adopts several attitudes towards feeding her baby:

Often she is emotionally volatile during the early postpartum period and is easily swayed by suggestion, even though her decision to breast-feed was made in pregnancy. If she lacks confidence and feels she cannot feed successfully, she may seek advice from the baby's father, or her friends or professional advisers. Such advice is always well meant, but not necessarily the best informed.

The father's attitude is extremely important, as his encouragement may be the only factor needed for successful nursing in the difficult stages after birth. He is also the best person to ward off criticism that might come from his side of the family. The doctor and nurse must be understanding, encouraging, knowledgeable and patient in their approach. If such an attitude is not forthcoming, they will not stand a chance against a well-meaning friend who decries breast-feeding because the milk looks "too watery" or "blue" or "too strong".

A mother needs to be shown the practical details of breast-feeding. Of necessity, this is time-consuming and is often avoided by the nurse handing over a bottle so that he or she can get on with other duties. Breast-feeding under such circumstances is doomed to failure.

Breast-feeding should be a joy to the mother, never a burden. If she is truly unable to breast-feed, any feelings of guilt or inadequacy should be allayed.

Fluid intake and diet

The feeding mother is best maintained on a diet adequate in protein, energy and vitamins. She will require one to two litres of fluid a day to maintain normal hydration and to replenish the fluid secreted from the breasts.

The technique of feeding

A mother must be shown the correct way to feed her baby in order to maintain normal lactation (see below).

TECHNIQUES OF BREAST-FEEDING

Time of the first feed

A baby can be put to the breast immediately after delivery. This enables the alveoli and ducts of each breast to be cleared of thickened colostrum and provides an early stimulus for milk secretion and drainage. It also aids the contraction of the uterus. The normal infant is allowed to suckle on demand.

One or both breasts

Optimum drainage of milk is achieved by using both breasts at each feed. The infant initially suckles the breast last used at the previous feed. This ensures that at least one side is completely emptied at each nursing session.

Duration of feeding

A baby should suckle long enough to promote the let down reflex. This ensures that sufficient fore- and hindmilk will be obtained. The duration of suckling varies and can range from about five minutes per breast on the first day to approximately 15 minutes by the third or fourth day.

The longer interval is favoured if the breasts are engorged. In most cases, the maximum volume of milk is taken within the first five minutes, and the time taken to ingest an adequate amount should rarely exceed 25 minutes. The initial vigorous sucking and swallowing becomes weaker and less frequent at the end of a feed. The nipple thereafter is used as a pacifier and weak sucking may continue until the baby falls asleep.

Demand-feeding

Feeding on demand does not disrupt hospital routine, and if it disrupts the occasional meal the food can be kept warm for the mother.

Put the baby to the breast whenever signs of hunger appear, such as sucking of fingers, rooting or crying.

A newborn may demand to be fed every two hours in the early days after birth. This is not unusual, especially as small volumes of colostrum are obtained on each occasion. Large infants may desire feeds more frequently. A convenient routine is usually established within four to five days. A baby may occasionally develop an inverted sleep pattern by demanding frequent feeds at night and sleeping during the day. A more peaceful night may be obtained by waking the baby for feeds every two hours in the day.

Daily requirements

Most babies are content with the small quantities of high-protein colostrum that are secreted during the first few days of life.

By the fifth day their average intake of fluid has reached 150 ml/kg per day, and this provides about 420 kJ/kg/per day.

The habit of offering bottle feeds to an infant before milk production is established cannot be condoned, as it:

- encourages a method of sucking which differs from that used on the nipple
- satiates the appetite and sucking is consequently less vigorous
- impairs adequate milk drainage due to poor sucking
- introduces a foreign protein, such as cow milk, and thus enhances the chance of allergy.

Note
Vitamin and iron supplements are not needed if the mother is well nourished.

Putting the baby to the breast
Make use of the rooting reflex. A baby will turn the head towards a stimulus applied to the cheek or to the corner of the mouth. If these areas are lightly touched with the nipple, the infant will grasp it with an open mouth. Do not attempt to push the baby's cheek towards the nipple as the infant will simply turn from the breast to the stimulus. The lips should cover the areola rim, as this overlies the duct sinuses.

Taking the baby off the breast
Any attempt to pull the infant off the breast will result in injury to the nipple.

Gently squeeze the nostrils, which prompts the baby to open the mouth, or slip a finger alongside the nipple into the baby's mouth to break the suction.

Position during feeding
A mother should feed in the position she finds most comfortable and relaxing for herself and the baby. She may wish to feed while lying or sitting in bed, or she may prefer to sit in a chair. She may support the nipple between the second and third finger to prevent the breast from obstructing the baby's nostrils. The baby should be kept warm during feeds.

Sitting in bed
A good support is necessary to enable the mother to lean forward. The infant can be fed while lying on a pillow or being held in her arms.

Lying in bed
Sitting may be uncomfortable, particularly if the mother has perineal sutures. She may feel at ease lying on her side with the infant alongside on a pillow.

Sitting in a chair
A low, comfortable chair with a good back support is required. The infant rests on the mother's lap and, by supporting her foot on a small stool, she can raise the baby to the breast on that particular side.

Care of nipples
The nipples may be washed with soap and water once a day, and with water only before feeding. Soap occasionally hardens the nipples, in which case it is best avoided. Care should be taken to dry the nipples after feeding and to keep them soft by massaging in a small quantity of lanolin. The breasts should be supported in a well-fitting bra, which must not compress the nipples. Cracked and painful nipples can be prevented by good antenatal care (p. 45) and by promoting the correct technique of sucking (p. 46).

Breaking wind
The baby is held upright against the mother's chest with its head resting on her shoulder. The baby's back is rubbed firmly with the palm of her right hand, which moves upwards from the small of the back towards the left shoulder.

Feeding twins

Twins can be fed simultaneously by using both breasts at a feed, or they may be fed one at a time. The breasts are alternated for the babies at each feed.

FEEDING PROBLEMS

Sore nipples

Mothers often experience a tingling sensation in the nipple when the baby starts to suck. This is normal. A truly sore nipple is red and may be cracked. This problem is more likely to occur in fair-skinned women.

In most cases soreness can be prevented by paying adequate attention to the nipples between feeds, and by the correct 'fixing' of an infant on the breast. Suction on the nipple should always be released at the end of the feed (p. 49).

Encourage healing by keeping the nipple dry and by massaging it with lanolin. Short exposure to sunlight or ultraviolet light will also aid healing. A cracked nipple should be rested for 24 hours. Milk can be expressed manually and given to the infant by cup and spoon.

Red, inflamed nipples can be the result of a *Candida albicans* infection. The fungus is usually present in the infant's mouth (p. 220). Apply Nystatin® ointment to the nipples after each feed and use Nystatin® drops to heal the mouth infection.

Breast engorgement

This may occur on the third or fourth day, especially in a primipara.

Signs

- The breast is full, heavy and painful.
- It may feel lumpy.
- The overlying skin becomes oedematous and red, and veins are prominent.
- The nipple becomes swollen and buried in breast tissue.

Treatment

In a mild case, advise the mother to take a hot shower before putting the infant to the breast. Iced cabbage leaves may be placed around the breast for relief. Encourage frequent feeding to empty the breast and maintain adequate milk drainage.

In a severe case, sucking may not be possible owing to swelling of the nipple and breast. Place warm compresses on the red and oedematous areas. Then attempt to express milk. Support the breast with one hand, and with the other hand gently massage the skin and underlying ducts towards the nipple. Then depress the areola with the fingers to empty the underlying sinuses.

Manual expression may not be possible if the breasts are grossly oedematous and painful. A rapid-acting diuretic can relieve tension and oedema. Give the mother a tablet of oxytocin citrate 200 units (buccal Pitocin®), which she places under her tongue, to stimulate the let down reflex. Gentle manual expression may now be attempted. If this is unsuccessful, empty the breasts using a mechanical pump.

Ultrasound therapy to the breasts can also relieve engorgement and promote milk drainage.

Inadequate lactation

Adequate lactation may take several weeks to establish. This is not an indication to discontinue breast-feeding.

Inadequate milk production can be associated with:

- the older mother
- maternal malnutrition
- contraceptive tablets
- anxiety
- poor sucking
- inadequate sleep
- incomplete emptying of the breasts.

Treatment

Frequent feeding, for example two-hourly, is encouraged to stimulate the release of prolactin from the anterior pituitary.

Adequate rest should be established. Encourage the mother to sleep while her infant is asleep and to appoint others to carry out household duties at these times.

Daily intake of fluid should be between one and two litres.

Factors causing anxiety, such as infant colic (p. 292), must be treated.

Contraceptives containing progesterone only should be prescribed, as they do not suppress milk production.

Factors associated with poor sucking must be treated (p. 46).

Complete emptying of the breasts ensures an adequate production of milk and this can reach 800 ml per day.

Drugs

Eglonyl® and Maxolon® can increase milk production, but their long-term side-effects are unknown and they are not necessary in the first week.

Mastitis

This condition is usually intramammary and results from stagnation of milk.

Signs
- A tender lump is palpable.
- The overlying skin is red and the axillary lymph nodes are enlarged.
- Pyrexia and rigors may occur.
- A staphylococcal infection is likely to cause an abscess if the obstruction is not relieved.

Treatment

Analgesics and local heat give symptomatic relief.

Prescribe an antibiotic, like cloxacillin, for a week.

Encourage frequent feeding to empty the breast. A mechanical pump may be necessary if sucking is too painful.

Note

Mastitis or a breast abscess is not an indication to discontinue breast-feeding.

Overfeeding

Most breast-fed babies can regulate their requirements accurately and it is doubtful whether overfeeding ever actually takes place. A rapid flow of milk may occur at the beginning of a feed and cause coughing or vomiting. The rate of flow can be controlled by compressing the areola of the breast between the second and third fingers and by leaning back during the feed.

Underfeeding

A poor gain in weight after the fourth day is the most accurate indication of underfeeding. In fact, it may be the only sign, as the infant may appear content after feeds.

Other features include persistent crying and sucking of the fingers and a reduction in the amount of stools and urine.

Signs such as the size and firmness of the breasts and the amount of milk that can be expressed before and after feeds are most unreliable. Factors that lead to underfeeding include engorgement of breasts; inadequate milk production, particularly in the first few days; and poor sucking owing to oversedation.

Determine the amount of milk taken by test-weighing the baby. This is done as follows:
- Weigh the fully clothed infant before and after a feed.
- Do not change the nappy during the feed whether or not it is soiled or wet.

The difference between the two weights indicates the amount of fluid taken by the baby. This varies from feed to feed and test-weighing should be done over several feeds to get an accurate estimation of the baby's intake of milk.

Treatment
The underfed infant will require extra fluid. If the problem is related to breast engorgement, give the baby expressed mother's milk. The oversedated baby will need treatment with naloxone if morphine, pethidine or barbiturate drugs are the cause (p. 302).

Drugs in breast milk: Drugs that can cross into milk and harm the infant should not be prescribed for a breast-feeding mother (p. 301).

Contraindications to breast-feeding
Absolute contraindications are rare, and include cases of HIV infection, breast carcinoma, eczema of the nipples and intractable nipple inversion.

The following circumstances may temporarily preclude breast-feeding, but do not exclude the use of expressed breast milk:
■ Prematurity.
■ Maternal illness, such as chickenpox, Coxsackie infection.

MILK BANKING
Breast milk can be collected from a healthy lactating woman and given to her preterm or ill baby who is unable to suck and would benefit from this source of nutrition.

Collection
Expression
Breasts can be emptied manually (p. 50) or mechanically (p. 50).

The milk should not be stored in a single container as this increases the risk of contamination. It is poured into sterile feeding bottles (50 ml) that are then capped and autoclaved (p. 57). They are stored in a refrigerator, and unused feeds are discarded after 24 hours.

Sterilisation destroys heat-labile proteins and cells in milk, but ensures sterility.

Note
Where facilities for sterilisation are inadequate, milk banking is not feasible and may in fact be hazardous in an environment of a high incidence of HIV infections.

INTRODUCTION OF SOLIDS
The contented breast-fed baby who is thriving does not need other liquids or solid food before six months of age.

The following scheme is useful:
■ 6–7 months: Cereal mixed with expressed breast milk.
■ 7–8 months: Freshly cooked vegetables and fresh fruit.
■ 8–9 months: Puréed meat and fish.
■ 9–10 months: Yolk of egg.
■ Thereafter: Suitable foods from the table.

Cereals
A home-cooked cereal, like oats, is suitable and must be strained. Many precooked products are now available. Rice and maize are recommended as they are unlikely to cause allergic reactions.

Vegetables and fruit
Freshly cooked vegetables – such as pumpkin, carrots, potato, green peas, etc. – are suitable, and fruit includes pear, apples and banana. These are sieved or blended.

Meat and fish
Home-cooked products such as meat must be blended or finely chopped and then sieved. Commercially packed vegetables, fruits and meats are available. They are free of preservatives, added sugar or salt. These products are convenient, but expensive, and their nutritional value does not exceed that of home-prepared foods.

General rules

Use a small spoon to place the food well back on the baby's tongue, otherwise it will be pushed out of the mouth.

Offer a new food in small quantities, such as one teaspoonful. Gradually increase this to about six teaspoons.

Introduce one food only. Allow a week to pass before trying another. This enables adverse reactions, for example allergy, to be detected.

Offer coarser foods at 7 to 10 months.

Do not force-feed – this can lead to rejection of food.

Breast milk remains the staple diet and is not replaced by solids.

The diet should not remain monotonous for weeks on end, as this encourages a taste for one food.

THE TERMINATION OF BREAST-FEEDING

In poor socioeconomic circumstances, breast-feeding provides an infant with the best chance of optimum growth and survival and should be continued for well over a year, preferably 18 months to 2 years. Earlier termination may be considered when breast milk accounts for less than half of the infant's milk requirements. Breast-feeding is phased out over several months in order to provide a gradual diminution in the amount of milk secreted.

First two weeks of weaning

Replace the afternoon feed (14h00) with milk in a cup or bottle.

Second to fourth week

Drop the morning (10h00) and evening (18h00) feeds in favour of the cup or bottle.

Fourth to sixth week

Omit the early morning (06h00) feed. Breast-feeds are still given during the night if necessary.

Lactation usually ceases about 40 days after the last feed.

Sixth to eighth week

Give all feeds by cup or bottle.

A mother will experience marked discomfort if feeding has to be terminated suddenly. If this is necessary, for example as a result of severe illness, it is advisable to bind the breasts tightly, prescribe analgesics and restrict fluids for several days.

Note

The following are not indications for the discontinuation of breast-feeding:

- Milk appearing 'watery' or 'blue'.
- Vomiting.
- Colic.
- Pregnancy, if the mother is well nourished.

CHAPTER 6

Artificial Feeding

Artificial feeding is a phenomenon of the 20th century and probably constitutes the largest uncontrolled nutritional experiment ever undertaken. Millions of babies have been reared in this manner, but the long-term effects are still entirely unknown.

The establishment of this form of feeding did not attract much criticism in industrialised countries as it coincided with a dramatic fall in infant mortality rates. Clean water, sterile milk products, refrigeration and cleanliness contributed towards the relative safety in affluent communities.

However, it remains a hazardous and expensive procedure among populations of low socioeconomic status.

COMPOSITION OF COW MILK

While cow milk has become accepted as an alternative to human breast milk, the two differ greatly in composition (Table 6.1).

Protein
Casein is the major protein, in contrast to lactalbumin in human milk. Cow milk proteins are allergenic and can cause sensitisation if undigested portions are absorbed from the gut (p. xxx).

Fat
Butter fat contains large amounts of saturated fatty acids, which are not digested as readily as the predominantly unsaturated fatty acids of human milk. The normal baby absorbs about 95% of breast-milk fat, in contrast to 75% of butter fat. Cow milk lacks the essential fatty acid gamma linolenic acid.

Carbohydrate
The lactose content of 4% is about half that in human milk.

Minerals
The high sodium content has been implicated in cases of hypernatraemia and the phosphorus load can result in hypocalcaemia and tetany.

Vitamins
The levels of vitamins A, D and C are lower than in human milk.

TABLE 6.1

Comparison of the constituents of human and cow milk

Quantity of nutrients per 100 ml (Information derived from various sources)

	Mature human milk	Cow milk
Energy (kJ)	280	260
Protein (g)	1,5	3,4
Casein	0,5	2,7
Lactalbumin	0,7	0,5
Lactoglobulin	0,2	0,2
Carbohydrate (g)	7,0	4,8
Fat (g)	3,8	3,7
Mineral salts (%)	0,2	0,7
Sodium (mmol)	0,7	2,5
Calcium (mmol)	0,9	3,2
Phosphorus (mmol)	0,48	3,3
Magnesium (mmol)	0,17	0,65
Iron (μmol)	trace	trace
Vitamin A (IU)	240	140
Vitamin D (μg)	1,0	0,15
Vitamin C (mg)	5,0	1,0
Thiamine (mg)	0,01	0,03
Riboflavine (mg)	0,4	0,17
Nicotinic acid (mg)	0,02	0,10
Vitamin E (IU)	0,5	0,1

Elements
The milk contains insignificant amounts of iron and fluoride.

pH
The mean pH of 6,6 is lower than that of human milk, which averages 7,3.

MODIFICATION OF COW MILK

Processed milk
Raw milk is unsuitable for infant feeding and can be partially improved by heating, acidification, evaporation or drying. These processes enhance the sterility and digestibility of the product, but do not alter the basic composition.

Modified/humanised milks
Cost is related to the degree of modification. Milk can be separated into its major components, which are suitably altered and reconstituted to resemble those of human milk:

Protein
The correct casein to lactalbumin ratio is obtained by mixing whey with skimmed milk.

Fat
Droplet size is decreased by homogenisation. The ratio of saturated to unsaturated fatty acids is adjusted by adding or substituting vegetable fats such as maize and coconut oil.

Carbohydrates
The sugar content is increased by adding lactose or another sugar.

Minerals
The excessive solute load is reduced by multichamber electrodialysis, using ion exchange resins.

Vitamins and iron
These are added to most products.

Examples of modified milks
- Nan.
- S26.
- Similac.

Milk substitutes
Certain milk substitutes are also available and include soya feeds, for example

Infrasoy, Isomil and meat-based extracts. These are used for cow milk allergy and lactose intolerance.

Note
No process of modification can reproduce the unique nutritional and immunological properties of human breast milk.

Various modified milks and substitutes that are used for full-term babies are listed in Table 6.2.

Choice of product
The selection of a milk depends on its composition and price.

Paediatric groups and associations in various industrialised countries recommend the modified products for infant feeding. This has to be tempered by the fact that these milks cost more than the less modified ones and consequently may not be available in all countries.

Subsidised products may be offered at various infant clinics. Powdered milks are used widely as they are less expensive than prepacked liquid feeds.

PREPARATION OF FEEDS
At home
Requirements
- Eight plastic feeding bottles and caps.
- Eight teats.
- One metal knife for levelling milk powder.
- One bottle brush.
- One large pot with lid.

Cleaning technique
Rinse all items immediately after use, invert the teats and squirt water through the holes to ensure patency. Scrub the bottles and teats once a day with detergent and then rinse with water.

TABLE 6.2

Modified milks and milk substitutes used for full-term infants from birth		
Product	*Type*	*Comments*
Nan 1	Mostley whey	a starter feed
Pelargon	Acidified milk;	starter feed
NanHA	Partially hydrolysed;	use to prevent cow milk protein allergy
Alfare	Extensively hydrolysed;	use for cow milk protein allergy
AL110	Lactose and whey free;	use for lactose intolerance, galactosaemia
Wyeth S26	Mostly whey;	starter feed
Infrasoy Soy	protein; lactose free;	use for cow milk protein allergy
Mead Johnson Nutramigen	Extensively hydrolysed;	use for cow milk protein allergy
Portagen	Fats, mostly medium-chain triglycerides;	use for fat malabsorption
Abbott Similac/iron	Mostly casein;	suitable for a very hungry baby
Isomil Soy	protein;	use for lactose intolerance, cow milk protein allergy
Nutricia Neocate	Amino acid product;	post necrotising enterocolitis

Sterilisation
Boiling
Immerse items in a pot of water and boil for 10 minutes. Remove them with tongs dipped in boiling water beforehand.

Antiseptic solution
An alternative method is to immerse all items in a weak solution of sodium hypochlorite (1 in 80 strength). Renew the solution each day to ensure its potency.

Milk powder
A scoop is provided with each tin of milk. It is specific for that product and may not be used for other milks. Fill the scoop and level the powder to the rim with a knife edge.

Do not compact the powder against the inner edge of the tin or with a knife as this will overconcentrate the feed.

Fluid
Boil water and let it cool. Then reconstitute the milk by adding a scoopful of powder to each 25 ml of warm (boiled) water. This ratio may alter in various countries, depending on the size of the scoop. Prepare feeds for the whole day if refrigeration is available. Store them at 4° C in capped bottles until required.

Example
A two-week-old baby weighs 4 kg and receives six feeds a day.
Daily fluid requirement:
  600 ml (150 ml/kg)

Quantity of each feed:
  100 ml (600 ÷ 6)

Number of scoops per bottle:
  4 (100 ÷ 25)

In hospital
Disposable items
Liquid prepacked feeds are convenient and require storage space only. A bottle of milk may be taken off the shelf and fitted with a disposable sterile teat. It is then ready for use.

These milks are expensive, but they dispense with elaborate sterilisation procedures and kitchen staff.

Milk kitchen
Feeds must be prepared in a milk kitchen if prepacked items are unavailable. The kitchen comprises two areas: a cleaning section and a section for preparing feeds. They are separated by a wall into which an autoclave is fitted. This device opens at either end and is the sole means of communication between the sections.

The cleaning section needs a working surface, bottle washer, racks and bottle carriers. The preparation section should be fitted with a working surface, washbasin, storage cupboards, large electric mixer, weighing scale and refrigerators.

The staff employed in a milk kitchen must be familiar with aseptic procedures.

Bottles and teats are washed thoroughly in the cleaning section before use.

It is most important to remove all particulate matter.

Cracked bottles and perished teats are discarded.

Bottles and teats are then autoclaved for 10 minutes at a pressure of 1,8 kg per sq. cm and a temperature of 135° C.

They are transferred to the preparation room when cool, and filled with the feeds. Each bottle is fitted with a teat and capped down to the neck with a plastic cover.

The bottles are packed in a rack and re-autoclaved for five minutes at a pressure of 0,7 kg/per sq. cm and a temperature of 110° C.

They are immediately transferred to a large refrigerator and cooled rapidly to 4° C. They remain in the refrigerator until required in the nurseries.

A feed list must be kept in both the nursery wards and the milk kitchen.

Each bottle must be identified with the baby's name or a number. This can be done with a Koki pen.

Samples of milk, teats and bottles should be sent weekly for bacteriological checks.

Other methods of feed preparation are not recommended in large hospitals.

In a small unit where no such facilities are available, bottles and teats may be soaked in a solution of sodium hypochlorite 1:80, for example Milton™.

It is essential to renew the solution each day.

Note
Never store salt in the preparation room as it may inadvertently be used in feeds.

FLUID REQUIREMENTS

Full-strength feeds are commenced within an hour of birth. An infant is satisfied with small amounts of milk at this stage and it is not necessary to offer more than 30 ml/kg on the first day. Additional amounts can cause vomiting.

The quantity is gradually increased to 150 ml/kg, which is reached by the fourth or fifth day and maintained at this level until five or six months of age, when mixed feeding is commenced. The daily requirement then declines to 70–85 ml/kg and need not exceed a litre of milk over 24 hours.

Number of feeds in 24 hours
Five to eight feeds may be required each day, depending on the demands of the infant. In hospital, a four- or three-hourly schedule is usually convenient.

Four-hourly feeds are offered at:
06h00
10h00
14h00
18h00
22h00

Three-hourly feeds are offered at:
06h00
09h00
12h00
15h00
18h00
21h00

At home, a three-and-a-half-hourly schedule is often more suited to family routine.

Feeds may be given at:
06h00
09h30
13h00
16h30
20h00 to 22h00

The 13h00 feed is given before the family has lunch, while the 16h30 feed enables a mother to accomplish her household tasks between 17h00 and 20h00.

Note
An infant may demand a feed in the early hours of the morning on any of the above schedules. This feed can usually be omitted after three or four months of age.

VITAMINS AND IRON

Most modified products contain sufficient vitamins and iron for normal growth. Daily vitamin supplements are essential if a non-fortified milk is used and are often given as water-soluble drops (p. 303). Iron drops (p. 304) are introduced after a month in the case of non-fortified milks and should be continued until the infant is on a mixed diet.

FEEDING TECHNIQUES

Hold the baby on your lap and support

the head on your elbow. Ensure that the milk is not too hot by dropping some on the back of your hand. It should feel comfortably warm.

At home an electric bottle warmer may be used to maintain a constant temperature.

WEANING (p. 53)

Solid food is not needed for the contented baby before five to six months of age. Most bottle-fed infants, however, are dissatisfied with milk only and scream to be fed within 1½–2 hours of a meal.

Solids may have to be introduced earlier (at three to four months) as there is a limit to the amount of fluid an infant can ingest.

There are certain disadvantages of early weaning and it cannot be recommended as a routine procedure. Solids increase plasma osmolality and hypernatraemia is likely to occur should an infant become dehydrated for any reason. The incidence of childhood obesity is greater in bottle-fed babies than in those who are breast-fed and the problem can be compounded by the early introduction of solids.

CHAPTER 7

Disorders of Maturation, Growth and Development

Infants who have deviated from the anticipated intrauterine pattern of gestational age, growth or development may develop significant complications after birth. These must be anticipated and treated to prevent handicaps or death.

THE PRETERM INFANT

Definition p. 8
Prematurity remains a major problem as it is associated with significant morbidity and mortality rates and is often not preventable.

Incidence
The likelihood of birth before 37 completed weeks of gestation varies throughout the world and ranges from under 6% in affluent populations to over 20% in poverty-stricken groups.

Classification
Mortality is related to birthweight. Infants can be grouped into these four categories for statistical purposes: 500–999 g, 1 000–1 499 g, 1 500–1 999 g, and 2 000–2 500 g.

Most preterm babies (60%) weigh more than 1 800 g and have a relatively good prognosis. Those of less than 1 000 g comprise a very small portion of the total, but contribute significantly to mortality and morbidity rates.

Aetiology
Numerous factors are associated with prematurity (Table 7.1), but usually the cause for early onset of labour is unknown. Amniotic fluid infection syndrome (p. 91) and bacterial vaginosis feature prominently, but their significance is uncertain.

TABLE 7.1

Factors associated with prematurity

Maternal
Age: Less than 16 years
    More than 35 years
Social: Low socioeconomic status
    Malnutrition
    Physical or emotional trauma
Illness: Urinary tract infection
    Heart and renal disease
    Acute febrile conditions
    Pregnancy-induced hypertension
Cervical pathology: Cone biopsies
    Fibrosis
Uterine abnormalities: Bicornuate uterus
    Fibroids
Amniotic fluid infection syndrome
Bacterial/Mycoplasmal vaginosis

Placental
Antepartum haemorrhage: Placenta praevia
    Abruptio

Fetal
Multiple pregnancy
Congenital abnormality
Infection, e.g. syphilis
Growth retardation

Iatrogenic
Incorrect assessment of gestation
Elective induction, e.g. Rhesus disease

Clinical features

Physical characteristics differ from those of the full-term infant. Several important features are as follows:

Head

Fontanelles are relatively small.
Skull bones are soft.
Ears are small and pliable.
Hair is silky and individual strands tend to adhere to one another.

Skin and subcutaneous tissue

Vernix caseosa is sparse.
Lanugo is plentiful.
Skin lacks keratinisation, and is red, smooth and thin. It is also easily traumatised.

Blood vessels are prominent and fragile.

Subcutaneous fat is scanty or absent and the underlying bony structure is prominent.
Hands and feet may be oedematous.
Nails are short and easily broken.
Skin creases are poorly developed.
Breast nodules are absent.

Respiratory system

Thoracic cage is relatively small.

Breathing is often irregular in rate and depth and may be periodic. Apnoea can occur.
Cough reflex is weak or absent.
Nostrils are small and easily blocked.
Crying may be weak.
Lung alveoli may lack surfactant and tachypnoea, and rib recession is common.

Gastrointestinal system

Sucking and swallowing are poor or absent.
The abdomen is relatively large and distended, and viscera can be palpated through the thin wall.
The bowel may lack movement (absent bowel sounds).

Genitalia

Males: Testes may be felt in the inguinal canal by 32 weeks and in the scrotum by 36 weeks.
Females: Labia majora are poorly developed. Labia minora are prominent and thick. The clitoris is prominent.

Neurological system

Reflexes: Sucking is present but weak before 32 weeks. Grasping, noted at 28 weeks, is well established after 34 weeks.
Posture: Before 32 weeks, the arms and legs are extended. From 32 to 34 weeks, the legs are flexed. After 34 weeks, the arms and legs are flexed.

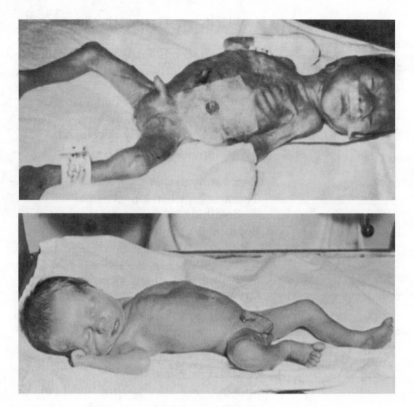

Fig. 7.1 *Preterm infant, 27 weeks, weight 700 g*

Fig. 7.2 *Preterm infant, 33 weeks, weight 1 500 g*

Abnormal neurological features may result from bleeding in the immature germinal matrix (p. 143) or from hypoxic damage to the cerebral white matter (p. 141).

Behaviour

The infant sleeps for the major part of the day. Stretching of limbs and yawning are well established after 32 weeks' gestation. Rapid eye movement (REM) sleep periods (p. 125) are frequent.

Management

Before birth

Threatened labour, intact membranes

Preterm labour is an obstetric emergency which should be handled in a maternity centre. The following queries need to be addressed:

- Is birth imminent?
- Is the fetus mature?
- What mode of delivery is preferable?

Birth is unlikely to occur if fetal breathing movements are detected on ultrasound examination or if fibronectin is absent in the vaginal secretions. In these cases an attempt is made to arrest labour for 48 hours through the use of various medications, such as Atisoban.

An amniocentesis is done to determine fetal lung maturity (p. 160). If this is not practicable, or if insufficient surfactants are detected in the amniotic fluid, then betadexamethasone is given to the mother (12 mg once a day over 48 hours). If labour can be prevented for this time, it will allow the fetal organs, such as the lungs, to mature.

Threatened labour, ruptured membranes

A decision must be made regarding the optimum time for delivery. The risk of infection is weighed against that of lung immaturity. Signs of intrapartum infection, like maternal pyrexia, or contamination, like bacteria in amniotic fluid, warrant antibiotic therapy.

Should the fetus show any signs of distress, such as tachycardia, abnormal cardiotocograph tracings or acidosis, then delivery by Caesarean section is indicated (p. 167).

At birth

A person experienced in resuscitation must be present, particularly if a very small baby (less than 1 500 g) is anticipated. Ensure adequate ventilation (p. 168) and provide warmth by immediately placing the tiny infant (< 1 000 g) into a plastic bag with a flap to cover the head, but not the nose or mouth. Dry a larger baby and transport the infant in a warm incubator to an intensive care unit. The extremely low birthweight infant or one with respiratory distress may be given nasal continuous positive airway pressure during the journey.

An ill or very small baby who is born at home or in a midwife obstetric unit can be warmed by kangaroo care (p. 65) and must be stabilised before transfer to a neonatal unit (p. 37).

After birth

The initial care and investigation of a premature baby is summarised in Table 7.2.

The most important considerations are: "Keep the infant warm, sweet (normoglycaemic), pink and aseptic". All care, be it primary, secondary or tertiary, centres around these cardinal rules. The smaller the infant, the more exacting is the need to apply them.

Body temperature

This determines the baby's chance of survival. When the skin temperature is persistently less than 35 °C or more than 37 °C the mortality is increased fivefold. The risk of dying is reduced significantly at a normal temperature of 36,5 °C.

TABLE 7.2

Initial management of a well preterm baby

Measurements: Measure weight, head circumference (p. 12)
Identification: Place nametags on two limbs (p. 32)
Vitamin K_1: Give 1 mg by intramuscular injection (p. 26)
Temperature: Use incubation or kangaroo care, and check the skin temperature (p. 64)
Respiration and colour: Place baby on an apnoea monitor and check oxygen saturation (p. 163)
Blood sugar: Obtain a sample of heel blood for blood sugar level (p. 262); recheck hourly until it is above 2,5 mmol/l
Gastric fluid: Aspirate a few millilitres for bubbles (p. 160), microscopy and culture
Infection screen: Ensure that mother's VDRL status is known; if not, obtain blood for syphilis screening (p. 228); collect blood for a white cell count if sepsis is suspected (p. 228)

Hypothermia

A small infant is likely to become cold because of:

- thin skin
- little or no subcutaneous fat
- inadequate amounts of brown fat (p. 268)
- a relatively large surface area, especially the head
- a rapid rate of breathing
- evaporation.

The ever-present risk is increased by exposure during:

- birth
- transportation
- weighing
- bathing
- procedures, such as an X-ray.

Hyperthermia

Small babies, especially if clothed, may overheat during phototherapy, incubation or radiant heating. This can result in apnoea and cyanosis.

Temperature measurement

Sites: The axilla or skin of the abdomen.

Record the axillary temperature on a low-reading mercury thermometer, or

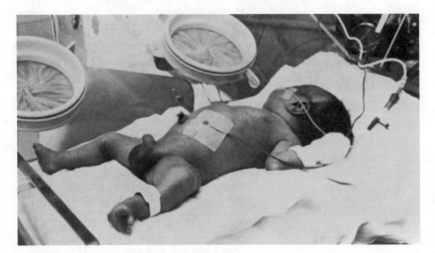

Fig. 7.3 *The measurement of skin temperature on the abdominal wall*

measure abdominal skin temperature with a thermistor probe. Attach this to the skin away from the liver area, as this may be warmer than other regions. Ensure that the probe does not lie between the infant and the mattress as this will give an erroneously high reading.

Keeping the baby warm
Babies who weigh less than 2 000 g cannot maintain a normal body temperature without additional warmth or insulation.

Incubators
The conventional single-walled incubator is suitable for most infants, providing its limitations are recognised. The temperature that keeps an infant in the thermoneutral state (p. 267) varies with the degree of humidity, the room temperature and the presence or absence of air currents.

Initially, set the incubator temperature at 34 °C and then adjust it to maintain the baby's skin temperature between 36,2 and 36,8 °C. Check and record the incubator and skin temperature half-hourly.

Suitable incubator temperatures for infants of various weights and ages are illustrated in Fig. 7.5. They range from 36 °C for newborn small babies (1 kg or less) to 32 °C for older and larger ones.

These measurements apply only to babies who are unclothed and nursed in a humidity of 50% and at a room temperature of 27 °C. They serve as a guide and have to be altered if the thermal environment changes.

Several incubators must be prewarmed and ready for use at all times.

Heat shield (Fig. 7.5)
A U-shaped perspex™ shield may be placed over the baby. This converts the incubator into a double-walled unit and maintains a stable environmental temperature by reducing the loss of heat from the air that surrounds the baby. It is recommended for infants of below 1 500 g in weight.

Servo-control
This device is fitted to an incubator and is used in conjunction with a thermistor probe. It adjusts the incubator temperature automatically to maintain the infant's skin temperature at a preset level, such as 36,5 °C.

Removal from incubator
Most preterm babies will benefit from incubation until they have reached

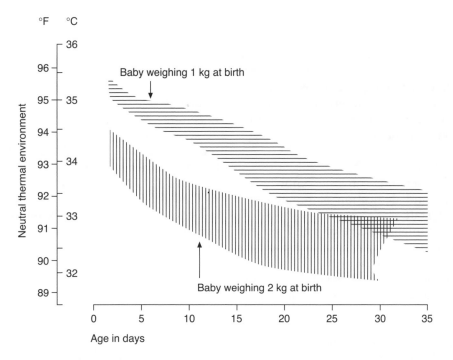

°F   °C

Neutral thermal environment

Baby weighing 1 kg at birth

Baby weighing 2 kg at birth

Age in days

Fig. 7.4 *Incubator temperatures that are needed to keep infants of different weights in a thermoneutral state* (*From Hey, E and Katz, G. 1970.* Archives of Diseases in Childhood, *45: 328*)

1 800–1 900 g in weight. At this stage they may be clothed and placed in a cot. Check skin temperature half-hourly for the first 24 hours and ensure that the head is adequately insulated with a thick cap. If kangaroo care is available, infants at a lower weight may be removed from incubators.

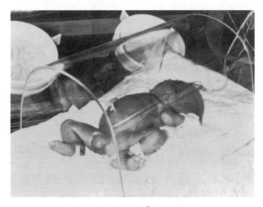

Fig. 7.5 *A perspex® heat shield*

Radiant heating

Intensive care cribs are popular. They consist of a radiant heater and a photo-therapy unit mounted above an open cradle. The infant's temperature is regulated by servo-control.

Advantages: The baby is accessible to staff and parents and can undergo various procedures without being moved. Hypothermia can be corrected rapidly.

Disadvantages: Insensible water loss is increased and extra fluid may be needed to prevent dehydration (p. 67), particularly in infants below 1 000 g. The problem can be minimised by covering the baby with a plastic sheet, which is thin and transparent. Transfer the infant to a closed incubator after the acute phase.

Kangaroo care

This form of ambulatory care keeps a preterm baby in intimate contact with the mother's skin. It ensures a constant body temperature, early and prolonged production of breast milk, less chance of serious infection, maternal confidence and timely discharge from hospital.

It can be used intermittently in an intensive care unit or continuously in a hospital or at home.

Requirements

Success depends on the knowledge, support and dedication of nursing and medical staff.

In the intensive care unit and nursery a comfortable chair and footstool are needed for the mother.

A designated area is essential for continuous kangaroo care. It must include facilities for sleeping, eating, ablutions and entertainment. Here a mother takes over responsibility for her infant under the supervision of knowledgeable nursing staff.

Technique

Remove the baby's clothes, except for the nappy and cap.

Secure the baby upright against the mother's skin, between her breasts. She does not require special garments, but a close-fitting cotton top will enhance support and permit her to walk about. The baby is maintained in this position throughout the day and night. The environmental temperature must be maintained above 20 °C.

The timing of kangaroo care depends on the experience of the staff. It can commence immediately after birth, after stabilisation of an infant, in an intensive care unit, or several weeks later when special care is not needed. Likewise, the weight at which this care is commenced is determined by staff experience. If an infant is weaned from an incubator at 1 500 g, continuous kangaroo care will be needed until 2 000 g. Part of this may be done at home, depending on the confidence of the parents and the progress of growth.

In the early stage, monitor the infant's heart and respiratory rate, temperature and oxygen saturation.

These should remain stable.

Feeding

Encourage a mother to express her milk as soon after birth as possible and to repeat this three-hourly. Breast milk may be given to her infant through a nasogastric tube (p. 71) or by cup (p. 70). The method depends on the state of the infant and the strength of the suck reflex. This can be enhanced by holding the baby's mouth on the mother's nipple during gavage feeding. It also promotes the let down reflex. Repeatedly attempt to get the infant to suck the nipple, thereby encouraging early breast-feeding. Feed hourly, then two-hourly until discharge.

Monitor the baby's weight daily. If weight gain is less than 15 g per day, supplementation will be necessary. Use a breast milk fortifier or other recommended additives (p. 69).

Discharge

The following factors are more important than actual weight: adequate feeding, the rate of weight gain, and a competent and confident mother who is willing to continue kangaroo care at home.

Follow-up

Check weight within three days of discharge and ensure regular assessments thereafter as with other preterm infants.

Alternative methods

Body warmth can be maintained by the following:

Clothing: Warm clothing is essential. Cover the baby's head with a woollen cap, as 30% of heat loss occurs from this site. Enclose the hands and feet in woollen mittens and cover the baby with at least two thick blankets.

Room temperature: The nursery may have to be heated to 28 °C if other methods are inadequate. This is uncomfortable for staff, but it ensures a consistently warm environment for babies.

Feeding

The nutritional requirements of a preterm baby are influenced by numerous physical and metabolic factors (Tables 7.3 and 7.4) and growth is more difficult to attain as gestation decreases. Significant losses of water, electrolytes and energy occur, and there is a risk of apnoea or aspiration during feeds.

Water loss

Body composition is related to gestation and the water content exceeds 80% in a baby of 1 000 g (Table 7.3). Water is lost in the stools and urine after birth. The renal loss can be accelerated by excessive glucose in the blood. Considerable amounts of water may evaporate from the respiratory tract and from the skin, which lacks a cornified epidermis. This evaporative loss is diminished in a humidified atmosphere.

TABLE 7.3

Body composition of preterm vs term infant		
	1 000 g	*3 500 g*
Water	86%	69%
Fat	1%	16%
Protein	8%	11%
Carbohydrate	0,5%	1%

The features of excessive water loss are:
- a significant fall in birthweight (up to 20%)
- hyperosmolar serum (over 300 mmol/l).

To ensure adequate water balance observe the following precautions:

- Nurse very small babies (800 g and less) in closed incubators with high humidity (60–80%).

  This allows a moderate intake of fluid and thus prevents a patent ductus arteriosus (p. 194).
- Check the blood glucose level three-hourly.
- Test the urine for sugar (Dipstix).
- Determine the osmolality of serum daily.
- Prevent overheating, for example during phototherapy.
- Provide an adequate intake of fluid (p. 68).
- Introduce fluid and energy within half an hour of birth to maintain hydration and a normal level of blood glucose.

TABLE 7.4

Factors that influence nutrition in the preterm baby	
Metabolic	Reduced stores of glycogen Reduced stores of iron and calcium Increased loss of sodium in urine Increased oxygen consumption
Gastrointestinal	Limited capacity of stomach Inadequate or absent gag reflex Inco-ordination of sucking and swallowing Poor gastro-oesophageal sphincter mechanism Diminished movements of bowel Decreased absorption of fat

Intravenous feeding

Ill babies and those under 1 500 g are less likely to develop complications if fed only by the intravenous route for the first 24–48 hours. Dextrose water 10% is suitable. A total of 60 ml/kg/day will cover basic metabolic needs, but is inadequate for growth. Avoid larger volumes in infants over 1 500 g at this stage, as fluid overload may occur. Check the blood sugar level three-hourly and maintain it above 2,5 mmol/l. If it exceeds 7 mmol/l, change the intravenous fluid to a 5% dextrose solution.

Nutritional reserves will be depleted within four days if milk feeding cannot be commenced. In this case intravenous supplementation is required with an amino acid/glucose solution (Vamin). This comprises 25% of total fluid intake and provides extra energy (p. 72).

The extremely low birthweight infant requires a larger initial volume of fluid to compensate for excessive evaporation from the immature skin – 120 ml/kg/day and the amino acid solution can be commenced earlier (on day two).

Oral feeding

Ill babies and those under 1 500 g may be fed orally as soon as bowel sounds are audible, meconium has been passed and the abdomen is not distended. This usually occurs within 48 hours of birth. Initially give 20% of the total volume of fluid orally. Expressed breast milk is suitable and can be run continuously into the stomach through a nasogastric tube. Control the rate of flow with a syringe driver or an infusion pump. Early feeding prevents excessive weight loss, reduces the risk of hyperbilirubinaemia, enhances gut motility, stimulates the release of gut hormones and enzymes, and promotes colonisation of the bowel with bifidobacteria.

Gradually increase the volume of milk and discontinue intravenous feeding when the daily intake of milk has reached 80–90 ml/kg.

Stop oral feeding if the abdomen distends, or vomiting occurs, or more than 3 ml of milk is aspirated from the stomach.

Healthy preterm babies over 1 500 g may start oral feeding soon after birth, provided the abdomen is not distended and bowel sounds are heard. Those with a strong suck reflex can be put to the breast.

Full fluid requirements (150–180 ml per kg per day) may be reached within days in larger babies, but can take weeks in smaller ones. Suggested weekly increases are shown in Table 7.5.

TABLE 7.5

Suggested fluid intake for the preterm baby over 1 000 g	
	(ml/kg/day)
1st week	60–90
2nd week	90–110
3rd week	110–130
Thereafter	150–180

These volumes apply only to infants in conventional single-wall incubators. Those who weigh less than 1 000 g or those under radiant heaters or phototherapy units may need extra fluid to compensate for insensible water loss. Also, many units prefer a more rapid progression, reaching 150–180 ml per kg per day within a week.

Phototherapy

Per se, this does not increase insensible water loss, but heat generated by some units may raise the baby's temperature with subsequent loss of fluid. An additional 15–20 ml per kg per day of fluid may be required.

Radiant heater

Babies may need 45–50 ml per kg per day of extra fluid.

Give this cautiously to avoid circulatory overload and patency of the ductus arteriosus.

Choice of milk

Human milk is suitable for all preterm babies and is the food of choice. Substitutes include products designed for the low-birthweight baby, for example Prenan,

S26 LBW. All breast milk substitutes contain bovine protein, which can be absorbed through the relatively porous gut to cause sensitisation and subsequent allergy. Avoid these products if there is a significant family history of allergy, such as asthma.

A mother's breast milk should be used for her preterm infant as it contains more protein, energy and sodium than does term milk.

Energy requirements

Preterm babies need approximately 480 kJ/kg/day for normal energy expenditure and growth. Human breast milk provides sufficient energy at a volume of 150–180 ml/kg/day. Additional energy must be supplied to babies who cannot tolerate this amount of milk, particularly those who weigh less than 1 500 g.

Breast milk fortifiers

These supplement breast milk with protein, minerals and energy. One such product (FM 85, Nestlé™) consists of hypoallergenic protein, maltrodextrin and minerals.

Its nutrient makeup is as follows:
- Per 5 g powder Protein 0,8 g
  Carbohydrate 3,6 g
  Calcium 51 mg
  Magnesium 2 mg
  Phosphorus 34 mg
  Sodium 27 mg

By adding 5 g of powder to 100 ml of breast milk, the energy of the latter is increased from 280 to 355 kJ.

If milk fortifiers are unavailable, you can consider the following additives: Caloreen™, a digestible glucose polymer, provides 16 kJ per gram of powder, and several grams may be added to feeds to give an additional 80–100 kJ per day.

Liprocil™, a readily absorbed mixture of medium chain triglycerides and essential fatty acids, provides 37,6 kJ per gram and can also be given in small amounts (5–8 g daily), depending on the estimated amounts of energy and fluid. Being a fatty solution it is recommended only for infants who have a nasogastric tube in place.

Example

A 10-day-old infant weighing 1 500 g is nursed in an incubator and is able to ingest 90 ml/kg of human milk each day.

Daily energy requirements: 480 kJ/kg
Actual energy intake: 288 kJ/kg
Shortfall: 192 kJ/kg

This is made up by adding:
Caloreen™ 5 g: 80 kJ/kg
Liprocil™ 4 g: 148 kJ/kg
Total: 228 kJ/kg

The infant will now receive 516 kJ/kg each day. The additional energy allows for wastage in stools and provides sufficient kilojoules for growth.

Sodium requirements

Excessive amounts of sodium are lost in the urine of babies who weigh less than 1 500 g. Hyponatraemia can be prevented by adding sodium bicarbonate to feeds. A total of 5 ml of 4% solution is mixed in 100 ml of breast milk to give an additional 2,5 mmol/dl of sodium.

The daily requirement of sodium is 4–5 mmol/kg.

Phosphorus

Additional amounts are required for normal bone development and growth. Add 15 mg phosphorus to each 100 ml of breast milk.

Frequency of feeding

Continuous feeding is favoured for ill babies and those who weigh less than

1 500 g, as it avoids abdominal distension and vomiting.

Commence intermittent feeding when the infant is able to tolerate more than 130 ml/kg/day. Milk is given at hourly, then two-hourly, and finally three-hourly intervals. The rate of progression depends on the size of the baby and may take several weeks to complete.

Weaning to breast or bottle

Co-ordination of sucking and swallowing is usually established between 34 and 36 weeks' gestation, and the breast, cup or bottle may be offered at this stage. The required amount of milk ought to be taken within 20–25 minutes' sucking time. Tube-feeding is maintained if this is not the case.

Sometimes the transition from tube to breast can be accelerated by non-nutritive sucking. Offer the baby a dummy or the mother's nipple during tube feeds. Additional factors that enhance the possibility of breast-feeding are close contact with the mother, as in kangaroo care, frequent expression of milk from her breasts, and the encouragement and assistance of skilled nursing staff.

A baby will need approximately eight feeds a day and the technique used to breast- or bottle-feed is similar to that for the term infant.

Cup feeding

This is helpful for infants who cannot complete a breast-feed because of a weak suck reflex. The method does not stimulate sucking and remains an interim procedure for establishing breast-feeding.

Support the baby's head upright and place the edge of a small plastic cup (the cover of a feeding bottle is suitable) on the lower lip. Tilt the cup so that milk trickles onto the infant's upper lip. With patience the baby will learn to 'lap up' the milk with the tongue.

Anticipated growth

Weigh babies daily to establish the adequacy of nutrition. On the above feeding schedule, growth is slower than that which occurs *in utero*. The rate of weight gain depends on the size of the infant at birth. Infants of less than 1 500 g lose approximately 5% of birthweight in the first week. They show a mean increase of 90 g during the second week and a subsequent weekly gain of 160–200 g. By 40 weeks' gestation, their weight averages 2 500 g.

The catch-up growth continues during the following months and normal size for age is attained within months or years, depending on birthweight.

The head circumference increases by approximately 1 mm a day.

Supplements

Iron (p. 304)

The preterm baby lacks adequate stores of this element and needs supplementation to prevent iron deficiency.

Daily requirements: 1,5–2 mg/kg of elemental iron. This can be obtained from an oral preparation, such as Ferrodrops™. Omit medication for the first month as it is considered to increase the risk of bacterial infection. Thereafter, continue with supplementation until the infant is on a mixed diet. Minor adverse effects include vomiting, constipation and dark stools.

Vitamins (p. 303)

Fat-soluble vitamins are poorly absorbed and deficiency states can result if supplements are not provided. Preterm babies are particularly susceptible to rickets during the stage of rapid growth. Those weighing less than 1 500 g may have the additional problem of folic acid and vitamin E depletion.

Recommended daily requirements of important vitamins are listed in Table 7.6. A solution such as ViDaylin™ drops contains most of these and is given shortly after birth and continued until the infant has been weaned.

TABLE 7.6

Daily requirements of certain vitamins	
Vitamin A	1 500 IU
Vitamin D	800 IU
Vitamin C	50 mg
Folic acid	0,35 mg
Vitamin E	5 IU

Nasogastric feeding
Requirements
- Sterile plastic feeding catheter, such as Pharmaseal™:
  - Size 8F for infants over 2 000 g.
  - Size 5F for smaller babies.
- Sterile plastic syringe, 5 ml.
- Stethoscope.
- Strapping, 4-mm wide Blenderm™.

Method
The length of tube to be passed into the stomach can be calculated by measuring the distance from the suprasternal notch to the xiphisternum, doubling this and adding 2,5 cm.

Support the infant's head to flex the neck slightly and gently insert the required length of catheter through a nostril into the stomach. Do not force the catheter down and try the other nostril if the passage is difficult.

Fix the catheter to the face with strapping. When 2 ml of air is rapidly injected into the tube, a loud noise can be heard in the stomach region through a stethoscope. This confirms the situation of the catheter tip. If the baby has just been admitted, withdraw a sample of gastric fluid to examine for pus cells and surfactant (p. 172).

Delivery system
A syringe pump is suitable for continuous or intermittent feeding. It delivers an accurate volume of milk within the required time and prevents fat from adhering to the wall of the syringe.

The following alternative methods can also be used.

Continuous: Milk is prepared in sterile 150 ml vacolitre bottles, which can be suspended from a drip stand. A bottle is attached to the nasogastric tube by a drip set and the rate of flow is regulated by a constant infusion pump. Vacolitres are changed every six hours and drip tubing is replaced three times a week. Attach a label marked 'gastric' to the line to distinguish it from intravenous lines that should be clearly identified by labels marked 'intravenous'. Renew nasogastric tubes weekly using the alternate nostril.

Intermittent: The bottle of sterile milk is connected to a drip set which is fitted with a two-way tap and 10 ml syringe. The required volume of milk is drawn into the syringe and injected through the nasogastric tube over 10–15 minutes.

To feed large babies attach the barrel of a sterile syringe to the nasogastric tube. Pour milk into the syringe and run it into the stomach by gravity over 5–10 minutes. Encourage sucking by offering the baby a teat during feeds.

Total parenteral nutrition
Nutrients can be given intravenously for days or weeks to those who cannot tolerate oral feeding after the third day of life. The main indications are:
- weight less than 1 000 g
- ileus
- necrotising enterocolitis.

Treatment is exacting and should be conducted only by experienced staff in an intensive care unit.

Requirements
A mixture, as listed in Table 7.7, provides sufficient energy, fat, protein, carbohydrate, electrolytes, trace elements

and vitamins for growth. The daily fluid requirement of 150 ml/kg should be attained within a week.

TABLE 7.7

Total parenteral nutrition with amino acids/glucose/ lipids ITN 1601A 150 ml pack (Isotec)	
Contents per: 100 ml	
Protein	1,97 g
Fat	1,75 g
Energy	58 kcal
Na	2,20 mmol
K	1,75 mmol
Mg	0,19 mmol
Ca	1,16 mmol
Phosphate	0,87 mmol
Trace elements	Zinc, copper, chromium, manganese, selenium
Multivitamins	
Other	Cysteine-HCl, carnitine

Method
Using a small sterile forceps, thread a 15-cm silicone catheter (Vygon™) through a 19-gauge winged needle into a peripheral vein and position it in a large vessel close to the heart. The catheter is immobilised and attached to a drip set. The procedure is done under aseptic conditions and the puncture site is covered with a dressing. In the absence of infection or thrombosis, the catheter can be left in a large vessel for two weeks.

Plastic cannulas may also be used, but the drip will need to be re-sited every 48 hours to prevent thrombosis or fluid leakage into tissues. Control the rate of flow with an infusion pump and use a drip set with a special in-line filter.

Potential complications are listed in Table 7.8.

TABLE 7.8

Complications associated with parenteral nutrition	
Drip site	Phlebitis Tissue necrosis Venous thrombosis Sepsis
Metabolic	Hypo-/Hyperglycaemia Electrolyte imbalance Mineral imbalance Metabolic acidaemia Uraemia Hyperammonaemia Hyperbilirubinaemia (cholestasis) Nephrocalcinosis (renal stones) Metabolic bone disease

Daily routine care
- Change drip packs and tubing to reduce the risk of infection and thrombosis.
- Weigh all wet nappies to measure urine output.
- Weigh the baby and measure head circumference to assess growth.
- Check blood glucose level and urine analysis.

Important investigations are summarised in Table 7.9.

Prevention of infection
The risk of bacterial infection is ever present and related to factors associated with prematurity (Table 7.10).

Pay particular attention to the following:

Hand-washing
This is the single most important factor in the prevention of cross-infection. All who enter a nursery unit must ensure that infants are touched with cleansed hands only (p. 31).

Infant
Amniotic fluid infection syndrome increases the likelihood of sepsis after birth and every preterm baby should

TABLE 7.9

Investigations during parenteral nutrition	
	Frequency
Blood	
Sugar	Daily (if stable)
Electrolytes	Weekly (if stable)
Acid base	Weekly (if stable)
White cell count	Weekly
Haematocrit	Weekly
Liver function tests	Weekly
Conjugated bilirubin	Weekly
Creatinine	Two-weekly
Ammonia	Two-weekly
Protein	Two-weekly
Triglycerides	Two-weekly
Trace elements	Two-weekly
Urine	
Glucose	Daily
Osmolality	Daily

be screened for contamination. This is characterised by pus cells or organisms in gastric fluid at birth and histological signs of chorioamnionitis in the placenta. Babies in this category require close observation for clinical and laboratory evidence of infection (p. 93).

Handle babies as little as possible and provide the following care:

Cord: Clean the umbilical stump three-hourly with methylated spirits to promote drying. Confine this to the cord and

TABLE 7.10

Factors that increase the risk of infection in the preterm infant
Disruption of protective barriers:
amniotic fluid infection syndrome
endotracheal intubation
vessel catheterisation
skin trauma
Inadequate immunity:
low level of IgG immunoglobulin
inadequate antibody response
reduced numbers of white blood cells
poor phagocytosis
low level of complement (C5)

do not apply alcohol to the surrounding skin.

Skin: See p. 74.

Feeding: Use breast milk to prevent gastroenteritis and necrotising enterocolitis and wipe the spigot of the nasogastric tube with spirits before it is opened.

Incubators

Wipe the external surfaces each day with methylated spirits. Clean the internal surfaces with a disposable wet cloth to remove urine or faeces. Keep the water bath empty to prevent colonisation with *Pseudomonas* and transfer the baby to a clean incubator each week.

High humidity is recommended for very small babies only, such as those less than 800 g. In this case, fill the water bath.

Method of cleaning

Remove unattached parts: cuffs, gasket, mattress, base and air filters.

Soak the cuffs in a detergent solution.

Do not remove the plastic cover from the mattress.

Wash all parts of the incubator with a detergent and then wipe them with methylated spirits.

If internal air filter strips are used replace them with clean ones.

External air filters are replaced two-monthly. The date of next change is noted on a label attached to the incubator.

Incubators require servicing every three months.

Visitors

Encourage parents, siblings and grandparents to visit and handle the baby frequently. Their presence affords the love and attention essential for the infant's well-being and does not increase the risk of infection.

Clothing

No restriction is placed on staff dress.

Staff selection

This is based on their desire to care for small babies and not on meaningless results of throat, nasal or rectal swabs! Those assigned to a nursery must not work in other wards of a hospital during this period. Staff with a flu-like illness, cold sores or skin infections are barred from the unit. They may be harbouring a Coxsackie, respiratory syncitial (RSV) or herpes virus, which can be fatal to newborn babies.

Nursing care

The intact survival of a premature baby depends primarily on the quality of nursing.

The distinction between nursing and doctoring tends to be blurred in a nursery, particularly in an intensive care unit, and a nurse must be prepared for every eventuality. Crises are often unpredictable and require immediate attention. Procedures like endotracheal intubation, assisted ventilation or venous catheterisation may have to be performed by a nurse. Thus practical skills must be encouraged in nurses in order for expertise to be maintained, especially if medical staff are unavailable.

Unlike a full-term infant, the premature one has a poor suck reflex and a paucity of body and limb movements. Therefore, pay attention to the following:
- *Mouth:* Crusts of mucus and epithelial cells collect on the lips. Gently remove them with water-impregnated swabs.
- *Eyes:* In a similar way, remove solid matter that may have accumulated at the nasal margins of the eyes.
- *Position:* p. 75.

Observation

Electronic devices play an essential but limited role in monitoring the well-being of a premature baby.

Signs like regurgitation, change in activity, abdominal distension, jaundice or seizures may reflect an impending disaster and can be detected only by the experienced eye. Therefore, constantly move from one infant to the next so as to notice the slightest deviation from normal.

The essence of care is observation. Remember, the change from apparent normality to severe illness can be very rapid. Keep a step ahead of an impending problem rather than attempting to rectify what could be a hopeless situation. You are given only one chance to prevent this, so heed any unusual feature (Table 7.11) and insist that the medical staff do likewise. Do not be lulled into a false sense of security by an electronic monitor, but rather stay in close physical contact with each baby.

Observe the pattern of breathing and count the rate, auscultate the heart and bowel, note the movements of the limbs and the response to pain or noise. Feel the warmth of the body and determine whether there is a discrepancy between that of the extremities and the abdomen. Look for characteristic features of REM sleep: the eyelids flicker, smiling is common and there are jerky movements of hands and feet. These are all important indications of normal neurological function.

Wherever possible, attune your care to infant cues. For example, do not disturb a sleeping infant, ensure quietness and relative darkness, feed the restless baby who sucks fingers, address the needs of an irritable or crying baby, avoid painful procedures unless they are essential, and ensure that medical staff utilise analgesia on such occasions.

Skin care

The fragile skin, particularly of an extremely premature infant, is vulnerable to trauma, infection, absorption of topical agents and fluid loss. To minimise

TABLE 7.11

Early warning signs of potential disease in the preterm infant	
Vomiting, abdominal distension, ileus	Necrotising enterocolitis
Umbilical skin flare, lethargy	Infection
Tachypnoea	Pneumonia, patent ductus
Tachycardia	Patent ductus, overheating
Watery stools	Gastroenteritis

complications, take the following precautions:

Bathing: Use cotton wool balls soaked in warm water. Do not apply soaps, oils, alcohol or lotions, and wipe off antiseptics with warm water after surgical procedures.

Avoiding trauma: Nurse the baby on a sheepskin that is covered with a sheet and change position every three hours. Follow and record a routine like lying the baby prone, then on one side, and then supine.

Also avoid multiple skin punctures. Collect blood for anticipated investigations from a single stab when possible, and ensure that the heel has been warmed first. Apply gentle pressure to control bleeding, not adhesive dressings.

Checking: Check skin colour and temperature frequently and note any redness, abrasions or oedema, particularly at sites of intravascular catheters.

Rotate the pulse oximeter attachment every six hours and use only gel-backed electrodes and thermistor probes.

Fluid loss: Nurse extremely small infants in a high humidity (> 80%) environment.

Records

Enter the details of monitoring and care on a daily chart. The details include:

- heart and respiratory rates
- infant and incubator temperatures
- oxygen concentration and saturation
- serum bilirubin level
- blood glucose levels
- the appearance of intravenous drip sites and skin
- all aspects of routine care, such as lips, eyes, cord and position
- daily weight
- volumes of fluid intake and output, including stools, urine, vomitus and gastric aspirates
- nature of fluid intake and feeding instructions
- medication details.

A more detailed record is needed for ill babies, especially those in ICU.

TABLE 7.12

Continuing care of a preterm infant			
TREATMENT	WEIGHT		
	< 1 500 g	1 500–2 000 g	> 2 000 g
Warmth Food Additives	Incubate Breast milk Caloreen™ Liprocil™ Sodium bicarbonate	Incubate Breast milk Caloreen™ Liprocil™	Cot, blankets and clothes Breast milk Nil
Frequency of feeds	Continuous Hourly	Continuous Hourly 2-hourly 3-hourly	3-hourly
Respiratory stimulant (p. 184)	Prophylactic	If indicated	Usually not necessary

The main aspects of management are summarised in Table 7.12.

Complications
The preterm baby is susceptible to numerous disorders (Table 7.13), some of which can cause irreparable brain damage or death. Establish the need for resuscitation, oxygen, intravenous feeding, respiratory stimulants, antibiotics and phototherapy as soon as possible after birth.

Discharge
Encourage a mother to spend most of the day with her infant once she has established breast- or bottle-feeding. In the case of kangaroo care, she will be with her infant all the time. By now she ought to be familiar with all aspects of mothercraft and should be able to handle her baby with competence and confidence.

Perform a full physical and neurological examination, chart weight and head circumference, and instruct the mother regarding feeds, clothing, vitamin and iron supplements, and immunisations. Ensure that BCG and polio drops have been given. Those prone to respiratory tract infection (< 1 000 g, chronic lung disease) should be immunised against RSV infection for several months. Record details on a 'road to health' chart and issue a letter of referral that contains the relevant details of the infant's hospitalisation.

Follow-up assessments are recommended to establish the pattern of physical and neurological development (p. 129). The frequency of examination will depend on the initial size and state of the infant. Very small babies (weighing less than 1 500 g) and those who were ill are assessed until well into junior school.

Prognosis
The overall outlook for preterm babies has improved greatly in recent years.

Those who weigh more than 1 800 g have the best prognosis, and their survival rate exceeds 90%. An intermediate group (1 500–1 800 g) also fare well if provided with adequate perinatal care. Morbidity and mortality rates rise significantly in those weighing less than 1 500 g and are particularly high in infants under 1 000 g. Neurological abnormalities are likely to occur in the latter groups and the risk is enhanced by complications such as hypoxaemia, hypoglycaemia, hypothermia and hyperbilirubinaemia.

A preterm baby is not precluded from attaining superior intelligence. Newton, Darwin, Victor Hugo and Winston Churchill were reputed to be preterm babies – and who would doubt their achievements?!

THE UNDERWEIGHT-FOR-GESTATION INFANT
Some babies fail to grow adequately *in utero* as a result of intrinsic or extrinsic factors. They are undersized at birth and are classified as 'small for gestational

TABLE 7.13

Complications of prematurity		
Respiratory	Birth asphyxia	p. 166
	Hyaline membrane disease	p. 172
	Recurrent apnoea	p. 184
	Pneumonia	p. 179
Cardiovascular	Patent ductus arteriosus	p. 194
Gastrointestinal	Vomiting	p. 203
	Abdominal distension	p. 213
	Malabsorption	
	Necrotising enterocolitis	p. 220
Metabolic	Hypothermia	p. 63
	Hypoglycaemia	p. 261
	Hyperbilirubinaemia	p. 104
	Hyponatraemia	p. 69
Neurological	Intraventricular haemorrhage	p. 143
	Periventricular leukomalacia	p. 141
	Kernicterus	p. 103
Eyes	Retinopathy	p. 155
Immunological	Bacterial infections	p. 90
Haematological	Anaemia	p. 226

age'. The problem is common in communities of low socioeconomic status.

Intrinsic causes

Severe prenatal disease is responsible for growth retardation in a small group of infants. Causes include the following:

Infections
Rubella
Cytomegalovirus

Noxious agents
Antimetabolite drugs
Radiation
Alcohol

Chromosome defects
Down's syndrome
Trisomy 13–15
Trisomy 16–18

Dwarf syndromes
Silver
Cornelia de Lange

The insult associated with impairment of fetal growth in these circumstances is often present at an early stage of pregnancy. This may lead to a reduction in the total number of cells in the body. Many such infants are learning-disabled.

Extrinsic factors

A fetus is likely to grow poorly during pregnancy if inadequately supplied with food substrates, energy or blood.

Maternal weight
Birth size is influenced by maternal nutrition and a woman who weighs less than 45 kg in early pregnancy is likely to produce a small baby, particularly if she gains less than 5 kg during pregnancy.

Other important factors
- Maternal addiction to cigarettes, alcohol, heroin

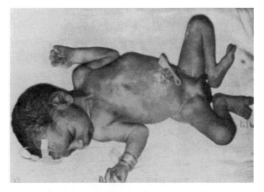

Fig. 7.6 *A growth-retarded infant. Note the lack of subcutaneous fat and the relatively large head*

- Severe toxaemia
- Hypertensive cardiovascular disease
- Multiple pregnancy

Extrinsic factors account for the majority of growth-retarded infants (over 90%), but a single cause may not be identifiable as multiple factors might be present.

Two extrinsic types of growth-retarded infants are described and probably depend on the timing of the insult *in utero*:

Type I: Symmetric growth retardation. Weight, length and head circumference are below normal and infants resemble miniature normal babies. Fetal growth has probably been suppressed throughout pregnancy. This type is commonly seen in infants born to malnourished mothers.

Type II: Asymmetric growth retardation. Weight is depressed more than length or head circumference, and growth has probably been impaired in the last trimester of pregnancy, when increased demands for energy cannot be met. This type is often associated with cigarette smoking or multiple pregnancy cases.

The following features are characteristic of asymmetric growth retardation:
- Weight is below the 10th percentile.
- Head circumference may be decreased yet disproportionate to weight.

- Skin may be dry and peeling.
- Vernix is sparse.
- The amount of breast tissue is diminished.
- Subcutaneous fat is lacking.
- Hair is sparse.
- Muscles are thin.
- Umbilical cord is thin and may be stained yellow.
- Placenta is small.
- Polycythaemia may be present.
- Congenital abnormalities may be detected, such as single umbilical artery, heart defect.
- Infants may be preterm or full-term.

Asymmetric growth retardation can also result from intrauterine weight loss in late pregnancy rather than from a failure to gain weight. Such an infant is usually full-term and is considered to be 'dysmature'. Subcutaneous fat is sparse. The skin is wrinkled and peels easily, and the umbilical cord, nails and skin may be stained with meconium. Birthweight is decreased, but may be within normal limits. Pregnancy beyond 40 weeks is extremely risky and hypoglycaemia is a major complication after birth.

Management
Impaired fetal growth owing to extrinsic factors can result in acute distress or sudden death *in utero* caused by depletion of glycogen in the fetal heart muscle. This is likely to occur during labour, when demands for energy are paramount.

Fetal well-being requires constant assessment before and during birth.

Assessment before birth
The diagnosis of intrauterine growth retardation is suspected on clinical criteria, such as diminished fundal height and reduced fetal size on palpation, and is confirmed by ultrasound measurements. In primary care units, serial fundal height measurements are important and a deviation from normal necessitates further investigation.

A mother can assist in checking the health of her growth-retarded baby by recording fetal movements. For example, starting at 9 a.m., she counts the number of movements until 10 movements have been recorded and then she enters the time on a chart. She repeats this daily and is instructed to contact the hospital should less than 10 movements be felt on two consecutive days.

Immediate admission is required if no movements have been felt for a day.

Serial ultrasound examinations also offer a guide to the state of the fetus based on breathing and body movements, tone, size of the skull and volume of amniotic fluid.

Diastolic blood flow velocity can be detected in the fetal aorta and umbilical vessels by Doppler ultrasound. Absent or reversed flow is ominous and needs immediate attention.

Any underlying disease, like hypertension, should be treated and bed rest may be necessary to improve placental blood flow. Smoking and alcohol consumption must be curtailed and diet should be ensured to be adequate.

Timing of birth
The risk of preterm delivery must be weighed against that of sudden intrauterine death, and the optimum time of birth ranges from 34 to 38 weeks. After 38 weeks, there is a risk of the baby dying *in utero*. Prior to 34 weeks, the risks associated with prematurity are significant.

An amniocentesis is performed before birth to determine lung maturity.

Prior to delivery, the fetal heart rate pattern is monitored by serial cardiotocography (CTG) (p. 167).

The pH of fetal scalp blood may be measured in labour when the cervix is sufficiently dilated (p. 167), but this procedure is avoided in southern

Africa because of the risk of HIV transmission.

Abnormal CTG recordings warrant delivery by Caesarean section in order to prevent fetal distress.

Assessment after birth
A growth-retarded fetus 'ripens' sooner than a normally grown one and the lungs, gut and brain are relatively mature at birth. There is a low incidence of hyaline membrane disease, ileus and intraventricular haemorrhage (Table 7.14).

The following complications should be anticipated and duly prevented or treated:

- Birth asphyxia (p. 166).
- Meconium aspiration (p. 178).
- Hypoglycaemia (p. 261).
- Hypothermia (p. 63).
- Polycythaemia (p. 226).
- Congenital malformations (p. 111).

Inadequate stores of glycogen and fat, impaired gluconeogenesis and perinatal hypoxia increase the likelihood of hypoglycaemia. All growth-retarded infants should receive intravenous feeding with dextrose water 10% for 24 to 48 hours, and blood sugar is monitored three-hourly during this period.

The subsequent management is similar to that for the preterm baby (p. 62).

Prognosis
Perinatal mortality
The chances of perinatal death are increased by 12 in babies who fall below the 10th percentile for weight. Most deaths are caused by hypoxaemia before, during or after birth.

Long-term outlook
The ultimate physical and neurological development is uncertain owing to numerous factors that influence growth before and after birth. Deprivations, for example, can be of a nutritional and social nature.

The earlier the onset of impaired fetal growth, the more severe is its consequence. Infants with symmetric growth

TABLE 7.14

Comparison of small-for-gestation and preterm infants		
	Small for gestation	*Preterm of normal size*
Gestational period	28–44 weeks	Less than 37 completed weeks
Birthweight	Below 10th percentile	Normal for gestation
Birthweight of siblings	Often low	Usually normal
Intrauterine death	****	*
Congenital abnormality	***	*
Congenital infection	**	*
Asphyxia neonatorum	****	**
Early metabolic acidaemia	***	*
Hypoglycaemia	***	*
Hypothermia	**	**
Jaundice	*	***
Recurrent apnoea	*	***
Intraventricular haemorrhage	*	***
Respiratory problems	Meconium aspiration	Hyaline membrane
Late physical growth	Uncertain	Normal
Late intellectual function	Uncertain	Usually normal

	Relatively low	*Moderate*	*High*	*Very high*
Incidence	*	**	***	****

retardation would be expected to fare less well than those with the asymmetric variety.

The mean IQ of five-year-olds who had ultrasound evidence of growth retardation before 26 weeks' gestation is less than that of children who showed impaired fetal growth at a later stage. The former have lower scores in writing, drawing and creative activities at school and their concentration span is short.

Perinatal complications play a significant role in the eventual outcome and infants subjected to asphyxia or symptomatic hypoglycaemia are likely to develop neurological deficits.

Differences between small-for-gestation and preterm infants are summarised in Table 7.14.

THE LARGE-FOR-GESTATION INFANT
Aetiology

Several factors are associated with the overgrowth of a fetus *in utero* (above the 90th percentile for weight). These include:

- maternal diabetes mellitus and pre-diabetes
- erythroblastosis fetalis
- transposition of the great vessels
- Beckwith syndrome (gigantism, macroglossia, exomphalos and various other congenital abnormalities)
- a familial tendency.

The large fetal size has been attributed to excessive amounts of insulin as a result of hyperplasia of the fetal pancreatic B cells.

The majority of overgrown infants are born to prediabetic or diabetic mothers (p. 278).

Complications
At birth

Size alone can cause a delay in delivery, such as impacted shoulders, and there is an increased risk of birth trauma or asphyxia.

After birth
Hypoglycaemia

This is a major problem in most overgrown infants irrespective of the underlying disease. In most cases, it appears to be caused by a transient increase in the levels of insulin.

Give a 10% dextrose solution intravenously to all overgrown babies immediately after birth. Use a total of 60 ml per kg for the first 24 hours. Early feeding diminishes the risk of hypoglycaemia and should be established before the intravenous therapy is discontinued. Monitor blood sugar levels hourly for six hours and then three-hourly for two days.

Polycythaemia

This is likely to occur in all groups of overgrown infants and may be associated with increased viscosity of the blood when the venous haematocrit is above 70%. A partial exchange transfusion using plasma may be indicated in some cases (p. 227).

Prognosis

The risk of death in the perinatal period is increased fivefold. This is owing mainly to intrapartum asphyxia, congenital defects or the complications of prematurity.

Summary of essential care for sick or small babies

- *Oxygenation:* Ensure prompt resuscitation, and thereafter maintain oxygen saturation between 89 and 92%. On occasion, this may require head box oxygen, nCPAP or assisted ventilation, depending on the circumstances.

- *Blood sugar:* Check the level after birth and maintain it above 2,5 mmol/l. This requires early feeding, which in the case of an ill or very small infant is by an intravenous solution of 10% dextrose water. Start oral feeds with breast milk as soon as bowel sounds are audible and meconium has been passed. Do not permit blood sugar to exceed 7 mmol/l. Use a 5% dextrose solution if this occurs.
- *Warmth:* Ensure protection from the moment of delivery by using kangaroo care or incubation, and remember that additional heat must be provided until the infant's weight exceeds 2 000 g.
- *Prevent infection:* Clean your hands before touching an infant. Identify the one who may have come from an infected birth canal (pus/bacteria in gastric aspirate), and watch for and treat one with suspicious signs of early infection, like umbilical flare. Prevent colonisation of the gut with pathogens by feeding breast milk. Promote kangaroo care.
- *Observations:* Remember that a change from apparent health to a moribund state can be rapid.
- *Extremely low birthweight:* The care of such a baby is too specialised to be addressed in detail.

Continually check vital functions and behaviour. Report any aspect that disturbs you.

MULTIPLE BIRTHS

The incidence of spontaneous multiple births is as follows:

Twins   1,6%
Triplets   0,01%
Quadruplets   0,002%

Multiple births can also be induced by gonadotrophin therapy for ovulation.

Twins

Twins may develop from one or two zygotes (fertilised ova).

Monozygotic twinning (*mono* = one) accounts for 25%, and dizygotic (*di* = two) for 75% of the total.

Monozygotic twins (identical)

Two inner cell masses form in the fertilised ovum (Fig. 7.7) at the blastocyst stage before implantation in the uterus. This is the commonest cause. It results in identical individuals who share a chorionic sac and a placenta, but have separate amniotic sacs.

The babies have:

- the same sex
- similar physical characteristics
- identical blood and histocompatibility groups.

Cell division before or after the blastocyst stage can also result in twins, but is rare.

Monozygotic twins have a 50% chance of dying before birth because of complications such as:

- discrepancy in size
- transfusion syndrome
- congenital abnormalities
- conjoinment.

Discrepancy in size

One twin may be significantly smaller than the other. This probably occurs during organogenesis and is permanent when the difference in weight exceeds 20%. The section of placenta that supports the growth-retarded fetus is smaller than the other portion and has fewer blood vessels (Colour plate V).

In gross cases, the smaller fetus may die and be resorbed to form a fetus papyraceous, that is, a parchment-like figure.

The smaller of the twins may not attain the physical and mental capacity of the other if the discrepancy in birthweight exceeds 25%.

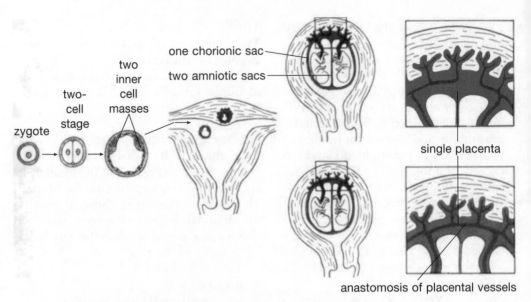

two-
cell
stage

two
inner
cell
masses

zygote

one chorionic sac
two amniotic sacs

single placenta

anastomosis of placental vessels

Fig. 7.7 *Most monozygotic (identical) twins are derived from two inner cell masses.*
They share one placenta and chorion, but have separate amnions (From Moore, K. 1977.
The Developing Human. *2 ed. Philadelphia: WB Saunders)*

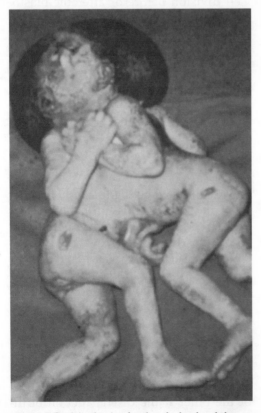

Fig. 7.8 *Conjoined twins fused at the head and thorax*

Transfusion syndrome (Colour plate V)
Numerous vascular connections occur in the circulation of diamniotic twins. This can produce a unidirectional flow of blood into one baby and cause polycythaemia or heart failure. The overtransfused infant is more likely to die than the anaemic one.

Congenital abnormalities
Twins derived from a split embryonic disc share one chorion, amnion and placenta. They may have abnormalities ranging from acardia (absent heart) to short umbilical cords.

Conjoinment (Fig. 7.8)
Conjoined twins result from an incomplete division of the embryonic disc. The fusion may involve skin, organs or circulations, and the connections can occur at the head, thorax, umbilicus or pelvis.

Some conjoined twins can be separated by surgery. The chance of success depends on the site of the fusion and the nature of the shared organs or tissues.

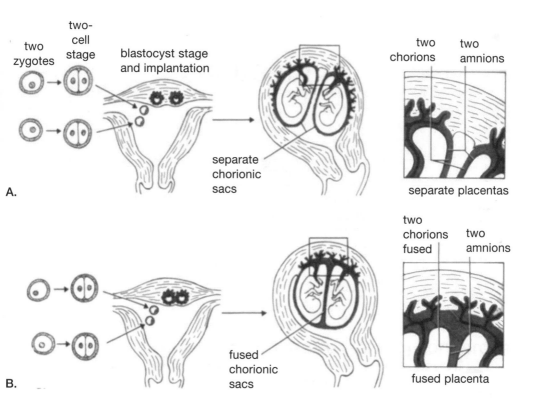

Fig. 7.9 *Two ova are fertilised to produce dizygotic twins. These have individual amnions and chorions, and the placentas may be separate or fused (From Moore, K. 1977. The Developing Human. 2 ed. Philadelphia: WB Saunders)*

Dizygotic twins (unidentical)

When two ova are fertilised by different sperms, the resultant twins always have separate amnions, chorions and placentas, although the chorion and placenta may be fused (Fig. 7.9). Sex and physical characteristics can differ.

Dizygotic twinning depends on the mother's inherited characteristics. It is common in black and in older women and recurs in families.

Complications

The following problems may occur, both in dizygotic and monozygotic twins:

Prematurity

Uterine enlargement can cause early onset of labour and the infants may develop the complications of prematurity (p. 76).

Intrauterine growth retardation

Growth rate declines after 35 weeks' gestation and one or both babies may show features of intrauterine growth retardation (p. 76). This increases the risk of birth asphyxia, meconium aspiration and hypoglycaemia.

Iron deficiency anaemia

Iron stores are inadequate and a deficiency state can develop during rapid postnatal growth.

CHAPTER 8

Infection

This chapter in outline:

PROTECTION AGAINST INFECTION

A baby is protected by a variety of factors.

Specific factors
Humoral antibodies
Three major antibody fractions – IgG, IgM and IgA – enhance the immunity of the fetus and newborn baby.

Immunoglobulin G (IgG)
Appreciable amounts of IgG are transferred across the placenta from the mother to the fetus in the last trimester. This fraction is found in both the vascular and extravascular compartments, where it neutralises bacterial toxins and binds micro-organisms to enhance phagocytosis.

This antibody protects a baby against infections to which the mother has been immunised. These include:
- viral illnesses, for example measles, mumps, poliomyelitis, smallpox and rubella
- bacterial illnesses, for example diphtheria, typhoid, tetanus.

This protection is termed naturally acquired passive immunity.

Note
An infant is not protected against these diseases unless the mother is immune.

Passive immunity is temporary and declines after four to six months of age.

Immunisation of a pregnant woman against tetanus in the last trimester confers immunity to the fetus.

A preterm baby shows less passive immunity owing to an inadequate transfer of maternal antibody.

The infant gradually manufactures IgG during the early months of life.

Immunoglobulin M (IgM)
This antibody has a high molecular weight and does not usually cross the placenta. It is produced by the infant after birth and is highly effective in agglutinating micro-organisms, especially Gram-negative bacteria. It is largely confined to the bloodstream.

Note
The fetus can produce IgM in response

to an intrauterine infection, for example congenital syphilis. Cord blood IgM is raised in most infants who develop infections before birth.

Immunoglobulin A (IgA)
This fraction does not cross the placenta. It is produced by an infant within the first few weeks of life and appears in the secretions of the gut and respiratory tract. The antibody is also found in the bloodstream. The secretory portion is active against certain viruses, for example poliomyelitis and various strains of *E. coli* organisms.

Note
The production of IgG, IgM and IgA by the baby after birth results in naturally acquired active immunity.

Cell-mediated immunity
T lymphocytes derived from the thymus and B lymphocytes from bone marrow protect an infant against many viral, fungal and enterobacillary infections.

The B lymphocytes respond to foreign antigens by migrating to lymph nodes and differentiating into plasma cells. These synthesise much of the circulating immunoglobulin.

The T lymphocytes mature in the thymus and are involved in cellular immunity. They initiate the body's response to bacterial invasion and destroy cells infected by viruses and fungi. These lymphocytes take up to two weeks after birth to gain full function.

General factors
Antenatal

Placenta
The intact placenta acts as a barrier to organisms during pregnancy and can filter out a number of viruses and bacteria.

The following significant micro-organisms can be transmitted across the placenta to produce illness in the fetus:

- Rubella virus.
- Toxoplasma.
- Cytomegalovirus.
- *Treponema pallidum.*

Amniotic fluid
Lysozyme, which destroys bacteria, and IgG antibody is found in the liquor.

Cervical plug
The operculum provides a mechanical barrier to organisms in the cervix and vagina. This protective factor may be absent when the cervix is incompetent.

Vaginal fluid
Quantities of IgG, IgM and IgA are found in the secretions during pregnancy.

Postnatal
Breast milk (Chapter 5)
Colostrum contains appreciable amounts of IgA antibody, which lines the mucosal surface of the infant's gut.

Mature milk has quantities of IgG, IgM and IgA antibody as well as macrophages and lysozyme.

The lactoferrin and transferrin in milk destroy Gram-negative organisms such as *E. coli.*

Breast-feeding promotes a bowel flora of bifidus and lactobacilli, and these bacteria adhere to the wall of the large bowel and inhibit colonisation with other organisms such as *E. coli* and *Klebsiella.*

Nursery care
The newborn infant is particularly susceptible to the following infections:
- *Gram-positive bacteria*, such as Group B streptococcus, *Staphylococcus aureus* and epidermidis.
- *Gram-negative bacteria*, for example *Klebsiella, Pseudomonas.*
- *Fungus*, for example *Candida albicans.*
- *Virus*, for example Coxsackie B and herpes simplex.

Outbreaks of these and other infections can be prevented by correct nursery techniques.

TYPES OF INFECTION
Infection is acquired from the following sources:
- Mother's blood.
- Mother's birth canal.
- Nursery staff or environment.

Infections from maternal blood
An infection such as syphilis is transmitted through the bloodstream to the fetus. This is a transplacental or antenatal infection. It is associated with significant morbidity and mortality in the fetus and newborn.

Important agents are:

Viral	Bacterial	Miscellaneous
Rubella	Listeria species	Treponema pallidum
Cytomegalo-virus		Toxoplasma gondi
Chickenpox		
HIV		

Presentation
Suspect an antenatal infection when there is:
- a characteristic history of maternal illness during pregnancy, for example rubella or HIV
- an unexpected intrauterine death or congenital abnormality, for example heart defect
- an abnormal placenta, for example gross enlargement, as in syphilis
- clinical signs of infection at birth, for example growth retardation, microcephaly, hepatomegaly or rashes.

Diagnosis
Clinical and radiological signs are discussed in the relevant sections.

Laboratory investigations
Total IgM in cord blood: The level of this antibody rises in the fetus in response to infection. An amount exceeding 40 IU/ml is suggestive of infection.
Specific IgM: The detection of this antibody, which is specific for a particular antigen, such as rubella, cytomegalovirus or syphilis, is strong evidence of that disease. The antibody persists in the infant's serum for a variable time, for example one month in rubella.
Serology: A fourfold rise in the titre of IgG antibody to a particular antigen indicates active infection.
Isolation of the agent: This is the most direct method. Specimens such as blood, urine, throat swab, cerebrospinal fluid and placenta are delivered to the laboratory immediately. They are kept cool and at a neutral pH. Viruses can be grown in tissue culture or identified by electron microscopy.

Human immunodeficiency virus (HIV-1)
HIV can be passed from a mother to her infant during pregnancy, labour or breast-feeding.

Over two-thirds of infections are acquired in labour and the overall risk of transmission without drug prophylaxis exceeds 35% in southern Africa.

The placenta plays a role in protecting the fetus *in utero*. This is attributed to cytokines like the leucocyte inhibiting factor (LIF) and human chorionic gonadotropin (hCG).

In labour, various maternal factors increase the risk of transmission. They include:
- Aids
- a high viral load
- a low CD4 lymphocyte count (< 200 cells/l)
- absent neutralising antibody
- other sexually transmitted diseases.

Intrapartum events that increase the risk are:

- artificial rupture of membranes
- prolonged rupture of membranes
- the use of forceps or a vacuum extractor
- fetal scalp lesions from pH sampling of blood.

Fetal risks are related to low birthweight (< 2 500 g).

The infected infant is usually normal at birth and after an incubation of four to six months may show signs of disease. These include recurrent infections such as pneumonia, meningitis, abscesses and diarrhoea.

Candida and pneumocystis are important organisms. Other features include hepatosplenomegaly, lymphadenopathy and failure to thrive. The disease is incurable, but many of its complications can be treated.

Of the infected infants, over one-third will have signs of disease by 6 to 12 months of age.

Only a few manifest the illness at birth or in the early weeks of life. These are likely to weigh less than 1 600 g and usually develop signs within a month. Their disease is characterised by hepatosplenomegaly and worsening pneumonia.

Identification of the infected infant

HIV-1 antibodies are transferred from mother to fetus and may persist in an infant for up to 18 months.

The presence of HIV antibody alone after birth is not diagnostic of infection.

Detection of HIV antigens is more reliable. This includes the P24 antigen and more specifically HIV ribonucleic acid (RNA). The latter can be demonstrated by the polymerase chain reaction (PCR).

Prevention of mother-to-child transmission
During pregnancy

Anti-retroviral therapy is necessary. A combination of two groups of drugs is recommended, namely, reverse transcriptase inhibitors and protease inhibitors. The former blocks a DNA copy of the virus RNA in the cell, and the latter prevents the assembly of particles that form a new virus to be spread from cell to cell. The following medications are prescribed when possible: Zidovudine (AZT), Lopinavir/Ritonavir and Lamivudine.

In labour or prior to delivery

A single dose of Zidovudine is given intravenously to reduce the risk of transmission.

A combination of antiprotease inhibitors and other retroviral drugs can reduce the rate of transmission in labour to less than 2%. Whenever possible, delivery should be by elective Caesarean section.

Infant prophylaxis: A combination of Zidovudine (2 mg/kg) four times a day for six weeks, and Lamivudine (2 mg/kg) twice a day for a week, is recommended. This should be started within 12 hours of birth.

During breast-feeding

The risk of acquiring infection from breast milk is increased by the following:

- A raised cell count in milk.
- Mastitis or a breast abscess.
- Multiple viral infections in the mother.
- Prematurity.
- Mouth ulcers in the infant.
- Early introduction of food other than breast milk.

An infected mother who has access to clean water and is familiar with the sterilisation of feeding bottles and teats is advised not to breast-feed her infant. This recommendation assumes that powdered milk will be supplied free of charge or is affordable.

If these requirements cannot be met, the risk of the baby acquiring the milk-borne virus must be weighed against that of the baby dying from gastroenteritis or pneumonia resulting from a lack of breast milk.

If the latter risk is great, then exclusive breast-feeding is the best option. No other dietary item should be introduced for six months in the hope of preserving an intact bowel wall, thereby deterring entrance of the virus. Infants who receive solids with breast milk in the early months are 10 times more likely to acquire HIV than those who are exclusively breast-fed.

Syphilis

This serious sexually transmitted disease is caused by the spirochaete *Treponema pallidum*. It involves many organs and can result in fetal death or characteristic disease, and an apparently normal infant may shows signs of infection only later.

The outlook is positive if maternal disease is detected and treated during pregnancy.

Antenatal diagnosis

A serological test (VDRL) can detect reagin antibodies in the mother. This indicates exposure to syphilis.

Clinical features after birth

Placenta: This is pale and bulky, and the villi are thickened.

Skin: A copper-coloured rash may be present. It is usually maculopapular and involves the palms, soles, perianal and nappy regions. Peeling is common.

Snuffles: Rhinitis causes a blocked nose and a watery or bloody discharge.

Rhagades: Excoriations and scars may appear at the angles of the mouth (Colour plate II).

Other signs: Oedema, jaundice, lymphadenopathy, hepatosplenomegaly, pneumonia, pallor and painful limbs.

X-ray signs

Destruction and reduced bone density occur in the metaphyses of long bones, and the periosteum may be thickened.

Laboratory findings

The spirochaete may be seen on dark-ground illumination of wet smears from the skin, placenta or mucous membranes. This is certain evidence of syphilis.

A specific 19S fraction of IgM antibody to *Treponema* (IgM FTA – ABS) also confirms infection.

In neurosyphilis, the cerebrospinal fluid has a raised leukocyte count, an elevated level of protein and a positive VDRL reaction.

An asymptomatic baby with positive serology (VDRL) poses a diagnostic problem. The VDRL antibody is acquired from the mother across the placenta. It indicates that she has been exposed to syphilis, but gives no indication of whether the disease is still active in her.

Each of the following would favour infection in the infant and would warrant treatment:

- A total IgM in excess of 60 IU/ml.
- A positive rheumatoid factor.
- Specific IgM antibody.
- X-ray features of disease.
- A VDRL titre that is four times higher than that of the mother.

Treatment

Infants with well-established clinical, radiological and/or laboratory features must be given procaine penicillin by intramuscular injection. The dose is 50 000 units/kg/day for 10 days. This ensures the eradication of neurosyphilis.

Infants who have normal clinical, radiological and laboratory findings, but whose mothers have been inadequately treated, may be given a single intra-muscular dose of benzathine penicillin (50 000 units/kg).

Outcome
The prognosis is excellent in infants who are treated early.

Note
Congenital syphilis is a notifiable disease.

Rubella
A fetus exposed to maternal infection during the first 16 weeks of pregnancy stands a 30% chance of abortion, stillbirth or defect. Thereafter, the hazard of fetal damage decreases and is rare after 24 weeks of pregnancy.

Clinical features
The majority of infected babies are growth-retarded and often show congenital abnormalities, for example:
- Heart lesions, such as patent ductus or septal defect.
- Perceptive deafness.
- Cataract.

Other abnormalities include the following:
- *CVS:* Myocardial necrosis, peripheral pulmonary artery stenosis.
- *CNS:* Full fontanelle, microcephaly, mental retardation.
- *Lungs:* Pneumonitis.
- *Bones:* Osteitis.
- *Blood:* Thrombocytopenia.
- *Liver:* Hepatosplenomegaly, jaundice.
- *Eyes:* Retinopathy, microphthalmia, glaucoma, cloudy cornea.
- *Skin:* Purpura, blueberry muffin spots (p. 260).
- *Other:* Adenopathy, hypogammaglobulinaemia.

Long bone X-ray
Coarse linear trabeculations may be present in the metaphyses.

Diagnosis
Suspect the disease if:
- there is a preceding maternal illness with rubella-like features
- cord blood IgM is raised (> 40 IU/ml)
- the infant has characteristic clinical and radiological features.

Confirmation is obtained by:
- a culture of the virus from the pharynx, CSF or urine
- a rise in antibody titre in the serum
- a specific IgM antibody.

Treatment
Symptomatic.

Note
A single lesion, for example deafness, may not be obvious at birth.

An apparently normal infant may have subclinical infection and later develops abnormal signs, for example deafness.

The infant excretes live virus for six months or longer after birth and is an infectious hazard to nursing staff and visitors who may be potential mothers.

Rubella is preventable and all children should be immunised before puberty.

Toxoplasmosis
Congenital toxoplasmosis may result from the haematogenous spread of *Toxoplasma gondii* across the placenta. The protozoon has a predilection for nervous tissue and frequently involves the CNS, retina and choroid.

The chances of transmission of the disease from mother to fetus increase from 15% in the first trimester to 60% in the third trimester. Most late infections are asymptomatic.

Clinical features
Only 20% of infected babies have clinical features of the disease. These include the following:

- *Eyes:* Choroidoretinitis, iridocyclitis, microphthalmia.
- *CNS:* Convulsions, hydrocephalus, facial palsy.
- *Liver:* Hepatosplenomegaly, jaundice.
- *Blood:* Thrombocytopenia.
- *Skin:* Maculopapular rash, purpura.
- *Other:* Ascites, lymphadenopathy, fever, growth retardation.

Skull X-ray
Intracranial calcification.

Diagnosis
Suspect if:
- cord IgM is raised (> 40 IU/ml)
- *Toxoplasma gondii* is identified in placenta.

Confirm diagnosis by:
- *Toxoplasma*-specific fluorescent IgM antibody in serum
- culture of *Toxoplasma* from CSF or organs.

Treatment
Sulphonamide.
Pyrimethamine.
Cortisone for choroidoretinitis.

Note
The primary infection affects only the offspring of that particular pregnancy, and not subsequent babies.

A pregnant woman should not eat raw meat and ought to avoid contact with kittens. Cat faeces is considered to be a source of the disease.

Spiramycin is the drug of choice during pregnancy.

Cytomegalovirus
This infection is relatively common in the pregnant mother, but it seldom produces clinical illness in the fetus. However, the incidence is increased significantly in the offspring of HIV-infected women. Fetal infection is most likely to occur in the first trimester.

The disease is characterised by interstitial inflammatory cells and giant cells which show cytoplasmic inclusions. Typical cytomegalic cells are found in the lungs, kidneys, salivary glands and brain.

Clinical features
- *CNS:* Microcephaly, choroidoretinitis, mental retardation, deafness.
- *Liver:* Hepatosplenomegaly, jaundice.
- *Blood:* Thrombocytopenia, anaemia, purpura.
- *Lungs:* Interstitial pneumonitis.
- *Other:* Growth retardation, oedema, hydrops.

Skull X-ray
Intracranial calcification.

Diagnosis
Suspect if cord blood IgM is raised.
Confirm by:
- specific IgM antibody
- culturing the virus from urine
- virus particles in urine
- cytomegalic cells with inclusion bodies in urine.

Treatment
A synthetic antiviral product, ganciclovir (p. 307), has been used with some success.

Infections from the birth canal
Pathogenic organisms in the vagina may spread into the cervical canal or uterine cavity. They can be acquired by the fetus before or during labour.

Most infections are caused by bacteria, for example Group B streptococcus, which cross weak or ruptured membranes.

The likelihood is increased ten fold when associated with:
- prolonged rupture of membranes (more than 24 hours)
- obstetric manipulation (Shirodkar suture)

- early onset of labour (before 34 weeks)
- a maternal pyrexia.

The resultant intrapartum infection may be local, for example conjunctivitis, or general, for example septicaemia.

Clinical signs are usually obvious within 72 hours of birth.

Important agents are:

Viral	Bacterial	Miscellaneous
Herpes simplex	Group B streptococcus Gonococcus	Chlamydia

Amniotic fluid infection

Organisms which enter the amniotic cavity from the vagina initiate a response from mother and fetus.

This shows:

Chorioamnionitis: The chorion and maternal side of the placenta produce neutrophils, which migrate into the amniotic cavity.

Funisitis: A similar inflammatory reaction may occur in the fetal vessels of the placenta and umbilical cord.

Products of inflammation, such as bacteria and neutrophils, may be swallowed or inhaled by the fetus. In most cases this is harmless; occasionally it causes infection. It is therefore wise to identify an infant who may be contaminated, that is, one who has been exposed to any of the risk factors above.

In such a case, insert a feeding tube into the infant's stomach after birth and withdraw sufficient fluid (1 ml) for examination. Neutrophils (more than five per high power field) and bacteria (Gram stain) indicate contamination.

Should a contaminated but healthy baby receive antibiotics to prevent infection? Only if the risk is high, for example Gram-positive cocci (possibly Group B streptococcus) plus the above risk factors.

In other circumstances, treatment is recommended only if there are early clinical signs, such as an umbilical flare.

Other important presentations of intrapartum infection include:
- gonococcal conjunctivitis (p. 154)
- chlamydial conjunctivitis and pneumonia (p. 154).

Group B streptococcal infection

This organism causes 50% of intrapartum infections. It colonises the vagina in 5 to 30% of pregnant women and may be transmitted to an infant before or during labour. In most cases contamination is harmless. Infection can present as an early or a late disease.

Early infection

This commonly occurs within 72 hours of birth and is prevalent in babies of low birthweight. Respiratory distress may be noted at birth and the illness can mimic hyaline membrane disease (p. 179).

A milder form of early infection is characterised by an umbilical flare, abdominal distension, ileus and jaundice.

The most severe infections are septicaemia and meningitis. However, these are uncommon soon after birth.

The following rapid laboratory tests distinguish Group B streptococcus infection from hyaline membrane disease:

Gastric aspirate: Pus cells and Gram-positive cocci are seen on a smear. The shake test for bubbles (p. 172) is usually positive.

Blood: Total white cell count is raised ($> 30 \times 10^9/1$) or lowered ($< 5 \times 10^9/1$). The ratio of band to total neutrophil is high ($> 0,2$).

Urine: Latex test (Wellcome™) for the streptococcal antigen is positive. Confirmation is obtained by culturing the organism from various specimens such as tracheal aspirate, urine, blood and cerebrospinal fluid.

Treatment: Ampicillin (p. 307) is given for 7 to 14 days, depending on the severity of the illness. Ceftriaxone (p. 307) may also be used.

Route: Intravenous for several days, then oral.

Outcome: The mortality exceeds 50% if septicaemia, shock or meningitis is present.

Late infection

This is probably acquired from cross-infection in the nursery. Meningitis is common after the first week and is usually caused by type III Group B streptococcus. Less common features include otitis media, pneumonia and skin infection. Late infection has a better prognosis than the severe early variety, but neurological sequelae can exceed 50% in cases of meningitis.

Other important presentations of intrapartum infection include:

- gonococcal conjunctivitis (p. 154)
- chlamydial conjunctivitis and pneumonia (p. 154).

Infections from the nursery

Cross-infection in a nursery may result from:

- contact, for example unwashed hands, venous catheter, urinary catheter, naso-gastric tube, endotracheal tube, skin abrasion and overcrowding
- ingestion, for example unsterile milk
- inhalation, for example exposure to influenza.

Unclean hands are the source of most postnatal infection.

Important causes are:

Viral	Bacterial	Fungal
Coxsackie B	*E. coli, Klebsiella*	Candida species
Hepatitis B	*Staphylococcus aureus*	
	Staphylococcus epidermidis	
	Enterococcus	
	Pseudomonas	

Presentation

The types of infection are similar to those acquired from the vagina, but they tend to occur later (after six days). Most are caused by bacteria and may be local or general.

Local

Conjunctivitis (p. 154), thrush (p. 220), omphalitis (p. 222) and skin pustules (p. 260) are common.

Affected areas are colonised by bacteria such as *Staphylococcus* or *Klebsiella*, and the signs are obvious.

These infections must be treated immediately, otherwise:

- they may spread to other regions, for example omphalitis can lead to septicaemia or meningitis
- an outbreak of cross-infection can occur, for example a baby has skin pustules and soon others may show similar lesions.

General

Significant infections include septicaemia, pneumonia (p. 179), urinary tract infection (p. 240), gastroenteritis (p. 221) and meningitis (p. 143).

Bacteraemia is the hallmark of systemic infection and likely organisms are *E. coli, Klebsiella, Staphylococcus epidermidis* and Group B or D streptococci.

Predisposing factors are:

- a source of infection, for example omphalitis
- disruption of a protective barrier, for example an indwelling venous catheter, endotracheal intubation, meningomyelocele.

Clinical signs

The early features are subtle and non-specific, and a change in behaviour, such as lethargy or poor sucking, is significant. No reliance can be placed on recognised signs such as pyrexia. This is often absent.

Important signs of systemic infection are tabulated on page 94.

Respiratory signs favour pneumonia, neurological signs indicate meningitis, and diarrhoea may be a feature of gastroenteritis. Abdominal distension, tenderness and ileus suggest peritonitis.

Prolonged jaundice or failure to gain weight may be the only presentation of a urinary tract infection. Signs such as a non-pitting oedema (sclerema) and persistent blanching of the skin on compression are late and ominous.

Laboratory investigations

Several rapid investigations ought to be done when sepsis is suspected. No single test offers an immediate or unequivocal diagnosis.

Important tests are:

■ White cell count (p. 228)

This simple investigation is available in most hospitals. Normal values do not exclude systemic infection, but abnormal ones are highly suggestive. An increase in the percentage of new polymorphs (band cells) is of great significance.

■ Urine

A clean specimen (p. 235) is obtained for two simple tests:
1. *Latex Group B streptococcus:* The antigen of this organism is excreted in the urine in systemic streptococcal infection.

    Filter the urine (0,22 μm millipore) prior to testing. This reduces the possibility of false positive results.
2. *Gram stain:* Organisms and pus cells may be detected in the urine sediment. If so, a sterile specimen is required for culture. This is obtained by a suprapubic puncture when the bladder is full (p. 236).

■ Cerebrospinal fluid

A lumbar puncture is necessary if meningitis is suspected (technique p. 150). Organisms detected on Gram stain indicate a bacterial infection.

■ Additional tests

Several investigations offer circumstantial or definite evidence of sepsis. They include:

C-reactive protein (CRP) – levels over 5 mg/dl favour infection

Blood culture

Cerebrospinal fluid culture

Urine culture

A decision to commence treatment cannot be based on cultures because of their long processing times. They provide a retrospective diagnosis and determine the duration and most effective type of treatment.

Treatment

Do not delay therapy if suggestive clinical and laboratory evidence is present. This is particularly important for preterm babies as they cannot mount adequate defences and may die within hours.

Antibiotics

The newer cephalosporins are active against most bacteria that cause sepsis. Ceftriaxone is a suitable choice. It maintains adequate levels in the blood for 24 hours, crosses the blood–brain barrier readily and is relatively free of side-effects. The drug is given once a day by intravenous or intramuscular injection (p. 307).

Additional or alternative antibiotics depend on the type and sensitivity of the organisms cultured from blood, urine, cerebrospinal fluid, or tracheal aspirate in the case of pneumonia. Suitable agents include vancomycin (ototoxic), gentamycin (ototoxic), imipenim and antifungal drugs like fluconazole.

Duration of treatment

Potential infection (negative cultures) is

treated for up to three days, septicaemia (positive blood culture) for 10 to 14 days, and meningitis (positive cerebrospinal fluid culture) for 14 to 21 days.

Most infants who receive antibiotics fall into the category of potential infection.

Supportive measures
Various complications of sepsis may need correction. They are:

■ anaemia – packed red blood cell transfusion (p. 309)
■ cyanosis – oxygen, assisted ventilation (p. 175)
■ thrombocytopenia – platelet transfusion (p. 230)
■ dehydration and shock – fresh frozen plasma or stabilised human serum (p. 309), inotropes
■ metabolic acidaemia – sodium bicarbonate 4% (p. 175)
■ seizures – phenobarbitone (p. 145)
■ hypoglycaemia – 10% glucose.

Other treatments have been used in severe infection, but their efficacy has not been established. They include corticosteroids, gammaglobulin, granulocyte transfusion and exchange transfusion.

Outcome
When late signs of infection are present, the mortality is up to 20%, especially in preterm babies. Survivors in this group have a high morbidity (up to 20%), especially after meningitis. Consequently, those with early signs of infection and those with doubtful diagnostic tests need immediate treatment to avoid these hazards.

Specific infections described in other sections include:
  Conjunctivitis (p. 154)
  Otitis media (p. 156)
  Thrush (p. 220)
  Pneumonia (p. 179)
  Skin (p. 260)
  Osteitis (p. 290)
  Omphalitis (p. 222)
  Meningitis (p. 144)
  Mastitis (p. 240)
  Urinary tract infections (p. 240)
  Rhinitis (p. 157)
  Gastroenteritis (p. 221)

Less common infections
Hepatitis B
The prevalence of hepatitis B virus varies throughout the world and is particularly high in Asia and Africa.

In a high-risk area, over 90% of infants born to HBeAg-positive mothers will become infected at or shortly after birth. The mode of transmission is uncertain and the risk of infection is unrelated to the type of delivery.

Most infected infants continue to harbour the virus into adult life.

Complications of the carrier state

TABLE 8.1

Signs of sepsis			
General	**Respiratory**	**Gastrointestinal**	**Neurological**
Lethargy	Cough	Vomiting	Tense fontanelle
Poor sucking	Tachypnoea	Abdominal distension	Apnoea
Unstable temperature	Rib recession	Ileus	Convulsions
Weight loss	Cyanosis	Diarrhoea	Hypotonia
		Hepatosplenomegaly	Hypertonia
Cardiovascular	**Haematological**	**Skin**	
Tachycardia	Petechiae	Jaundice	
Hypotension	Purpura	Sclerema	
Decreased capillary filling time	Bleeding		

include hepatitis and possibly carcinoma of the liver.

Prevention
Hepatitis B vaccine – 0,5 ml at birth, repeated at one and six months of age.

Hepatitis B immunoglobulin – 0,5 ml (50 IU) at birth.

When these are given in combination within a week of birth, over 90% of infants born to HBeAg-positive mothers can be protected. In an endemic area, babies should also be treated when the mother is HBeAg negative, but HBsAg positive.

Note
Hepatitis B vaccine is now given to all infants as part of the immunisation programme.

Herpes simplex
Herpes infection can be acquired from a labial lesion at the time of a vaginal delivery. It is most likely to be caused by the herpes virus 2 (HSV-2).

An acute maternal infection is more hazardous for the infant than a chronic one, which initiates antibodies that cross the placenta to protect the baby.

The disease has an incubation period of 6 to 12 days and can present as a local or disseminated illness. Vesicles may appear on the skin, on the conjunctivae or in the oral cavity, and the central nervous system may be involved in the disseminated variety.

Antiviral agents, such as acyclovir (p. 306), are effective and should be used to treat the infected infant.

Note
In an acute maternal infection, delivery by Caesarean section is recommended.

Scalp trauma, for example electrode clip, increases the risk of infection.

Tuberculosis
This disease is rarely transmitted across the placenta, but an infant can become infected after birth from droplet spread.

Prevention
Normal infant of a mother who is receiving anti-tuberculosis treatment
Immunise baby with BCG and assess for several months.

Encourage breast-feeding.

Normal infant of an untreated mother (prophylaxis)
Give baby isoniazid (INH), rifampicin and pyrazinamide (Rimcure paed) for two months. Dosage is based on weight, for example 1 kg = quarter tablet, 2 kg = half tablet, 4 kg = one tablet (crushed). Then do a Heaf test. If the test is negative, stop treatment and immunise with BCG. If the test is positive, continue therapy for six months.

Do not separate mother and baby and encourage breast-feeding.

BCG immunisation (p. 34)
Babies in a community at risk for tuberculosis should receive BCG vaccine shortly after birth. The vaccine offers reasonable protection against the disease, especially meningitis.

Listeria monocytogenes
This uncommon infection is produced by a Gram-positive pleomorphic bacillus that is transmitted to the fetus across the placenta or into the amniotic cavity from the cervix. The fetus may be stillborn with evidence of hepatitis, purpura and granulomata.

The amniotic fluid is often brown.

The liveborn baby may show signs of meningoencephalitis at birth, or the disease may manifest several days later with diarrhoea, vomiting, hepatosplenomegaly, jaundice, anaemia, pneumonia and purulent meningitis.

Diagnosis
Culture of the organism from blood and urine.

Treatment
Ampicillin for 14 days.

Outcome
The mortality rate is high, particularly in cases of early infection.

Chickenpox
Varicella can be transmitted from a mother to baby before or after delivery. In early pregnancy it can cause defects such as scarring, limb hypoplasia and cortical atrophy, though this is extremely rare.

Maternal infection 5 to 21 days before delivery can be associated with disease in the infant before or after birth. The course is mild, probably due to the transfer of maternal immunoglobulin.

Maternal infection four days before or two days after delivery can be associated with severe infection in the infant. Lesions appear 5 to 10 days after birth and disseminated varicella has a 30% mortality rate.

Treatment
Give the infant zoster immunoglobulin (ZIG) within 72 hours of birth to prevent or to attenuate the disease (p. 308).

Isolation
Infected babies
Isolation wards are usually removed from the area of intensive care and are not necessarily staffed by senior personnel.

This is a major disadvantage for babies who may be extremely ill and isolation should be restricted to those whose disease may cause epidemics such as:
- gastroenteritis
- myocarditis
- skin sepsis.

Mother and infant are preferably kept together, but this depends on the baby's condition and on available facilities.

Normal babies of infected mothers
Healthy babies should not be in contact with mothers who have an acute infectious disease such as:
- hepatitis
- Coxsackie infection
- chickenpox
- herpes simplex.

Keep the infant in the nursery during the infectious phase of the maternal illness.

Jaundice

Jaundice is common and implies yellow staining of the skin owing to hyperbilirubinaemia. It is usually temporary and benign, but may be viewed with undue concern by parents if they do not have a clear understanding, or do not receive a clear explanation, of the condition.

There is a difference between physiological and pathological hyperbilirubinaemia.

BILIRUBIN PHYSIOLOGY

Metabolism in the fetus
Red blood corpuscles are broken down continuously in the fetus, and this process is intensified after birth. The haemoglobin that is released from these cells is taken up by the reticuloendothelial system, especially the spleen, where it is converted to the pigment unconjugated bilirubin. This is bound to albumin and a portion is transported across the placenta. It is attached to the mother's serum albumin and excreted through her liver. The remainder goes to the fetal liver, where it is converted to bilirubin diglucuronide

and discharged into the fetal gut. Here the enzyme beta glucuronidase reconverts a portion to unconjugated bilirubin, which is reabsorbed into the bloodstream, thus completing the enterohepatic circulation of bilirubin.

Metabolism in the infant (Fig 9.1)
In its unconjugated form, bilirubin is potentially toxic to brain cells. After birth it is detoxified solely in the liver and is conveyed to this organ by serum albumin. One gram of albumin can bind 250 μmol of bilirubin, and this prevents the toxic pigment from penetrating the normal blood–brain barrier to damage neurons.

Conjugation in liver
Bilirubin is released from albumin, taken up by ligandin molecules in the liver and transported to the endoplasmic reticulum of the hepatocytes. Here a significant reaction takes place. Two molecules of glucuronic acid are added to bilirubin to render it non-toxic and water-soluble. The enzyme involved in this process is

glucuronyl transferase, and the resultant product is bilirubin diglucuronide, or conjugated bilirubin.

glucuronyl transferase
unconjugated ⟶ conjugated
bilirubin   bilirubin

Excretion

Conjugated bilirubin then flows through the bile ducts into the duodenum. It is reduced to urobilinogen by bacteria in the lower intestine and is excreted in the stools as stercobilin.

The early introduction of feeds promotes

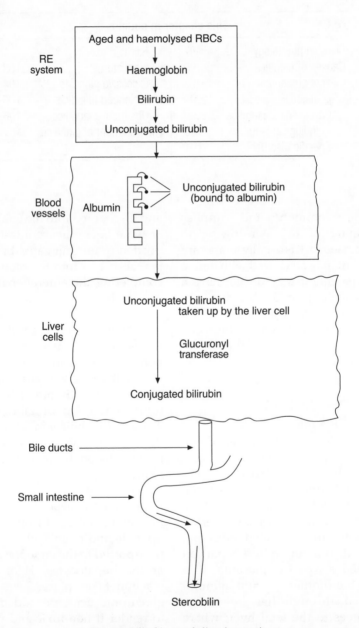

Fig. 9.1 *Bilirubin metabolism (see text)*

colonisation of the gut with bacteria and thus aids the excretion of bilirubin.

Bilirubin terminology
The laboratory reports serum bilirubin as follows:
▪ Total bilirubin.
▪ Unconjugated bilirubin.
▪ Conjugated bilirubin.

The values are expressed in μmol/l.

When serum bilirubin is determined by a micromethod, such as the bilirubinometer, only total bilirubin (conjugated + unconjugated) is reported.

The differences between the two types of bilirubin are as follows:

	Unconjugated bilirubin	Conjugated bilirubin
Synonym	Indirect	Direct
Water-soluble	No	Yes
Excretion in urine	No	Yes
Toxic to brain cells	Yes	No

CAUSES OF JAUNDICE

Bilirubin may accumulate in the blood as a result of:
▪ an excessive destruction of red blood cells

▪ defective conjugation in the liver
▪ impaired excretion into the bowel.

Haemolysis and conjugation abnormalities result in an unconjugated hyperbilirubinaemia. This is common but potentially harmful because of the toxic bilirubin pigment. Causes are listed in Table 9.1.

Factors that obstruct the passage of bilirubin into the bowel are uncommon and cause a conjugated hyperbilirubinaemia. Causes are listed in Table 9.2.

CLINICAL PRESENTATION OF JAUNDICE

Jaundice is the commonest problem in the first week of the baby's life. It may be physiological or pathological, and sometimes requires treatment.

Physiological jaundice (Fig. 9.2)
Cord blood contains less than 35 μmol/l of unconjugated bilirubin. After birth, the serum level rises, peaks on the fourth day and then declines. This temporary accumulation of bilirubin probably results from the destruction of red blood cells. A baby requires fewer red cells for oxygen carriage after birth. A level of bilirubin over 120 μmol/l is sufficient to stain the tissues and jaundice is noticeable in 40% of normal babies.

TABLE 9.1

Causes of unconjugated hyperbilirubinaemia			
Excessive haemolysis			*Defective conjugation*
Blood group incompatibility	ABO		Prematurity
	Rhesus		Drugs, possibly oxytocin
	Kell, Duffy		Hypoxaemia
			Hypoglycaemia
Familial spherocytosis			
Red cell enzyme deficiency	G6PD, Pyruvate kinase		Crigler-Najjar syndrome
			Cretinism
Haemoglobinopathies			Infection
Enclosed haemorrhages	Subaponeurotic bruising		
Polycythaemia			
Swallowed blood			
Increased enterohepatic circulation	Bowel obstruction		

TABLE 9.2

Causes of conjugated hyperbilirubinaemia		
	Hepatocellular disease	Bile obstruction
Infection	Syphilis	Atresia of bile ducts
	Toxoplasmosis	Inspissated bile syndrome
	Cytomegalovirus	Cystic fibrosis
	Herpes simplex	Choledocal cyst
	Rubella	
Metabolic disorders	Galactosaemia	
	Tyrosinosis	
	Hypermethionaemia	
	Alpha-1 antitrypsin deficiency	

Physiological jaundice in the full-term infant has the following features:

- It appears after 36 hours of age.
- The peak level seldom exceeds 275 μmol/l.
- It fades within 10 days.
- Babies remain well, gain weight and pass yellow stools.

Pathological jaundice (Fig. 9.3)

Jaundice in the full-term infant is abnormal when:

- it occurs within 24 to 36 hours of age
- bilirubin level exceeds 275 μmol/l
- it persists beyond the 10th day.

A baby with significant jaundice has a 99% chance of unconjugated hyperbilirubinaemia, but there are times when the level of conjugated bilirubin must be determined. This is discussed under 'obstructive jaundice' (p. 106).

Early onset jaundice

Jaundice that appears within 24 to 36 hours of birth is usually owing to an excessive destruction of red blood cells. It requires urgent investigation and treatment to prevent an accumulation of toxic unconjugated bilirubin.

Immediate steps

- Check the mother's blood group.
- Start phototherapy (p. 107).
- Check the level of serum bilirubin four-hourly.

If the mother's blood group is O, a likely cause is ABO incompatibility.

Following investigations

- *Blood groups:* mother and baby.
- *Direct Coombs test:* to reveal antibodies on infant's red blood cells.
- *Blood smear:* To detect numerous nucleated red cells and abnormal-shaped red cells, like spherocytes.

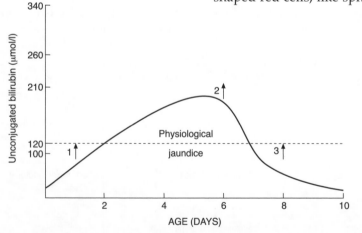

Fig. 9.2 *The physiological rise in bilirubin after birth. Pathological hyperbilirubinaemia is indicated by points 1 (early onset), 2 (too high for age) and 3 (prolonged) (From Odel, GB. 1976. The Neonate. Young, D; Hicks, J (eds). New York: Wiley)*

Further tests are usually unnecessary, but in unexplained cases the following may be helpful:

- *Haematocrit:* to detect anaemia.
- *Cord bilirubin level:* to confirm haemolysis before birth.
- *Reticulocyte count:* to reveal increased production of red blood cells.
- *Immune antibodies in mother's serum:* to detect maternal sensitisation.

Red cell enzymes, haemoglobin electrophoresis and osmotic fragility of red cells are helpful tests for obscure cases (Table 9.1).

Specific disorders
ABO incompatibility
This blood group incompatibility is the commonest cause of haemolytic disease in the newborn. In the majority of cases, the mother is group O and the fetus is group A. Serum of a group O adult contains natural anti-A and anti-B antibodies. These are produced in response to the absorption of A- and B antigens from food and bacteria in the gut.

During pregnancy, fetal red cells (group A or B) may cross into the maternal circulation to stimulate the production of immune antibodies. These, together with the natural antibodies, like anti-A, cross the placenta if they are of the IgG class, and adhere to fetal red cells. The resulting haemolysis is variable.

Clinical signs
An affected infant is normal at birth, but may become yellow within 24 to 36 hours. Jaundice is more intense than the physiological type and serum bilirubin can reach pathological levels. Mucous membranes may be pale, owing to anaemia. Some sensitised infants never develop jaundice.

The following features are characteristic:

- *Mother:* Group O.
- *Baby:* Group A, occasionally B.
- *Direct Coombs test:* Positive or negative.
- *Peripheral blood smear:* Spherocytes, many nucleated red blood cells.
- *Haematocrit:* normal or low.
- *Reticulocyte count:* Over 5%.
- *Bilirubin:* Mostly unconjugated.

Treatment
Consider jaundice of early onset to be ABO incompatibility if the mother is group O. Treat promptly with phototherapy and then confirm the diagnosis. Phototherapy alone is effective in the majority of cases.

Exchange transfusion is rarely needed, but may be necessary for hyperbilirubinaemia in a late admission.

A transfusion of packed red cells is indicated if anaemia is severe (p. 223).

Outcome
ABO is less severe than Rhesus incompatibility and the prognosis is usually excellent.

In midwife obstetric units, babies are often sent home with their mothers within six hours of birth. To ensure that ABO incompatibility is not missed, a serum bilirubin level is obtained on infants whose mothers are group O. Those with levels exceeding 80 μmol/l at six hours of age receive phototherapy.

Rhesus incompatibility
The Rhesus (Rh) antigen of red cells consists of three major proteins, termed C, D and E. These are inherited in varying combinations with other minor factors.

The D antigen is the one of concern as it readily stimulates the formation of anti-D antibodies, which are responsible for 99% of cases of clinical Rhesus disease.

People with the D antigen on their red cells are considered to be Rh positive. Those who lack the D antigen are usually regarded as Rh negative, since the C, E and minor Rhesus antigens rarely stimulate antibody production. However, there are exceptions to this statement.

Rh antigens are not found in food or bacteria so that anti-D antibodies do not appear spontaneously in the blood of people who lack the Rh factor. They develop only after Rh antigen has entered the body in large quantities, such as a transfusion with Rh-positive blood.

Initial sensitisation

Fetal red cells which contain the D factor may cross the placenta and enter the circulation of a Rh-negative mother during her first pregnancy. Antibody production takes several months, or may not occur if too few fetal cells are present. It is more likely to follow a substantial leakage of red cells at delivery.

The firstborn infant therefore does not show signs of haemolytic disease.

Repeat sensitisation

A sensitised Rh-negative mother produces anti-D antibodies rapidly and in large quantities in subsequent pregnancies when challenged with small numbers of Rh-positive fetal red blood cells.

Incidence

Sensitisation of a Rh-negative woman is preventable (p. 103) and rarely seen with good ante- and postnatal care.

Diagnosis

Rhesus disease should be anticipated if anti-D antibodies are detected in the serum of a Rh-negative woman during pregnancy. The following laboratory results are characteristic after birth:

- *Mother:* Rhesus negative.
- *Infant:* Rhesus positive.
- *Direct Coombs test:* positive.
- *Bilirubin:* mostly unconjugated.

Clinical presentation

Clinical features depend on the degree of haemolysis before and after birth and the disease may present as:

- haemolytic anaemia

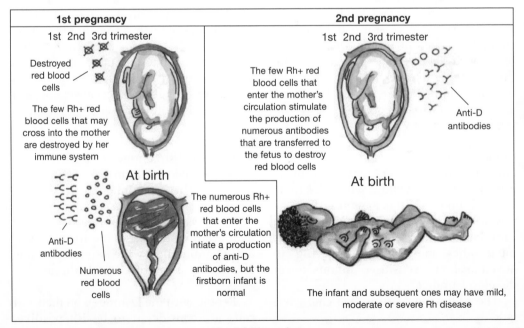

Fig. 9.3 *Rhesus factors*

- icterus gravis neonatorum
- hydrops fetalis (Colour plate III)
- intrauterine death.

Haemolytic anaemia is a mild form with moderate jaundice and anaemia after birth.

Icterus gravis neonatorum, as the name implies, is a severe variety. Excessive haemolysis causes early jaundice, which is potentially hazardous because of the risk of kernicterus. Anaemia is an associated complication that can progress for approximately six weeks.

Hydrops fetalis literally means oedema of the fetus. This is the most severe form of the disease. Amniotic fluid, vernix and umbilical cord are stained yellow and the placenta is pale and grossly enlarged. Generalised oedema, hepatosplenomegaly, jaundice and pallor are consistent findings, and petechiae may be present. The pleural and peritoneal cavities are filled with fluid, which can impair breathing, and heart failure is usually present.

Hydrops fetalis may result in intrauterine death. The outlook after birth is grave even with treatment.

Complications of hyperbilirubinaemia
Kernicterus is more likely to occur in Rhesus disease than in any other form of hyperbilirubinaemia.

Treatment
The management of Rhesus disease depends on the degree of haemolysis and hyperbilirubinaemia.

Phototherapy plays a limited role and is likely to be effective only in mild cases, that is, those with a cord bilirubin level of less than 60 μmol/l. Light therapy is commenced as soon after birth as possible and may be needed for up to 10 days.

Phototherapy can also be used for severe cases in conjunction with exchange transfusion, but is never a substitute for the latter.

Indications for exchange transfusion are listed on p. 109.

A straight transfusion of blood may be required for anaemia within the first six weeks.

Prevention of Rhesus sensitisation
Give concentrated human gamma globulin (IgG) containing 200–300 μg of anti-D antibody to Rh-negative mothers who have delivered their first Rh-positive infant. This prevents maternal production of natural anti-D antibodies, but the mechanism is uncertain. In order to be effective, the injection should be given within 72 hours of delivery. Repeat it after subsequent births of Rh-positive infants.

In rural areas, and in midwife obstetric units, the blood group of an infant may not be identifiable for several days, in which case anti-D globulin should be given to all Rh-negative mothers after birth.

The injection may be given during pregnancy if there is a significant risk of sensitisation. This is likely to occur with complications such as abruptio or bleeding associated with amniocentesis. The only known side-effect is a positive Coombs reaction of fetal red cells. The antibody crosses the placenta and adheres to these cells, but does not destroy them.

Other indications for immunisation include abortion and ectopic pregnancies.

Bilirubin toxicity (kernicterus)
Unconjugated bilirubin can damage brain cells irreparably should it cross the blood–brain barrier. This is known as kernicterus, which literally means yellow-stained nuclei of the brain (Colour plate IX).

The mechanism whereby bilirubin enters the brain is uncertain, but is probably related to excessive permeability of the blood–brain barrier and displacement of unconjugated bilirubin from serum albumin.

Certain factors are known to increase the risk of kernicterus (Table 9.3).

A correlation exists between kernicterus and the level of unconjugated bilirubin in serum. The upper limit of safety is uncertain. In Rhesus disease an appreciable risk occurs when serum bilirubin exceeds 340 µmol/l, but haemolytic conditions such as ABO incompatibility appear to be safe up to 400 µmol/l.

Risk factors necessitate a lowering of the upper safety levels by at least 60 µmol/l or more in the case of very small babies, that is, less than 1 500 g.

Clinical features of kernicterus
The signs of encephalopathy usually occur after 36 hours of age. The jaundiced infant becomes listless, sucks poorly and has a weak Moro reflex. Eyes lose their normal conjugate movement and roll down to show a 'setting sun' appearance. The head and neck may arch excessively to give optisthotonic posturing. Pyrexia is common.

The presentation may not be specific in preterm babies, who often develop apnoeic attacks.

The brain damage caused by kernicterus cannot be corrected by any known therapy.

TABLE 9.3

Risk factors associated with kernicterus	
Prematurity	*Drugs:*
Hypoxia	Ceftriaxone
Acideamia	Salicylates
Low serum albumin	Sodium benzoate
Excessive fatty acids (NEFA)	Sulphonamides
Hyperosmolality	

Course
Fifty per cent of infants die. Those who survive may present in later life with any combination of the following:

- Athetosis.
- High-tone deafness.
- Cerebral spasticity.
- Mental retardation.
- Green teeth.

These hazards must be averted by the timeous treatment of unconjugated bilirubinaemia.

Excessive jaundice (after 36 hours)
After the second day, a level of bilirubin that exceeds 250 µmol/l requires investigation.

At this age the most likely associations are:

- an exaggeration of physiological jaundice (idiopathic)
- prematurity
- bruising or other haemorrhages
- a bacterial infection.

Immediate steps
Examine the baby to exclude obvious signs of infection or enclosed haemorrhages, such as bruising.

Examine urine for pus cells, bacteria and the Group B streptococcus antigen.

Obtain a white cell and band cell count (p. 228).

Ensure that the blood groups of baby and mother are not incompatible, such as ABO.

Start phototherapy.

Check the serum level of bilirubin daily.

Idiopathic jaundice
Healthy full-term babies may develop excessive jaundice in the absence of obvious pathology. In fact, most babies who require phototherapy fall into this category. Jaundice is considered to be an exaggerated physiological event.

The following can increase the possibility:

- A delay in feeding.
- Breast milk.

- Labour-induction agents, for example oxytocin.

Prematurity

Glucuronyl transferase and ligandin levels are probably reduced in the preterm infant and bilirubin conjugation is delayed. This transient problem corrects itself within a week or so.

Extravasation of blood

Red blood cells are broken down following the collection of blood in various sites. Haemolysis is not as intense as in blood group incompatibility and jaundice usually occurs after 48 hours.

Causes are: bruising, subaponeurotic or intracranial bleeding and, occasionally, cephalhaematoma.

Polycythaemia

Jaundice may occur when the haematocrit exceeds 65%. It usually presents after 48 hours of age.

Infection

Organisms such as Group B streptococcus can cause hyperbilirubinaemia. Signs of infection, like omphalitis, should be sought in all cases of jaundice.

Prolonged jaundice (longer than 10 days)

Jaundice which persists beyond the 10th day may be caused by an obstruction to the excretion of bilirubin, such as bile duct atresia. This is an ominous cause as it can result in liver failure, but it is certainly not a common one.

Prolonged jaundice is more likely to be associated with:

- prematurity
- breast-feeding
- urinary tract infection
- hypothyroidism.

Initial steps

Examine urine for colour, pus, bacteria and reducing substances (see Galactosaemia p. 273).

Note the colour of the stools – they ought to be yellow and not white.

Ensure that thyroid-screening tests are normal (p. 276).

If these investigations are normal in a breast-fed baby then breast-milk jaundice is the likely explanation.

Breast-milk jaundice

Some breast-fed babies remain yellow for several weeks. The level of unconjugated bilirubin rarely exceeds 180 μmol/l.

These are the usual features:

- Jaundice does not increase.
- Babies are well, and thrive.

The condition is benign, yet the reason for hyperbilirubinaemia is unknown. Breast milk contains the enzyme beta glucuronidase and it may convert conjugated bilirubin in the bowel to the unconjugated form, which is reabsorbed into the circulation.

The mother should continue to breast-feed her infant.

Congenital hypothyroidism

Persistent jaundice is a feature of this endocrine deficiency. It may be the only early sign of the disease and appropriate studies for thyroid function (TSH, T4) should be done if jaundice persists beyond the third week. Failure to detect and treat hypothyroidism at this age can result in the infant being mentally retarded.

The primary defect is probably one of conjugation, which results in a mild and persisting unconjugated hyperbilirubinaemia.

Urinary tract infection

Prolonged jaundice may be the only manifestation of a urinary tract infection caused by *E. coli* organisms. The endotoxins of these bacteria can cause cholestasis, as well as haemolysis of red blood cells.

Examine the urine for pus and bacteria in each case of prolonged jaundice.

Appropriate antibiotic therapy is required.

Obstructive jaundice

Chronic liver disease and congenital abnormalities of the bile duct prevent the excretion of conjugated bilirubin into the bowel. Prompt diagnosis and treatment can avert hepatic failure.

Presentation

The causes of obstructive jaundice are listed in Table 9.2.

Suspect obstruction when:

- jaundice persists beyond three weeks
- the stools are pale and the urine is dark
- hepatosplenomegaly and other signs of congenital infections are present.

Any of these warrant the following tests:

- *Serum:* Level of conjugated bilirubin, total serum IgM for infection, liver function tests.
- *Urine:* Clinitest for reducing substances.

Further investigations will depend on the suspected disease.

Hepatocellular disease

Various infections and metabolic defects listed in Table 9.2 can cause chronic hepatocellular disease.

Clinical features include hepatosplenomegaly, pale stools and dark urine. The liver function tests are abnormal and a conjugated hyperbilirubinaemia is present.

In many cases, like syphilis, the primary cause is treatable, but prolonged hepatitis can result in giant cell infiltration of the liver and hepatic failure. The mortality rate is 25%.

Bile duct obstruction

The excretion of bile can be impaired by intra- and extrahepatic bile duct atresia or a choledocal cyst.

Clinical and laboratory features are similar to those of hepatitis and an abdominal mass may be palpable in the case of a choledocal cyst.

Biliary obstruction must be distinguished from hepatitis, as extrahepatic duct atresia and choledocal cyst are treatable by surgery. Failure to make a distinction within eight weeks can result in hepatic fibrosis, which is fatal.

Extrahepatic duct atresia is treated by the Kasai operation. This provides drainage of bile from the liver through a hepato-jejunal anastomosis and is successful in up to 90% of cases.

A distinction between hepatitis and bile duct atresia may be difficult on routine clinical and laboratory investigations and the following special tests are helpful:

- *Ultrasonography:* This can detect a choledocal cyst.
- *Radiopharmacology:* This can detect obstruction to the flow and excretion of the bile, such as p-butyl-IDA, colloid.
- *Liver biopsy:* Differences present in the early stages are listed below.

	Hepatitis	Biliary atresia
Bile ducts	normal	hyperplastic
Giant cells	numerous	scanty
Fibrosis	minimal	marked
Bile plugs	absent	present

Investigations for other unusual causes of obstructive jaundice include the following:

- *Amino acid chromatography:* tyrosinosis.
- *Sugar chromatography:* galactosaemia.
- *Alpha-1 antitrypsin:* antitrypsin deficiency.
- *Sweat sodium:* cystic fibrosis.

Nutrition support

In obstructive jaundice, bile salts fail to reach the bowel and fat absorption is impaired, with resultant malnutrition. Ensure an adequate supply of fat by using medium chain triglycerides, such as Liprocil™, which do not depend on bile salts for absorption. Water-soluble vitamins A and D will have to be substituted for the fat-soluble ones.

THE TREATMENT OF JAUNDICE

Phototherapy

When a jaundiced infant is exposed to light of 400–500 nm waveband, the molecular structure of unconjugated bilirubin in skin capillaries is altered. It becomes water-soluble (lumirubin) and is readily excreted in urine and stools. A small amount of bilirubin is photo-oxidised to biliverdin and tetrapyrolles, which are also easily eliminated from the body. These products do not appear to be toxic to neuronal cells. The peak absorption wavelength of light at which bilirubin is broken down is 458 nm.

Phototherapy avoids an exchange transfusion by reducing the level of unconjugated bilirubin.

No long-term side-effects have been described, but the risk of hyperbilirubinaemia should always outweigh unknown hazards. The level of bilirubin at which phototherapy is recommended varies with the gestation and age of an infant. Indications for light therapy in normal term and preterm babies are shown in the accompanying graphs (Fig. 9.4). Use prophylactic phototherapy from birth in haemolytic disease and if any of the complications listed in Table 9.3 are present.

Side-effects (Table 9.4)

Minor adverse effects may occur during phototherapy. Some are related to light *per se* and others to the environmental circumstances.

Retinal cells of piglets can be damaged by intense light, and although this hazard has not been described in humans, it is advisable to cover a baby's eyes during phototherapy.

Method

Remove clothes, except for the nappy, and place the baby in a cot or incubator under a phototherapy unit. This consists of a series of fluorescent light tubes mounted on a platform approximately 50 cm above the infant. The efficacy of treatment depends on the waveband of light and alternate blue and white fluorescent tubes may be used. They are changed after 1 000–2 000 hours of continuous use as their therapeutic effect (light intensity) decreases.

A more efficient system uses light-emitting diodes (LED). The advantages include thousands of hours of effectiveness, and the absence of ultraviolet and infrared radiation so that the light unit can be placed close to an infant without compromising safety. However, long-term effects are not known.

Cover the baby's eyes with clean gauze pads, kept in place with Micropore adhesive tape. Check the axillary temperature hourly and remove the baby from the light source for feeds.

Exposure may be continuous or intermittent. Continuous therapy results in a

TABLE 9.4

Complications of phototherapy	
Side-effects	*Causes*
Skin rashes	Photosensitisation of skin
Diarrhoea	Possibly lactose intolerance from breakdown products
Bronzing of skin	Polymerisation of porphyrins with obstructive jaundice
Hypothermia	Exposure of naked infant
Hyperthermia	Absorption of light energy
Conjunctivitis	Eye pads do not permit observation of eyes
Nasal obstruction	Dislodgement of eye pads
Crying spells	Separation of mother and baby

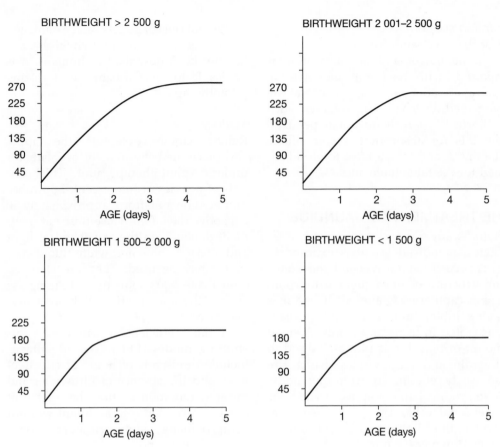

Fig. 9.4 *Use phototherapy when the bilirubin level is above the line in the relevant graph*
(Adapted from Cockington, RA. 1979. A guide to the use of
phototherapy in the management of neonatal hyperbilirubinaemia. J Pediatr 95: 28–5)

fall of serum bilirubin of about 50 μmol/l per day in nonhaemolytic disease.

Liver enzyme induction

Phenobarbitone is considered to stimulate the production of glucuronyl transferase and has been used to treat infants with high levels of unconjugated bilirubin.

Phenobarbitone is not as effective as phototherapy and may lead to drowsiness and difficulty with sucking, particularly in preterm babies. It can be used with phototherapy if the bilirubin exceeds 300 μmol/l.

Dose 3 mg/kg, given once.

Exchange transfusion

Purposes

To remove excess bilirubin and prevent kernicterus.

To correct anaemia.

To remove sensitised red cells.

Indications

These are listed in Table 9.5.

Method

The blood of an infant is partially exchanged for that of a donor. Donor blood has to be:

- Rh negative – preferably group O
- compatible with the blood of the mother

- fresh, that is, no older than 48–72 hours
- anticoagulated with citrate
- warmed before use
- pH-corrected.

Preparation

Place the baby in an incubator or open crib to regulate body temperature.

Immobilise the arms and legs. They can be fitted into lengths of stockinette tied to the underlying frame.

Pass a nasogastric tube into the stomach and aspirate its contents. Omit feeds during the transfusion. Insert a cannula into a peripheral vein and use 10% dextrose for energy requirements.

TABLE 9.5

Indications for exchange transfusion	
At birth	Cord unconjugated bilirubin of over 70 μmol/l Cord haemoglobin of 10 g/dl or less Hydrops fetalis
Later	A rise of unconjugated bilirubin in excess of 17 μmol/l per hour. A total unconjugated bilirubin level of: 340 μmol/l (Rhesus and G6PD deficiency), approximately 400 μmol/l (ABO)

These levels are reduced by approximately 60 μmol/l when complications listed in Table 9.3 are present

Attach ECG leads to the chest and monitor the cardiac rate and complexes continuously. Fit an oximeter probe to an ear lobe or foot for oxygen saturation readings. Measure skin temperature from an abdominal probe or from a thermometer in the axilla. Ensure that oxygen tension, temperature and acid-base values are normal before commencing the exchange.

Blood exchange

Warm the pack of donor blood in a blood warmer or place it in a water bath at 36 °C for 30 minutes, then attach it to a burette and drip set. Fill this to the 100 ml mark with blood and add 2 ml of sodium bicarbonate 4% to prevent acidaemia.

Clean the umbilicus with Hibitane in spirits, then dry and drape the area. Cut off the cord about 1 cm above the skin. Attach an end-hole umbilical catheter (size 5 or 8F) to a two-way stopcock and fill it with heparinised saline from a 10 ml syringe.

Insert the catheter into the umbilical vein, that is, thin wall vessel, with a fine forceps. Apply gentle pressure to the syringe plunger and halt the advance of the catheter when a free flow of blood is obtained. The catheter tip is probably in or close to the inferior vena cava. Immobilise it by tying a cord around the umbilical base. If the umbilical cord has been cut flush with the skin, insert a purse-string suture around the vein and tighten it when the catheter is sited correctly.

Attach a glass manometer to the side-arm of the stopcock and measure the venous pressure at the level of the heart (normal 6–12 cm of blood). Fit a second stopcock in series with the first. Attach the proximal one to a line from the donor blood and the other to a waste receiver.

Withdraw 10 ml of blood from the infant and replace it with 10 ml of donor blood. Repeat this using 10 ml or 5 ml aliquots, depending on the size and state of the baby. When the amount of blood in the burette is down to 10 or 20 ml, add 1 ml of 10% calcium gluconate, to prevent hypocalcaemia. This is may be given for each 100 ml of blood. Use a total of 160 ml per kg body weight of donor blood.

This should exchange approximately 80% of the infant's blood. Check the venous pressure after each 100 ml of exchanged blood and do not exceed a rate of 2 ml/kg/min for the procedure.

A nurse should record the:
- heart rate quarter-hourly
- temperature quarter-hourly
- oxygen saturation quarter-hourly
- blood volume of each extraction and replacement

amounts of sodium bicarbonate and calcium gluconate used.

Halt the exchange in the event of:
- cyanosis
- cardiac arrhythmias
- tachycardia (over 180/min)
- bradycardia (less than 100/min)
- vomiting
- raised venous pressure.

Post exchange
Measure the venous pressure and if necessary return it to normal by withdrawing or adding sufficient donor blood. Take a sample of the infant's blood for bilirubin level, culture and cross-matching (in the event of a second transfusion). Remove the catheter and occlude the vein by tying the cord or tightening the purse-string suture. Apply a sterile gauze dressing to the umbilicus.

The prophylactic use of antibiotics is not recommended after the first exchange transfusion, but it can be considered for subsequent exchanges.

Complications
They are reactive hypoglycaemia, overloading of the circulation, hypovolaemia with shock, air embolism, hypokalaemia, hypocalcaemia, cardiac arrhythmias, thrombosis, infection, necrotising enterocolitis, portal vein hypertension.

The mortality rate of exchange transfusion, providing all precautions are taken, is less than 1%.

Post-exchange procedures
Check the level of bilirubin three-hourly.

Determine the level of blood sugar (Dextrostix) hourly.

Recommence milk feeds.

Estimate the level of haemoglobin weekly for two months.

Examine the baby at intervals for five years to exclude cerebral damage or deafness from hyperbilirubinaemia.

CHAPTER 10

Congenital Abnormalities

This chapter in outline:

Definition

A defect in body structure or function at birth is referred to as a congenital abnormality. It may be obvious, for example meningomyelocele (p. 135), or occult, such as coarctation of the aorta.

An abnormality transmissible from one generation to another is said to be inherited and is always congenital as it is present at birth.

Examples:

Structural: Achondroplasia (p. 282).

Functional: Phenylketonuria (p. 272).

Many congenital abnormalities are not inherited and result from known or unknown factors that impair embryo or fetal development.

Example: Fetal alcohol syndrome (p. 113).

Most functional abnormalities, such as metabolic disorders, are inherited. They are discussed on page 270.

STRUCTURAL ABNORMALITIES

Classification (Table 10.1)

Malformation

This results from the abnormal development of an organ or tissue. It occurs at fertilisation or during organogenesis and may be generalised, like fetal alcohol syndrome, or confined to a particular area, such as a cleft lip.

Disruption

A breakdown of a previously normal organ or tissue results in a disruption. This may be caused by a vascular insult, such

TABLE 10.1

Classification of structural abnormalities			
Type	*Time of onset*	*Cause*	*Reversibility*
Malformation	Zygote/embryo	Defective chromosomes or genes Teratogenic factors	No
Disruption	Embryo/fetus	Amniotic bands Infections	No
Deformation	Fetus	Mechanical constraints	Yes

as small bowel atresia, or by a mechanical one, like amniotic band syndrome.

Deformation
Mechanical forces can alter the shape or position of normal tissues in fetal life, for example oligohydramnios can cause malalignment of the feet, such as in calcaneovalgus (p. 285).

Incidence
Recognisable abnormalities occur in 2% of newborn babies. The incidence rises to 4% within a year, with detection of occult lesions such as heart defects.

Together with accidents and malignancy, congenital abnormalities account for the majority of childhood deaths in industrialised countries.

The incidence is influenced by the following factors:

Sex
Certain lesions occur more frequently in boys, for example harelip, hypertrophic pyloric stenosis, hydrocephalus and club feet. In girls, there is a higher incidence of anencephaly, spina bifida and dislocation of the hip.

Geography
Various countries have a high incidence of specific conditions, for example dislocation of the hip is particularly common in Israel and Italy.

Age of mother
Mothers over 30 years of age have a relatively high chance of producing infants with abnormalities, such as Down's syndrome, heart defects, spina bifida, anencephaly, hydrocephalus, harelip and cleft palate. The chance of a malformation increases threefold if the mother is over 45 years of age.

Multiple birth
Monozygotic twins have a greater percentage of defects than singletons.

Consanguinity
Inbreeding enhances the chance of unfavourable traits.

Maternal illness
There is an increased risk of congenital abnormalities in the offspring of diabetic women.

Drugs
Women who ingest a variety of common medicines during early pregnancy, such as aspirin, antibiotics and iron, may have a higher chance of producing malformed babies than those who do not consume such agents.

Alcohol consumption is hazardous for the embryo and fetal alcohol syndrome is prevalent in wine-producing regions of southern Africa. It is characterised by microcephaly, growth retardation, microphthalmia, absent philtrum and heart defects

Malformation
Aetiology
Environmental and genetic factors account for 30% of malformations, whereas the rest are associated with unknown causes.

Environmental factors
The developing human is most susceptible to teratogenic (*tera-tos* = a monster) agents during organogenesis. Important factors include:

- microbial agents
- drugs
- radiation
- hyperpyrexia.

Microbial agents
The rubella virus can cross the placenta in early pregnancy and cause malformations

such as patent ductus and septal defects (p. 193). Toxoplasmosis (p. 89) and cytomegalovirus infections (p. 90) are also implicated.

Drugs

A relationship between drugs and malformation was established several decades ago. Thalidomide, hailed as a safe sedative and antiemetic, caused severe limb defects such as phocomelia (p. 284) when used in early pregnancy.

Several other medications are known to be teratogenic and no drug is safe for girls of child-bearing age. Many women are unaware of being pregnant in the critical stage of organogenesis.

Radiation

Fetal damage can be caused by X-radiation of the pelvic region during pregnancy. This hazard was recognised in 1925 and complications from this source are rarely encountered. Excessive radiation can produce abortion, microcephaly and microphthalmia.

Some microcephalic infants were born to women pregnant at the time of the atom bomb explosions in Nagasaki and Hiroshima. Subsequent pregnancies did not show an increase in the incidence of abnormalities.

Hyperpyrexia

Hyperpyrexia in early pregnancy has been implicated in various facial and neurological abnormalities.

Genetic factors

Role of chromosomes and genes

The nucleus of each cell contains fine threads of chromosomes (Gr. *khroma* = colour + *soma* = body) that are considered to be responsible for the form of all life. These structures are composed of proteins and DNA (deoxyribonucleic acid). The DNA molecule resembles a spiral staircase, with sugar and phosphate forming the framework, and linkages of adenine with thymine, and cytosine with guanine, forming the steps.

Genes represent varying numbers of such 'steps', called nucleotides. They are the basic units of heredity and a single gene might contain 2 000 steps.

Each gene carries the instructions for the amino acid sequences of proteins. The 46 chromosomes are estimated to contain up to two billion steps and can be regarded as a series of genes in linear order. The human is estimated to have 40 000 genes.

The complex DNA staircase keeps life going in two ways. It reproduces itself and it manufactures the proteins that cells need in order to function properly. An alteration in a single step, or nucleotide, may cause a mutation in the DNA molecule and result in a defective protein.

Arrangement of chromosomes

Autosomes

The 46 chromosomes consist of 23 pairs. In 22, the paired chromosomes are identical in size and shape and are known as autosomes. Each chromosome consists of a pair of chromatids joined at the centromere and they are numbered from 1 to 22, depending on characteristic transverse bands (Fig. 10.1).

Sex chromosomes

The remaining pair consists of two sex chromosomes. In the female, the members of the pair are identical, being two large X chromosomes. In the male, these structures differ, one being an X chromosome, the other a much smaller Y chromosome. The X chromosome contains approximately 1 000 genes and about half are expressed in the brain.

Note

The cells of the female contain 22 pairs of autosomes and one pair of X chromosomes (46, XX). The cells of the male have

22 pairs of autosomes and one X and one Y chromosome (46, XY).

Cell division
Body cells
When a normal cell is about to multiply, each chromosome of a pair splits lengthwise. The original and its copy move to opposite ends of the cell, which then divides. The two cells resulting from this mitosis are identically equipped with a full set of paired chromosomes.

Gametes
The formation of an ovum or sperm differs in that each new cell receives only one member of a chromosome pair through a process of meiosis. A sperm cell therefore contains 22 autosomes and either an X or a Y sex chromosome, while an ovum consists of 22 autosomes and a single X chromosome.

Embryo
When sperm and ovum unite to form a zygote, the full number of chromosomes is restored. The physical characteristics of the fetus are determined by the combined action of genes inherited from the parents and preceding generations. A female fetus is formed when an X chromosome is transferred from the sperm, whereas a

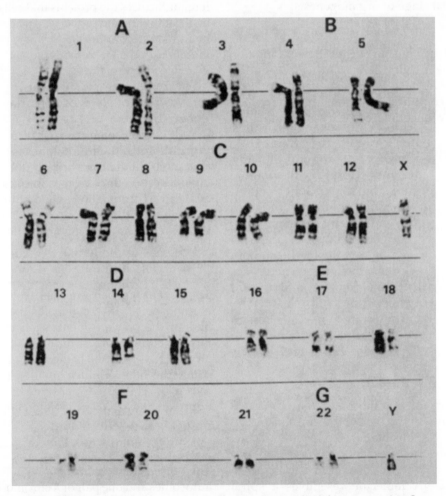

Fig. 10.1 *Chromosomes of a normal male. The autosomes are divided into groups A to G*

male will result from the introduction of a Y chromosome.

Only the sperm nucleus enters the ovum so that DNA from other sources, like mitochondria, is passed to the embryo solely through the egg.

Some genes function properly only if donated by the father, others must come from the mother. An incorrect distribution can cause malformations, for example some cases of Prader-Willi syndrome are caused by chromosome 15 receiving two copies of maternal genes. It thus lacks a paternal contribution, whereas Angelman syndrome results from the same chromosome receiving two copies of paternal genes.

Homozygous and heterozygous
Since chromosomes are paired, the genes are also paired, and the two members of a pair may carry similar or different instructions regarding the trait they determine, such as colour of eyes. If both members of a gene carry similar instructions, the trait is said to be homozygous. If the instructions differ on each pair, for example brown vs blue eyes, the trait is termed heterozygous. In this case, the particular trait will be determined by whichever gene is dominant, that is, brown eyes, while the message conveyed by the recessive gene, that is, blue eyes, remains repressed.

Gene disorders
Gene abnormalities are responsible for up to 1,7% of all malformations. They can be classified into the following groups:

Polygenic
Multiple genes are defective and in association with adverse environmental factors may cause an abnormality, like a cleft palate. Knowledge of this group is still incomplete.

Monogenic
A single gene is defective. This group can be subdivided into dominant and recessive conditions.

Dominant trait
The specific gene can be present on one or on both members of a chromosome pair. A heterozygote can be abnormal.

Recessive trait
The specific gene must be present on both members of a chromosome pair. Only a homozygote will be abnormal.

Autosomal dominant abnormalities
The individual who exhibits an abnormal trait usually carries one dominant pathologic gene and one normal gene, and is therefore heterozygous. When such a person conceives with a normal partner, the chances of the offspring developing the trait are one in two. The unaffected children are genetically normal (Fig. 10.2).

If an affected adult conceives with a normal person, the chances of transmitting the abnormal gene remain at 50%.

The children who do not show the trait will have healthy offspring, provided their partners are normal. Examples of autosomal dominant traits include polydactyly and achondroplasia.

Abnormal dominant genes show considerable variation in their degree of penetrance and a defect can occasionally be transmitted by an individual who exhibits no clinical signs of the abnormality. The defect may also skip several generations.

Autosomal recessive abnormalities
Common: If an apparently normal individual who carries a pathologic recessive gene conceives with a person who is similarly heterozygous, the chances of producing a homozygous child who exhibits the abnormal trait is one in four for each

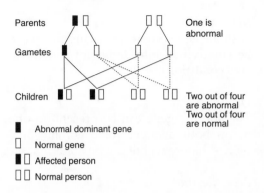

Parents — One is abnormal

Gametes

Children — Two out of four are abnormal
Two out of four are normal

■ Abnormal dominant gene

☐ Normal gene

■☐ Affected person

☐☐ Normal person

Fig. 10.2 *Dominant heredity (heterozygote)*

pregnancy (Fig. 10.3). Consanguineous conceptions favour the appearance of such recessive traits.

Examples of recessive abnormalities include cystic fibrosis (p, 216) and adrenogenital syndrome (p. 275).

Uncommon: If a homozygous-affected individual conceives with a heterozygous carrier, 50% of the offspring will be homozygous and exhibit the abnormal trait, while the remaining 50% will be carriers.

Sex-linked dominant abnormalities

These are rare. An affected male who conceives with a normal female can transmit the mutant gene only to daughters, whereas an affected female who conceives with a normal male can transmit the defect to both sons and daughters.

Such abnormalities are often lethal to the developing male fetus and after birth tend to occur more frequently in females, for example X-linked hypophosphataemic rickets.

Sex-linked recessive abnormalities

Certain recessive traits can appear in the males of a family. The females, however, show no evidence of the disease, but carry the trait.

Reason: A recessive gene located on the X chromosome of the male can produce an abnormality as it is not matched by a corresponding normal gene on the Y chromosome.

On the other hand, a recessive gene on the X chromosome of a female can be checked by a corresponding normal gene on the opposite X chromosome.

Common: If the female carrier of an abnormal trait, such as haemophilia, conceives with a normal male, half the sons can exhibit the disease and half can be genetically normal. Half the daughters can carry the pathologic gene and half can be genetically normal (Fig. 10.4).

Chromosome disorders

Structural or numerical abnormalities can occur in autosomes and sex chromosomes. These affect large numbers of genes.

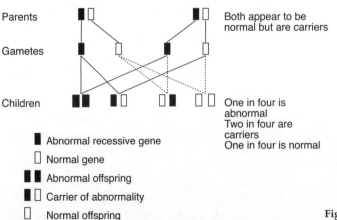

Parents — Both appear to be normal but are carriers

Gametes

Children — One in four is abnormal
Two in four are carriers
One in four is normal

■ Abnormal recessive gene

☐ Normal gene

■■ Abnormal offspring

■☐ Carrier of abnormality

☐ Normal offspring

Fig. 10.3 *Recessive heredity*

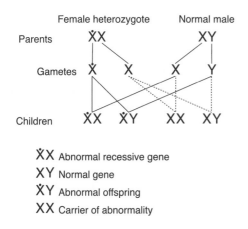

Parents   Female heterozygote   Normal male
          X̌X   XY

Gametes   X̌ X   X   Y

Children X̌X   X̌Y   XX   XY

X̌X Abnormal recessive gene
XY Normal gene
X̌Y Abnormal offspring
XX Carrier of abnormality

Fig. 10.4 *Sex-linked heredity*

Autosome defects

These produce characteristic physical abnormalities with some degree of mental retardation. Most defects are caused by an extra chromosome (trisomy) in the cells of an infant.

Note

Chromosome abnormalities are found in 25% of early abortions and account for about 0,5% of congenital malformations in liveborn babies.

Important abnormalities in the liveborn include the following:

- Trisomy 21 – Down's syndrome.
- Trisomy 13 – Patau syndrome.
- Trisomy 18 – Edward syndrome.

Trisomy 21

Down's syndrome (mongolism) is the most common chromosome defect and occurs in about 1 in 600 births.

Non-dysjunction: The abnormality usually arises during the development of an ovum. A pair of number 21 chromosomes may fail to separate during meiosis. This is termed non-dysjunction – and one egg receives two 21 chromosomes instead of one. After fertilisation a third 21 chromosome is added to the zygote. Non-dysjunction can also occur during mitotic division of the zygote after fertilisation, though this is extremely rare.

Down's syndrome owing to non-dysjunction is mostly age-related and occurs in 1 in 60 infants born to mothers over 40 years of age. The cells of the infant will contain 47 chromosomes.

Uncommon causes of Down's syndrome include mosaic and translocation defects of chromosomes.

Mosaicism: Non-dysjunction can occur in one of the cells of the early embryo during mitosis. The descendants of that cell contain an extra 21 chromosome, while the other cell lines have the normal complement. Babies may have features of mongolism or they may be virtually normal.

Translocation: A 21 chromosome can become attached to a 15 chromosome in the ovum or sperm. During meiosis the translocated chromosome is transferred to the same cell as the normal 21 chromosome. At fertilisation a third 21 chromosome is added and results in Down's syndrome, with a complement of 46 chromosomes. This may occur in young and old women. Other chromosomes rarely translocate.

The mother with a 15 to 21 translocation defect has a one in three chance of producing a Down's syndrome child.

The father with a similar defect has a 1 in 20 chance. The reason for this difference is not known.

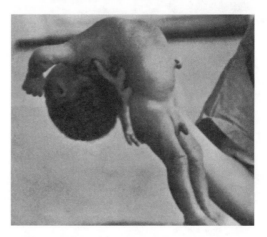

Fig. 10.5 *General hypotonia in Down's syndrome*

Clinical

Characteristic physical signs are usually recognisable at birth.

General: Hypotonia is a constant feature and the baby may feel floppy when picked up (Fig. 10.5). The hair and skin are smooth and silky.

Skull: The head is small and the circumference may be below the third percentile. The occiput is flattened.

Eyes: Palpebral fissures slant upwards. Inner epicanthic folds are prominent (Fig. 10.6). Strabismus may be present. The iris can be speckled, especially if the eyes are blue (Brushfield spots).

Face: The nasal bridge is flat. The nose is small. The ears are small and malformed. The tongue tends to protrude.

Neck: This appears shortened. Excess folds of skin are present posteriorly.

Hands and feet: The extremities are broad, with shortened digits. A wide gap may be present between the first and second fingers and toes. The small finger is often hypoplastic and in-turned. The palmar crease may be single. The palmar axial triradius is situated distally.

Genitalia: The testes are underdeveloped and often undescended.

Associated abnormalities

Heart: Atrioventricular communis, ventricular septal defect.

Gastrointestinal tract: Duodenal atresia.

Prognosis

The rate of development is slow: the average baby sits at 12 months and walks at 25 months. Toilet training may be established at three-and-a-half years. Mental retardation is constant and the IQ rarely exceeds 50. Normal schooling is not feasible, but the child may cope with work of a simple and repetitive nature in a special class or in a school for the learning-disabled.

The child is usually well behaved and happy, and particularly enjoys music. A home upbringing is advisable.

Males are considered to be infertile, but females do menstruate and can reproduce.

Respiratory tract infections, especially rhinitis, are common. The incidence of leukaemia is 10 times higher than in the normal population, and hypothyroidism may occur at any stage.

Physical disability and death may result from associated defects such as congenital heart disease.

Trisomy 13 (Fig. 10.7)

Incidence is 1 in 5 000 births.

This rare syndrome is associated with an extra chromosome 13 of the 13–15 group and exhibits defects of the midface, eye and forebrain.

Clinical signs include mental retardation, microphthalmia, cleft lip and palate, polydactyly, flexion of fingers, hyperconvex nails, rocker bottom feet

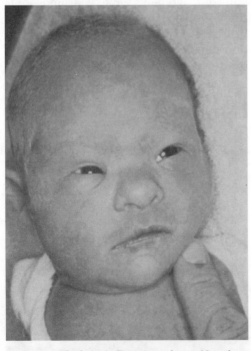

Fig. 10.6 *The facies in Down's syndrome. Note the slanting of eyes and epicanthic folds*

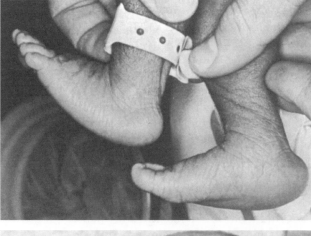

Fig. 10.7 *Rocker bottom feet*

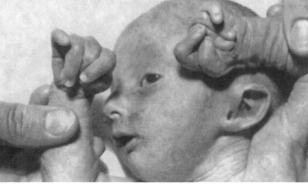

Fig. 10.8 *Trisomy 18. Note the low-set ears and overlapping of the fingers*

(Fig. 10.7), capillary haemangiomas and heart defects. The majority of infants die within six months of birth.

Trisomy 18 (Fig. 10.8)

Incidence is 1 in 3 000 births.

Clinical features are characterised by growth retardation, a prominent occiput, mental retardation, micrognathia, clenched hands, lapping of index finger over third, hypoplastic nails, umbilical hernia, cryptorchidism and cardiac defects. Most infants die within the first six months. Cytogenetic examination reveals 47 chromosomes, the extra chromosome being a number 18 in most cases.

Sex chromosome defects

Fragile X 46, XY
Klinefelter 47, XXY
Double Y 47, XYY
Triple X 47, XXX
Turner 45, XO

Fragile X syndrome

This is one of the commonest forms of inherited mental retardation. It is an X-linked recessive condition with unstable DNA elements at the end of the long arm of the X chromosome. It involves the FMRI gene and occurs in 1 in 5 000 males. Features may be difficult to identify at birth, but they become prominent later.

Protruding ears, a long face, prominent jaw, flat nasal bridge, hypertelorism, epicanthic folds and an anti-mongoloid slant are characteristic facial features. In childhood, the behaviour is often hyperactive with autistic tendencies. Temper tantrums are common, and development is delayed.

Klinefelter syndrome

This has an incidence of 1 in 1 000 births.

Small testes and penis may be the only abnormal features at birth.

Cytogenetic studies show an XXY sex chromosome pattern and there may be up to four X chromosomes. Despite this, the sexual characteristics of the infant are still determined by the Y chromosome.

The buccal smear is positive for sex chromatin and shows a fluorescent Y chromosome.

Childhood problems include mental retardation, gynaecomastia and infertility.

Double Y and triple X syndromes

Infants with XYY and XXX sex chromosomes usually appear normal at birth. The XYY male may grow relatively tall and exhibit behaviour problems, whereas some of the XXX females are considered to show aberrant behaviour or mental retardation. Serial follow-up is essential.

Turner syndrome (Fig. 10.9)

Incidence is 1 in 5 000 births.

An XO constitution, which results from the absence of the Y sex chromosome, or a mosaic pattern, for example XO/XX, can present the following clinical signs:

General: Most infants are growth-retarded and their stature remains small after birth. They are usually mentally normal.

Gonads: Hypoplastic ovaries are present and there is no sexual development at puberty.

Lymphatics: The dorsum of the hands and feet may be swollen at birth owing to lymphoedema (Fig. 10.10).

Chest: The nipples are widely spaced and hypoplastic.

Neck: The hairline is low at the back and the neck may be webbed.

Arms: Cubitus valgus is common.

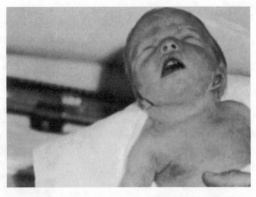

Fig. 10.9 *Turner syndrome. The neck is webbed*

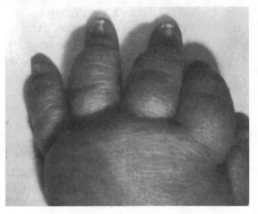

Fig. 10.10 *Turner syndrome. Oedema of the dorsum of the hand*

Cardiovascular system: Coarctation of the aorta may be present.

Note

Webbing of the neck, coarctation of aorta and lymphoedema are rarely present in mosaics.

All girls with short stature should be suspected of having Turner syndrome.

Treatment

If ovaries are absent the woman will be sterile, but the secondary sex organs can be developed by oestrogen therapy.

Disruption

A breakdown of normal fetal tissue is likely to be associated with the amniotic band syndrome.

Amniotic band syndrome

The amniotic sac may rupture in early pregnancy and cause the fetus to enter the space between the amnion and chorion. The fetal limbs, cranium or bowel can be entrapped by mesodermal bands, which arise from the amnion. The resultant defects are listed in Table 10.2.

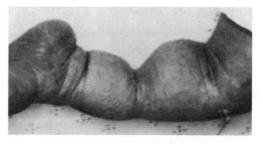

Fig. 10.11 *Defect owing to amniotic bands*

TABLE 10.2

Amniotic band syndrome	
Limb defects	Constriction rings (Fig. 10.11) Amputations Clubbed feet
Craniofacial defects	Anencephaly Encephalocele Cleft lip, palate
Visceral defects	Gastroschisis Omphalocele

Deformation

Deformations are likely to result from mechanical constraint in late pregnancy and usually involve the musculoskeletal system. They may be associated with maternal or fetal factors such as uterine malformations, fibroids, oligohydramnios or multiple pregnancy.

Important types of deformations are listed in Table 10.3.

Most deformations improve with time and the involved tissue returns to its normal shape and function.

TABLE 10.3

Types of deformations
Asymmetry of head, nose, mandible or ears
Torticollis
Scoliosis
Calcaneovalgus, overriding toes
Dislocated hips
Lung hypoplasia

GENETIC COUNSELLING

Genetic factors account for a third of malformations of known origin and counselling plays a major role in identifying families at risk. It offers an understanding of the ways in which that risk can be handled and the information affords parents various options. They may elect to proceed with further pregnancies despite the risks, or wish to forgo pregnancy and instead adopt, or opt for abortion following the prenatal diagnosis of an abnormal fetus. The counselling also offers information that can allay guilt and blame.

DIAGNOSIS OF FETAL ABNORMALITIES

Numerous metabolic and structural defects of the fetus can be detected during pregnancy, but few are treatable at this stage.

Antenatal diagnosis allows for immediate therapy after birth in selected cases, for example oesophageal atresia and adrenogenital syndrome, or abortion for others, as in the case of neural tube defects. Future therapeutic advances will hopefully avert the latter crude method of "removing a patient from the disease".

Methods of investigation:

- Chorionic biopsy.
- Amniocentesis.
- Maternal blood.
- X-ray.
- Ultrasound.
- Amnioscopy.

Chorionic biopsy

The placenta is not fully developed until 12 weeks of gestation. Its loosely anchored chorionic villi can be sampled through a transcervical catheter or a transabdominal needle guided by ultrasound. A biopsy can be obtained as early as seven weeks to detect various metabolic and genetic disorders.

Diagnostic amniocentesis

Amniotic fluid, an ultrafiltrate of maternal and fetal serum, contains amniotic and fetal cells as well as non-fetal stem cells. The small quantity of fluid before 12 weeks gestation increases to 100–150 ml between 14 and 16 weeks. It reaches approximately one litre at 34 weeks and then decreases till term.

A sample of amniotic fluid is obtained as soon as it is technically feasible, that is, between 14 and 16 weeks.

Indications for diagnostic amniocentesis include the following:

- Previous chromosome disorder, such as Down's syndrome.
- Inherited metabolic disorder, such as galactosaemia.
- Previous severe congenital defect, like neural tube defect.
- Known carrier of disease, for example haemophilia.
- Maternal age above 35 years.
- Recurrent abortions.

The following studies can be done on the sterile amniotic fluid:

Uncultured amniotic cells and fluid

Chromatin pattern: A single X chromosome is needed for normal cell function in both sexes. In the female, the second X chromosome is thought to fuse with the nucleus to form a deeply staining mass termed a Barr body. The number of Barr bodies in a nucleus will be one less than the number of X chromosomes for that individual, that is, a normal female (XX)

has one Barr body and is termed chromatin positive. A normal male (XY) has no Barr bodies and is termed chromatin negative.

Fluorescent Y body: The Y chromosome in the male can be demonstrated by a staining technique that causes this chromosome in the nucleus to fluoresce. The fluorescence is detected by microscopy.

These methods are relatively simple and rapid and enable the sex of the fetus to be established.

DNA probes: Genetic disorders like thalassaemia can be detected in the DNA of fetal cells from amniotic fluid, chorionic villi or maternal blood by recombinant DNA technology. Most single gene defects have been identified in this way. DNA is readily obtained as it is present in all cells. The relevant section of DNA to be studied can be amplified by the polymerase chain reaction (PCR). This augmented section will adhere to a complementary DNA probe, which contains the gene of interest. In the fluorescent *in situ* hybridisation test (FISH), a single strand DNA probe that has been conjugated with a fluorescent dye will combine with its complimentary fetal DNA sequence.

A variety of other sophisticated molecular genetic techniques are also used to identify various gene or chromosome defects.

Alpha fetoprotein: This protein is manufactured by the fetus and can be detected in amniotic fluid. The levels are significantly raised when a fetus has an open lesion covered by a thin membrane, such as a meningomyelocele or omphalocele.

Reduced amounts of alphafetoprotein occur in Down's syndrome. The test is non-specific, but can be used to screen pregnancies at risk, for example as in the case of previous neural tube defect.

Cultured amniotic cells

Chromosomes can be examined by a laboratory test known as a karyotype. Each chromosome has characteristic bands that enable detailed studies to be made of localised areas.

The following information can be derived:
- Number of chromosomes.
- Deletion or duplication of chromosomes.
- Sex of fetus.

Biochemistry: Cultured fibroblasts release various products into the surrounding medium that can provide information of particular enzymatic malfunction.

Types of abnormalities that can be identified on cell culture and fluid biochemistry include the following:
- Chromosome defects, such as trisomy.
- Enzyme deficiencies, for example:
  - Hunter syndrome.
  - Galactosaemia.
  - Tay-Sachs disease.
- Biochemical abnormalities, such as adrenogenital syndrome – raised levels of 17 ketosteroids are suggestive; anencephaly, meningomyelocele and exomphalos – raised levels of alphafetoprotein are present.

Amniocentesis is the method used most widely for early detection of metabolic and chromosomal disorders. Other techniques can give more accurate information of structural defects at a later stage of pregnancy, that is, over 20 weeks.

Maternal blood

The following biochemical tests can be used to screen for Down's syndrome in the first trimester: Alpha fetoprotein (reduced), unconjugated oestriol (reduced) and human chorionic gonadotropin (raised). Fetal cells can be separated from maternal blood and cultured.

X-ray

In the second and third trimesters, skeletal abnormalities such as anencephaly, microcephaly and achondroplasia may be detected. Indications for X-ray include polyhydramnios, oligohydramnios and persistent abnormal lie.

Ultrasound (Fig. 10.12)

Sector scanning provides a clear outline of external features such as fetal limbs, male genitalia and the umbilical cord. It can also demonstrate the size and shape of internal organs such as heart, kidneys, spine and vertebrae. The procedure is considered to be safe for mother and fetus.

In addition it is used to guide needles inserted into the amniotic cavity.

Echocardiography

When used with colour flow Doppler, this can demonstrate various structural and rhythm abnormalities of the fetal heart.

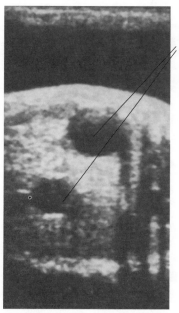

The two dark areas represent accumulations of amniotic fluid in the stomach and duodenum

Fig. 10.12 *Ultrasound detection of duodenal atresia in the fetus.*

Amnioscopy

A fibreoptic scope inserted into the amniotic cavity in early pregnancy can visualise and photograph lesions of the fetal limbs, head and back. Amniotic fluid, fetal blood and skin, and placental chorionic tissue may be sampled for investigation.

Neurological Disorders

NEUROLOGICAL EXAMINATION

A normal baby interacts with the environment in a predictable manner, but considerable experience is needed to interpret deviations from the expected pattern. Temperature, sound, light, state of arousal, gestational age and drugs greatly influence the reactions of a baby, and repeated examinations may be necessary before the neurological status can be established.

The neurological examination incorporates three major assessments: infant behaviour, motor function (posture, tone, movements) and primitive reflexes.

Behaviour

Newborn babies demonstrate characteristic patterns of behaviour while awake and also during sleep. These cerebral reactions provide invaluable information regarding normal brain function.

Observation is the essential keyword. Do not disturb a sleeping baby or one who is awake and alert. Watch the facial expressions and body movement before undressing the infant, and listen to the cry of the upset baby.

Deep sleep

This state is characterised by closed eyes, very little movement of limbs and regular shallow breathing. The abdomen rises as the diaphragm moves downwards. Many a mother has been alarmed by the absence of chest movement and thinks her baby has stopped breathing!

Rapid eye movement (REM) sleep

The eyes flicker beneath closed lids and

they may be seen to 'roll around' should the lids open. This is a period of 'dreaming' and characteristic facial movements occur, such as smiling, grimacing and sucking. Breathing is irregular and the limbs may jerk intermittently. Rapid flicking movements of fingers and toes may be seen. This state occupies up to 50% of total sleeping time and recurs every 45 to 50 minutes.

Awake

Various waking states have been described. A baby may wake of necessity, for example dirty nappy or hunger, in which case sleep recurs once the unpleasant factor has been removed. The infant may also awaken out of choice and wish to be stimulated. This phase of alertness is seen more frequently in those who are kept at their mother's bedside than in those who remain in a nursery.

The open eyes scan the environment and show conjugate movement. They give the impression of alertness and may fix on the mother's face or on a bright object such as a red ball. This may be followed through an arc of 180° in the horizontal plane (p. 152).

Note

Cranial nerves II, III, IV and VI are involved in these functions.

Visual and auditory responses can be assessed in this state. Offer the infant a nipple or teat to suck and briefly shine a bright light into the eyes. The infant blinks or startles and momentarily ceases to suck. A similar cessation of sucking occurs when a rattle is shaken close to the baby's head (cranial nerve VIII). Repetitive stimuli of this nature result in termination of the response, called habituation. The brain of a normal baby soon shuts off reactions to unpleasant stimuli.

Other characteristic patterns of behaviour may be seen. A hungry baby may be calmed temporarily by sucking a finger and a similar calming effect may follow the soothing appeals of the mother.

Smell (cranial nerve I) and taste are well developed, but not tested routinely. Feeding depends on the muscular activity of cheeks and tongue (cranial nerves V and XII) and on co-ordination between sucking and swallowing (IX, X, XI).

Taste buds develop from eight weeks' gestation and an infant prefers sweet liquids to those that are bitter or sour. Discrimination for salt is considered to be poor. Taste involves branches of cranial nerves V (anterior portion of tongue) and IX (posterior tongue).

Skin receptors for touch are very sensitive. Stroking or patting a crying or irritable baby usually has an immediate calming effect and constant stimulation of the touch sense is essential for normal bonding. This is of particular importance in the care of premature infants with the use of skin-to-skin contact between baby and parents. Whenever possible ensure that a baby is held during feeds.

Crying

The normal cry is vigorous and sustained, unlike that associated with neurological abnormalities in which the sound may be high-pitched, cat-like, weak or short-lasting. The eyes close tightly during a spell of crying and facial features remain symmetrical (cranial nerve VII).

Motor function

Posture

The normal full-term baby adopts characteristic postures when lying in the supine or prone positions.

Lying supine (Fig. 11.1)

The head is turned to one side.

The legs and arms are semi-flexed.

The following spontaneous movements may occur:

- Intermittent fisting of fingers and abduction of thumbs.

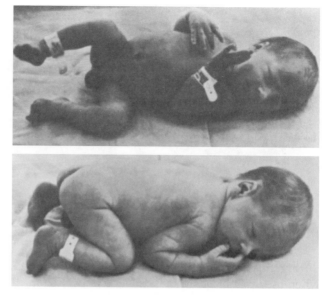

Fig. 11.1 *The full-term baby lying supine. Head turns to one side, arms and legs are flexed*

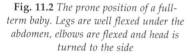

Fig. 11.2 *The prone position of a full-term baby. Legs are well flexed under the abdomen, elbows are flexed and head is turned to the side*

- Alternate flexion and extension of limbs.
- Stretching of limbs with arching of the back.
- Yawning, sneezing and hiccupping.

Paucity of movement should arouse suspicion.

It can be related to:
- oversedation
- prematurity
- birth injury, for example fractured clavicle
- floppy syndrome (p. 148).

Voluntary movements commence after three months of age when flexor tone in the limbs starts to diminish.

Lying prone (Fig. 11.2)
The head turns to one side and can be briefly lifted off the surface.

Arms are flexed at the side of the body.

Hips are flexed and tucked under the abdomen.

The pelvis is held high with the buttocks in the air.

Muscle tone
This is assessed in several positions.

Lying supine
Extend the baby's elbows and release the arms suddenly. They immediately spring back to a flexed position.

Similar flexion is noted in the knees and hips when the legs are extended and rapidly released.

Pull-to-sit (Fig. 11.3)
Gently lift the baby by the hands or shoulders to a sitting position. The head lags

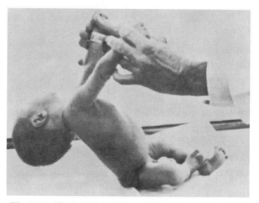

Fig. 11.3 *The initial head lag of a full-term baby lifted into the sitting position*

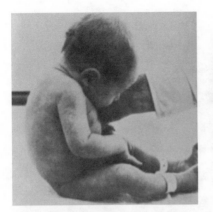

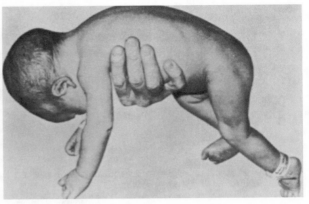

Fig. 11.4 *The sitting position of a full-term baby. Back is curved and head is flexed forward*

Fig. 11.5 *Prone suspension*

during this movement. It bobs forward when the upright position is reached and the chin comes to rest on the chest (Fig. 11.4).

Suspended prone (Fig. 11.5)
When the infant is lifted and supported under the abdomen, the spine and limbs remain semi-flexed.

The neck may momentarily extend.

Reflexes

Many primitive reflexes are present at birth. They are used to assess gestational age and to determine overall neurological well-being. A number of easily elicited reflexes may be used in the neurological examination.

Suck
This is well established in the normal full-term baby and is best assessed when an infant suckles the breast. The powerful suck uses cheek and tongue muscles and is associated with swallowing. Biting is abnormal and so is a weak suck.

Grasp (Fig. 11.6)
The infant will firmly grasp a pen or a finger that is pressed against the palm of the hand or the sole of the foot. This reflex persists for two to three months.

Moro (Fig. 11.7)
A startle response can be produced by grasping the infant's hands, extending the arms and suddenly releasing them. An alternative method is to lift the head in the palm of the hand and allow it to fall back about 2 cm.

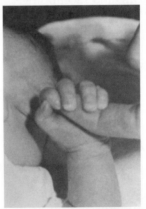

Fig. 11.6 *Palmar grasp*

Fig. 11.7 *The Moro reflex*

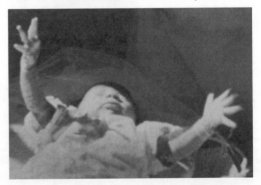

TABLE 11.1

Moro reflex	
Type of abnormal response	*Comment*
Weak, incomplete or absent reflex	May indicate gross immaturity, i.e. less than 28 weeks' gestation Cerebral or spinal cord birth injury (p. 146) Kernicterus (p. 103) Neuromuscular diseases, which cause floppiness (p. 148)
Asymmetrical reflex	May indicate birth injuries, e.g. fractured clavicle (p. 289), Brachial plexus lesions (p. 147), Cerebral haemorrhage
Overactive reflex	May indicate meningitis (p. 143) Drug withdrawal syndrome (p. 150)
Reflex present after 6–8 months of age	May indicate immaturity at birth

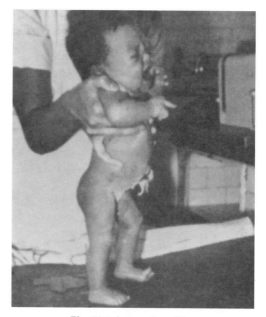

Fig. 11.8 *Automatic walking*

The hands fly open and the arms fling out.

The legs may extend and the eyes may open widely.

This stage is followed by a slow return to the flexed position. The response is symmetrical and persists for three to four months. An abnormal response is helpful in outlining a variety of conditions.

Walking reflex (Fig. 11.8)

Support the baby in the standing position with the feet on a surface. When the head and shoulders are tilted forwards the baby may attempt to walk by lifting a foot and placing it in front of the other. The raised foot often gets caught behind the knee of the opposite leg.

This reflex is variable and depends on the state of arousal. It persists for about six weeks.

ASSESSMENT OF DEVELOPMENTAL MILESTONES

Neurological examinations should be repeated during infancy under the following circumstances:

Preterm infants, especially less than 1 500 g weight.

Small-for-gestation infant
Congenital abnormality
- Structural, that is, abnormally large or small head.
- Metabolic, that is, phenylketonuria.

Perinatal complications
- Maternal infection, that is, rubella, toxoplasmosis, cytomegalovirus.
- Maternal illness, that is, diabetes mellitus.
- Hypoxaemia, that is, birth asphyxia, respiratory distress.
- Hypoglycaemia, that is, symptomatic.
- Hyperbilirubinaemia, that is, bilirubin above 340 μmol/l.
- Birth injury, that is, cerebral haemorrhage.

Family history of neurological abnormality
Abnormal neurological signs
These may be associated with the above complications and include:

TABLE 11.2

		Six-week-old baby	
System	*Test*	*Normal response*	*Suspicious response*
Motor	Lying supine on table or on mother's lap	Limbs are flexed, movements active and bilateral	Constant immobility Asymmetry of movement Legs maintained in extension
	Pull-to-sit position	Initial head lag; some control when baby reaches 45°	Complete head lag to upright position; buttocks slide forward or infant rises up on to feet
	Supported sitting	Head momentarily controlled then bobs forward	Head immediately bobs forward
	Prone suspension (Fig. 11.10)	Limbs are flexed; head kept in plane of body or momentarily elevated	Limbs droop; head droops
	Lying prone (Fig. 11.9)	Head turns to one side; hips are partially extended on surface	Head fails to turn; knees remain flexed under abdomen; pelvis remains elevated
Primitive reflexes	Moro	p. 128	Depressed, asymmetric
	Grasp	p. 128	Absent
Social behaviour	Stroked under chin	Smiles in response	Absence of a smile
Vision	Object or light moved across vision 20–30 cm from eyes Mother bends over and talks to baby	Follows object to midline or to other side Fixes on mother's face and watches her intently	Nystagmus, squint, ptosis, lack of interest Absence of fixation
Hearing	Loud noise, bell, high-pitched rattle, mother's voice	Quietens with sound Startles, blinks, cries or grimaces	Constant absence of a response
Speech		Baby noises; occasional cooing	Too quiet

- coma
- convulsions
- bulging fontanelle
- persistent nystagmus
- failure to suck
- defective muscle tone, for example neck retraction, floppiness, persistent fisting of thumbs, persistent flexion or extension of limbs
- lack of spontaneous movement.

Motor function, manipulation, social behaviour and special sense are reassessed in these circumstances. Examinations are recommended at the following ages:

- Six weeks.
- Six months.
- Ten months.

A scheme which serves as a guide to development at the specified ages is presented in Tables 11.2, 11.3 and 11.4.

The following factors must be considered when developmental milestones are assessed:

- Infants should be physically well and co-operative at the time of examination.
- Due allowance must be made for gestational age at birth, for example a 32-week preterm infant aged eight months is assessed at a six-month level.
- Abnormality in any one field of development, for example motor function, does not necessarily imply mental retardation.

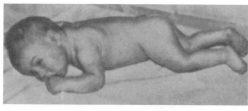

Fig. 11.9 *Prone lying: six weeks*

(Figures 11.11 to 11.14 from Illingworth, R. 1975. Development of the Infant and Young Child: Normal and Abnormal. 6 ed. Edinburgh: Churchill Livingstone)

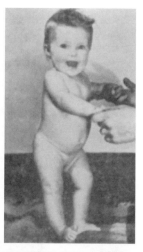

Fig. 11.12 *Walking development: 24 weeks*

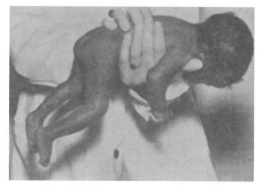

Fig. 11.10 *Prone suspension: six weeks*

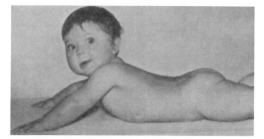

Fig. 11.11 *Prone lying: 24 weeks*

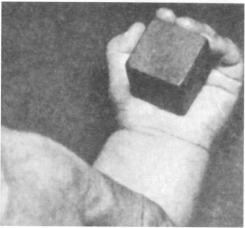

Fig. 11.13 *Manipulation: 24 weeks*

- Note must be taken of familial tendencies, for example late onset of speech.
- Persistent abnormal responses, particularly if asymmetrical, increase the likelihood of an underlying neurological abnormality.

These developmental examinations serve as a screening process only.

Infants who show persistent or gross deviations from the normal pattern must be referred for expert assessment and treatment.

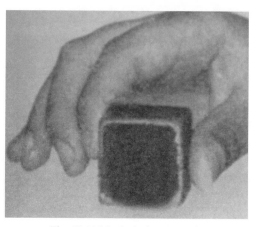

Fig. 11.14 *Manipulation: 44 weeks*

TABLE 11.3

		Six-month-old baby	
System	*Test*	*Normal response*	*Suspicious response*
Motor	Lying supine	Lifts head, rolls to prone position	Lack of movement, unable to lift head
	Pull-to-sit	Lifts head, flexes elbows, no head lag	Initial head lag, slides forward on bottom, rises on to feet
	Supported sitting; sway body from side to side	No head wobble	Considerable head wobble
	Sitting position	Sits momentarily	Falls immediately
	Lying prone (Fig. 11.11)	Takes weight on hands, extends arms, rolls to supine	Lies with flexed arms caught under body
	Support standing (Fig. 11.12)	Knees straighten, bears weight	Knees buckle; unable to straighten knees
Manipulation	Lying supine; object dangled within easy reach	Reaches forward, usually with one hand	No interest in reaching for object
	Sitting on mother's lap	Reaches forward, with one hand. Palmar grasp; secure grasp; brings cube to mouth; begins to transfer cube from one hand to the other	Lack of interest
	2,5 cm cube placed on table within reach (Fig. 11.13)		
	Sitting on mother's lap; raisin or small object placed on table	One hand extends forward; clumsy grasp which usually fails	Lack of interest
Social behaviour		Alert and interested; smiles and laughs; holds out arms to be picked up; begins to imitate	Persistent lack of interest; limited smiling and laughing
Vision	Lying supine; object dangled in front of face	Follows object from side to side and up and down	Squint, nystagmus / Lack of interest
	Raisin or small object held in examiner's hand	Inspects object	Lack of interest
	Held in front of mirror	Smiles, vocalises	Lack of interest
Hearing	Lying supine; noise is made out of vision about 45 cm away and level with ear; bell, crinkle paper, spoon stroked in cup	Head turns to noise	Failure to respond
Speech	Mother's voice	Coos, hums, laughs, interested in producing different sounds	Too quiet; makes too few sounds

TABLE 11.4

	Ten-month-old baby		
System	*Test*	*Normal response*	*Suspicious response*
Motor	Lying supine Lying prone Sitting	Rolls to sit Creeps forwards or back- wards on belly Good control; maintains bal- ance on turning; protective response if pushed; pulls up on to knees and sometimes stands	Unable to roll over Unable to move Poor control; unable to sit unsupported; absent protec- tive response
Manipulation	Sitting on mother's lap; raisin placed on table 2,5 cm cube placed on table (Fig. 11.14)	Index finger approach; picks up raisin accurately between tip of index finger and thumb Picks up cube and transfers to other hand; matches 2 cm cubes, one in each hand; occasionally carries objects to mouth	Ataxia, tremor, lack of interest or clumsy; Palmar grasp Palmar grasp
Social behaviour		Helps with dressing; feeds self with biscuit; chews biscuit; plays 'clap hands'; waves bye-bye	Failure to chew; no bye-bye
Vision	Sitting on floor; roll small ball	Follows objects in all direc- tions; follows rolling ball	Squint, nystagmus, lack of interest
Hearing	As for six months	As for six months; babbles; imitates sounds, "Dadda", "Mamma", one other word	Lack of vocalisation

Developmental screening for large groups

Population norms have been established for sitting, walking, single words and sentences, as reported by mothers (Fig. 11.15). These milestones can be determined at a health clinic without the aid of sophisticated training or equipment. They are of practical value for the early detection of mental retardation and should be established in each baby who attends a health clinic. The infant who deviates from the normal range should be referred to a paediatric centre for developmental assessment.

Definitions

Sitting unsupported: Infant sits for at least one minute without support of hands.

Walking unsupported: Infant takes at least 10 steps unaided.

Single words: Infant uses three or four words with correct meaning.

Sentences: Infant puts three or four words together with meaning.

CONGENITAL MALFORMATIONS

Neural tube

The nervous system develops from the medullary plate, a thickened area of dorsal ectoderm in the embryo. The edges fold over to form a neural groove and fuse to produce the neural tube. Fusion begins in the thoracic region, extends towards the head and tail, and is complete by the fourth week.

Failure of fusion at various sites can produce the following defects:

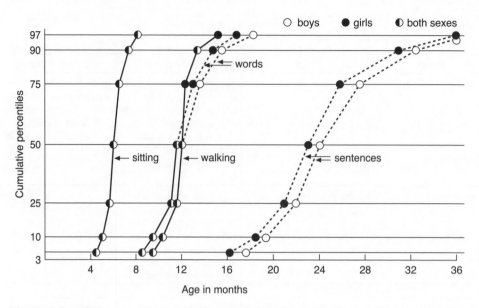

Fig. 11.15 *Cumulative percentile curves for four standard developmental milestones (From Neligan, G and Prudham, D. 1969.* Development Medicine and Child Neurology *11: 413–22)*

- Anencephaly.
- Cranium bifidum – encephalocele, meningocele.
- Spina bifida occulta.
- Spina bifida cystica – meningocele, meningomyelocele.

Aetiology

These malformations occur between the second and fourth weeks of gestation. There is a familial tendency as the chance of a subsequent baby having a neural tube defect is slightly more than 3%. After two affected children the incidence increases to 10–15%.

Vitamin deficiencies, particularly folic acid, play a role in the aetiology, as the expected incidence in high-risk women has been reduced significantly by supplementing their diets with folic acid before and during subsequent pregnancies.

Prenatal diagnosis

An excessive amount of alpha fetoprotein accumulates in amniotic fluid and maternal serum when neural tube defects are not covered by skin. The protein is manufactured by the fetus and possibly transudes across the exposed lesion into the amniotic cavity. It is also found in high concentrations in Turner syndrome, duodenal atresia and omphalocele.

The test may be offered at 14 weeks' gestation to women who have the following risks:

- Previous infant with a neural tube defect.
- Type 1 diabetes mellitus.
- Drug exposure, for example Valproic acid.

When the alphafetoprotein concentration is excessive, high-resolution ultrasonography might detect a specific lesion.

Anencephaly

This lethal malformation is characterised by absence of the vault of the cranium and a partial or total lack of cerebrum and cerebellum (Fig. 11.16). Most infants (80%) are stillborn and the remainder die within hours or days of birth. Associated abnormalities include spina bifida and club feet.

Anencephaly is three times more common in girls than in boys and the incidence varies throughout the world. In England and Wales, the prevalence declined from 4,2 per 1 000 births in 1972 to 1,2 per 1 000 births in 1990. This occurred before prenatal diagnosis was an established investigation.

Cranium bifidum

A portion of the posterior midline of the skull may fail to fuse and cranial contents can herniate through the defect.

These uncommon lesions occur anywhere along the midline of the skull from the bridge of the nose (Fig. 11.17) to the nape of the neck (Fig. 11.18). The majority (80%) are situated in the occipital region. They vary from the size of a pea to an orange.

Meningocele: This refers to a defect that contains meninges only.

Encephalocele: This lesion contains brain tissue.

A brain scan determines the size and contents of the lesion and the appearance of the ventricles.

Treatment

Minor lesions have an excellent prognosis and surgical repair is performed soon after birth.

Large lesions have a variable prognosis. Meningoceles are treatable, but hydrocephalus may develop later.

Large encephaloceles may not be amenable to surgery if they contain extensive amounts of brain tissue.

Spina bifida

Posterior defects can occur along the vertebral column with or without protrusion of the spinal contents.

Spina bifida occulta

A hairy patch or pigmented birthmark in the midline of the lower back may be the

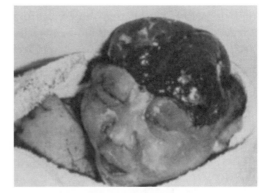
Fig. 11.16 *Anencephaly*

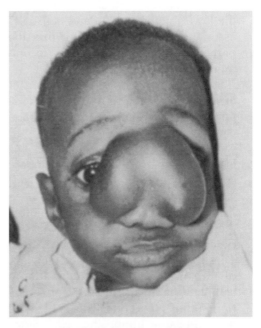
Fig. 11.17 *Cranial encephalocele*

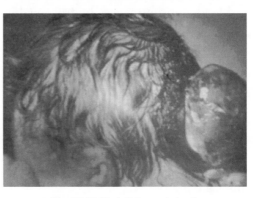
Fig. 11.18 *Occipital encephalocele*

only external sign of this malformation. X-ray examination reveals absent vertebral arches, but symptoms are uncommon and treatment is usually unnecessary.

Spina bifida cystica
This lesion of the laminar arches may be associated with the protrusion of meninges (meningocele) or neural components (meningomyelocele) through the defect.

Meningocele: The herniation consists of meninges and cerebrospinal fluid and is often covered with skin. It occurs in the lower lumbar region and is usually associated with normal motor function of the legs. Retention of urine is uncommon and usually not debilitating.

Surgical correction is done soon after birth as the long-term prognosis is good. Hydrocephalus is an occasional complication.

Meningomyelocele (Colour plate VII): This is a serious malformation as part of the spinal cord is contained within a sac, which may or may not be intact.

The lesion occurs 10 times more often than a meningocele and is always associated with neurological abnormalities. These vary from motor and sensory disturbances of the legs and bladder to complete paralysis and lack of sensation in the lower body. This is likely to occur in large lumbo-thoracic lesions and is often associated with bowel and bladder incontinence, hydrocephalus, mental retardation, club feet and other congenital abnormalities.

Investigation and treatment
A full neurological examination, X-ray of spine and skull, and a brain scan are performed as soon as possible to establish the extent of the lesion.

The best form of treatment is still not known and the following recommendations are offered.

Surgical closure is done as soon as possible for small lesions, which have minimal neurological deficits.

Surgery is not advised for large open defects with associated head enlargement and total paralysis of the lower body and legs. The chances of survival are poor, irrespective of the type of treatment.

Intermediate defects present a dilemma and parents must discuss the implications of closure of the lesion with a neurosurgeon.

Adequate medical and nursing care is given to each baby, whether or not surgery has been performed.

Long-term management is essential for survivors and may include orthopaedic, urologic, neurologic, physiotherapy and developmental assessments. The following problems may need attention:

- Hydrocephalus.
- Urinary and bowel incontinence.
- Pressure sores.
- Club feet.
- Abnormal gait.
- Learning difficulties.
- Psychological disturbances.

Failure of the neural tube to fuse can be associated with other rare defects. They include:

- *holoprosencephaly:* abnormal development of the midline face and forebrain
- *diastematomyelia:* a split in a segment of the spinal cord.

Hydrocephalus ('Waterhead') (Fig. 11.19; Colour plate VI)

This implies an excessive accumulation of cerebrospinal fluid in the ventricles of the brain. It is usually caused by an obstruction inside or outside the ventricular system and can result in head enlargement, raised intracranial pressure and brain compression.

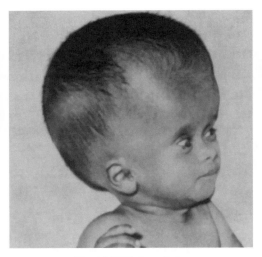

Fig. 11.19 *Hydrocephalus*

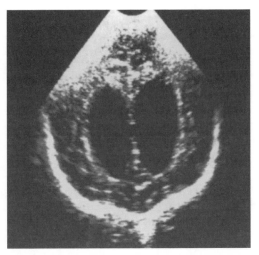

Fig. 11.20 *Ultrasound features of severe hydrocephalus*

Aetiology

Congenital varieties may be owing to the following:

- Stenosis or forking of the aqueduct of Sylvius.
- Atresia of the foramina of Magendie and Luschka.
- The Arnold-Chiari malformation. This accounts for 40% and is characterised by elongation of the cerebellar tonsil and protrusion of the medulla oblongata through the foramen magnum.
- Sex-linked type, which occurs in males and is associated with a defective LICAM gene.

Acquired forms may be owing to intrauterine or postnatal complications such as:

- toxoplasmosis
- cytomegalovirus
- intracerebral bleeding.

Clinical features

The head is enlarged, with a circumference above the 97th percentile, and the fontanelles and sutures are widely separated.

The infant may be asymptomatic or show irritability, poor sucking, vomiting and failure to thrive.

Severe hydrocephalus is associated with a 'setting sun' appearance of the eyes, high-pitched cry, delayed milestones, mental retardation and blindness.

Investigations

Ultrasonography may detect the dilated ventricles and head enlargement *in utero*. It tracks the progression of hydrocephalus and its effect on cortical size (Fig. 11.20). Transillumination of the skull in the dark shows an increased light reflex.

Treatment

To alleviate compression of brain tissue the cerebrospinal fluid is drained from the ventricular system into the peritoneal cavity by a shunt.

The timing of the procedure depends on the state of the infant, the thickness of the cortex and the rate of increase in head circumference.

Hydranencephaly

This is caused in early fetal life by a loss of cerebral tissue supplied by the anterior cerebral circulation, that is, from the internal carotid arteries. Tissue, such as thalamus and brainstem, which is perfused by the posterior circulation – that

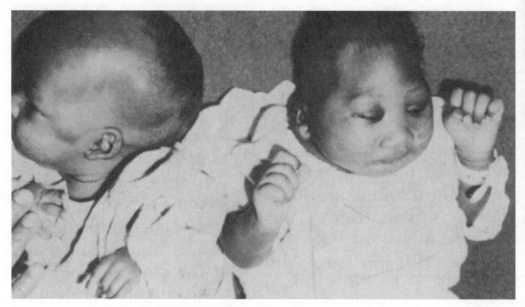

Fig. 11.21 *The infant on the right has microcephaly*

is, the vertebro-basilar system – is preserved.

The cerebral cortex and corpus callosum are absent and replaced by a sac filled with CSF. The head may be of normal size at birth, but enlarges thereafter. It shines like a lantern when transilluminated in the dark (Colour plate IX).

The diagnosis is confirmed by a brain scan. Babies are learning-disabled and blind, but may have a good sucking reflex. Most are dead by three months of age.

Megalencephaly

An excessively big brain can cause the head to enlarge.

This is often familial, so check the head size of parents before you label the infant as abnormal. It is usually associated with normal neurological development and the rate of head growth is not excessive.

Learning-disablement and seizures may accompany megalencephaly when it is related to various abnormalities, for example Tay-Sachs disease.

Ultrasonography is essential to establish the size of the ventricles and to rule out hydrocephalus.

Microcephaly (Fig. 11.21)

The head is smaller than normal and continues to grow at an abnormally slow rate. The occipito-frontal circumference is below the third percentile at birth and rarely reaches more than 43 cm later in life. Microcephaly becomes more noticeable as the face enlarges.

Head size alone cannot be used to predict mental function. Caution must be exercised, particularly when an underlying cause is not identified at birth. Cigarette smoking, for example, can depress fetal head growth *in utero*, but this is rapidly corrected after birth. This temporary impairment is not associated with long-term mental deficits.

Aetiology

Genetic: Various genetic factors are associated with an undersized and underdeveloped brain. They include chromosomal abnormalities such as Down's syndrome, trisomy 13 and trisomy 18. The forehead may be flattened, the anterior fontanelle is small or absent, and the ears may be prominent. Neurological abnormalities can be present, such as abnormal cry and changes in muscle tone.

Acquired: Drugs such as alcohol and diphenyhydantoin (p. 112) can impair brain growth. Intrauterine infections such as rubella, toxoplasmosis and cytomegalovirus can do the same.

Perinatal asphyxia and meningitis can damage the brain sufficiently to impair its growth.

Investigations and treatment

Serial head circumference measurements are essential before a definitive diagnosis of microcephaly can be made. This is important when an obvious underlying cause is absent.

A brain scan indicates the size of the cortex and ventricles and an X-ray of the skull may detect calcification in diseases such as cytomegalovirus infection.

Treat an underlying cause where possible.

ACUTE INSULTS TO THE BRAIN

Perinatal insults, such as ischaemia, hypoxia, haemorrhage, infection or hypoglycaemia, can cause temporary or permanent dysfunction of the brain.

Hypoxic-ischaemic encephalopathy

In primary care units, birth asphyxia and hypoxic-ischaemic encephalopathy (HIE) are the cause of most neonatal deaths in full-term infants. Spastic quadriplegia is the main disability in survivors.

Aetiology

HIE is often preceded by fetal distress in labour. This probably results in hypoxaemia and ischaemia of the fetal brain to cause cerebral infarction, oedema, necrosis, apoptosis and eventual atrophy.

Areas in the cortex distal to the origin of blood vessels are the most vulnerable. In full-term babies the cerebral cortex and adjacent subcortical white matter may become haemorrhagic, necrotic, cystic or atropic. Other susceptible areas are the internal capsule and basal ganglia.

Damage is not confined to the brain and can affect the heart, lungs and kidneys as well.

The reason for fetal hypoxaemia is unknown.

In industrialised countries there is little evidence to link intrapartum ischaemia to HIE. Consequently, the term 'hypoxic-ischaemic' has been dropped in favour of 'acute neonatal encephalopathy'. In South Africa, HIE is particularly common in black babies. They appear to be more vulnerable than others.

Clinical features

Most infants have abnormal neurological signs at birth. However, brain function may remain normal for several hours, depending on the timing of the insult in labour.

Suspect HIE in a baby who has abnormal neurological features on the day of birth, particularly when they are preceded by fetal distress and birth asphyxia. The presentation is characterised by:

- increased tone in the limbs
- a floppy neck
- a tense or full fontanelle
- an increase in head circumference
- a poor or absent suck reflex.

The state of consciousness depends on the severity of cerebral derangement and varies from hyper-alertness to coma. Seizures may occur on the first or second day after birth.

Important clinical features are listed in Table 11.5 (p. 140). Severity is graded as mild, moderate or severe, and an infant may progress from one stage to the next.

Ischaemic damage to other organs presents the following features:

TABLE 11.5

	Severity of hypoxic-ischaemic encephalopathy					
	Behaviour	*Pupils*	*Muscle tone*	*Moro reflex*	*Suck reflex*	*Seizures*
Mild	Conscious and stares	Normal	Normal or increased	Normal or exaggerated	Normal	No
Moderate	Lethargic	Small	Decreased	Weak	Weak	Yes
Severe	Coma	Dilated No reaction	Floppy	Absent	Absent	No

- *Kidneys:* oliguria, anuria, haematuria.
- *Heart:* cardiomegaly, hepatomegaly, tachycardia, bradycardia.
- *Lungs:* tachypnoea, rib recession, cyanosis.

Investigations
The effects of ischaemia and hypoxia on the brain can be clearly defined by nuclear magnetic resonance, infrared spectroscopy, pressure monitoring and technetium brain scans.

These aids are unlikely to be available in areas where HIE is prevalent and reliance is placed on clinical features, brain scanning (ultrasound, CAT) and electroencephalography (EEG).

Brain scanning: In the early stage cerebral oedema is prominent and leads to compression of the ventricles. Sequelae such as cysts, cerebral atrophy and ventricular dilation can be demonstrated later.

Electroencephalography: Seizures can be detected even in the absence of clinical signs. Characteristic patterns are described, but may be difficult to interpret. Voltage is low and bouts of electrical activity alternate with periods of suppression.

Urine: Blood and protein may be detected on Dipstix.

Blood: The levels of urea, creatinine and unconjugated bilirubin are raised, while those of glucose, magnesium and calcium may be reduced. A metabolic and respiratory acidaemia may be present.

Differential diagnosis
Intracranial haemorrhage and hypoglycaemia cause abnormal neurological signs at or soon after birth. Ensure that a blood sugar level is obtained as soon as possible. An ultrasound brain scan will detect cerebral haemorrhage.

Other acute brain insults like meningitis, kernicterus and inherited metabolic defects should be considered, but are likely to present later.

Treatment
The following factors may have to be controlled:
Hypoxaemia: Oxygen, assisted ventilation (p. 175).
Cerebral oedema: Controlled ventilation
Seizures: Phenobarbitone (p. 144).
Oliguria, anuria: Fluid restriction (p. 241).
Hyperbilirubinaemia: Phototherapy (p. 107).
Hypoglycaemia: 10% dextrose (p. 263).
Hypomagnesaemia: Magnesium sulphate (p. 264).

Recently attempts have been made to reduce the extent of cerebral damage by cooling the brain. The efficacy is yet to be fully established. It is likely to be of assistance in mild rather than severe cases.

Infants require meticulous nursing care to compensate for their impaired defence mechanisms, such as inadequate sucking and swallowing, paucity of movements, obstructed airways, poor response to painful stimuli, lack of blinking and urine retention.

Clean the mouth, moisten the lips, protect the eyes, clear the airways and express the bladder frequently. Assess the neurological state, measure urine output hourly, monitor blood pressure continuously and record head circumference daily. Ensure that blood glucose level remains normal.

Outcome
Infants with mild signs have a good chance of recovery. Those with moderate signs also have a good outlook provided the EEG is normal within five days of the insult. Poor prognostic features include persistent seizures, flaccidity and unconsciousness. These are usually associated with diffuse damage to basal ganglia and white matter. Failure to suck at seven days of age is a particularly ominous clinical sign. Thirty per cent of infants with severe signs die and the others are left with permanent neurological impairment, mainly spastic quadriplegia and microcephaly.

Periventricular leucomalacia (PVL)
This is probably the equivalent of HIE in a preterm infant and occurs in up to 25% of those under 32 weeks' gestation.

It is characterised by necrotic areas in the white matter on both sides of the brain adjacent to the lateral ventricles. This symmetry distinguishes it from the sequelae of periventricular haemorrhage (p. 142). Like the latter it is probably caused by inadequate cerebral perfusion, and the two constitute the most common brain lesions in preterm infants. It may occur during or after birth.

Risk factors include:
- chorioamnionitis
- hypo- or hypertension
- hypocarbia
- hypoxaemia
- maternal cocaine addiction.

Clinical features
Initially the infant may be asymptomatic and later develop any of these features: decreased lower limb tone, increased neck tone, apnoea, bradycardia, irritability, lethargy, seizures.

Diagnosis
The lesions can be detected by ultrasound. The characteristic features are periventricular echo-densities or cysts.

Treatment
Risk factors should be addressed to prevent the complication. Once PVL is established, treatment is merely symptomatic.

The long-term sequelae include intellectual impairment; cerebral palsy, particularly spastic diplegia; and visual disorders.

Cerebral oedema
This implies an increased water content of the brain. It may be intracellular, extracellular or interstitial in origin.

Intracellular oedema is caused by an accumulation of sodium and water within brain cells and commonly occurs in hypoxic-ischaemic encephalopathy. Less common causes include inappropriate antidiuretic hormone (ADH) secretion, water intoxication and hexachlorophene poisoning.

Extracellular oedema results from an extravasation of plasma through damaged vessels in the blood–brain barrier and may occur with intracranial haemorrhage, cerebral infarction and meningitis.

Interstitial oedema is rare.

Clinical features
Cerebral oedema results in swelling of the brain and is characterised by tenseness of the fontanelle, separation of sutures, an increase in head circumference and deterioration in neurological status. Suspect it when these signs are present. The types

of oedema are indistinguishable on clinical features.

Investigations
Cerebral oedema causes intracranial pressure to rise and a transcutaneous electrode positioned over the fontanelle can monitor pressure.

Brain scanning may detect cerebral oedema and compression of blood vessels and ventricles, but cannot measure intracranial pressure.

Treatment
Treat the underlying problem, for example meningitis, and ensure that blood pressure is kept normal to maintain adequate perfusion of the brain.

The following methods are used to control brain swelling, but their efficacy is uncertain, particularly if intracranial pressure cannot be monitored:
- *Fluid restriction:* 60 ml/kg/day.
- *Diuretics:* Mannitol (p. xxx).
- *Dexamethasone:* Useful in extracellular oedema.
- *Hyperventilation:* Reduces PCO_2 and cerebral blood flow.

Intracranial bleeding
Haemorrhages may be:
- subdural
- subarachnoid
- intracerebral
- intra- or periventricular.

Brain scanning can identify and localise most haemorrhages and should be done whenever intracranial bleeding is suspected.

Subdural haemorrhage
Blood can accumulate in the supratentorial or posterior fossa regions from tears in the tentorium, dural sinus, falx cerebri or bridging veins. In a full-term baby this is caused by birth trauma, for example breech delivery, or forceps or vacuum extraction.

Lethargy, vomiting, seizures, hypotonia and pallor are important signs. An enlarged head, a tense fontanelle and separated sutures indicate raised intracranial pressure. The signs can occur after delivery or several days later. They may be delayed for weeks if a haematoma is replaced by an enlarging effusion in the supratentorial region.

Investigation
Brain scanning (ultrasound/CAT) can identify most haemorrhages and is essential wherever this complication is suspected.

Treatment
Many haematomas and effusions resolve spontaneously. Some may have to be tapped if intracranial pressure is raised. Cerebral oedema (p. 141), blood loss (p. 224) and respiratory failure may also require treatment.

Subdural bleeding is rare if the following are addressed:
- Antenatal diagnosis and assessment of cephalopelvic disproportion and abnormal lie of the fetus.
- Elective Caesarean section when indicated, for example primip breech.
- Frequent assessments of the progress of labour.
- Selective episiotomy.
- Expert application of forceps or vacuum cup.
- Vitamin K_1 to infants after birth.

Subarachnoid haemorrhage
This complication is likely to occur in a preterm baby who has been subjected to intrauterine hypoxia or birth asphyxia. Underlying hypoxic brain damage may be more significant than the actual haemorrhage (p. 141). Apnoea, seizures and pallor are features of extensive bleeding. Lumbar puncture reveals red blood cells in the CSF and treatment is symptomatic. Hydrocephalus is a likely complication.

Intracerebral haemorrhage

Bleeding can extend into the brain substance, particularly in association with intraventricular haemorrhage. This complication is likely to occur in preterm babies of less than 32 weeks' gestation and can be catastrophic.

Peri- or intraventricular haemorrhage

This occurs in over 50% of infants of less than 32 weeks' gestation and is a frequent cause of death in those with severe hyaline membrane disease (p. 177).

Neuropathology

Bleeding originates in the microcirculation of the germinal matrix. This embryonal tissue surrounds the ventricular system and is rich in immature blood vessels. Haemorrhage usually occurs in the region of the caudate nucleus and may extend into the ventricles or white matter of the brain.

Aetiology

The cause of bleeding is poorly understood and may be related to the following:

Hypoxia: Severe hypoxia often precedes bleeding and is thought to increase venous and capillary pressure in the brain by abolishing the autoregulation of cerebral perfusion. The bleeding often occurs when arterial hypotension has been corrected.

Brain shrinkage: Hyperosmolar solutions, such as sodium bicarbonate, can accentuate brain shrinkage when given as a bolus injection.

Raised intracranial pressure: Pneumothorax, crying and straining may increase the risk by raising the pressure inside the skull.

Bleeding tendency: A low platelet count or a decreased prothrombin time are also considered to be aggravating factors.

Clinical presentation

Mild bleeds are often asymptomatic and may be detectable only on daily ultra-

sound scanning of the brains of small infants.

Episodes of apnoea or lethargy can occur in this variety.

Extensive bleeding often presents as a catastrophic event on the second or third day of life. There is usually a preceding history of severe hypoxia related to fetal distress, asphyxia or apnoea.

Signs include:

- apnoea
- shock
- pallor
- seizures
- abnormal eye movements
- hypotonia
- bulging fontanelle
- reduced haemoglobin level and presence of metabolic acidaemia.

Diagnosis

Ultrasound scanning is the most satisfactory method of detection.

Lumbar puncture reveals red cells in the CSF if bleeding has extended into the ventricles.

The extent of bleeding correlates with prognosis and has been graded as follows:

Grade I – bleeding is confined to germinal matrix.

Grade II – bleeding extends into the ventricles, which are not dilated.

Grade III – intraventricular bleeding has occurred and ventricular dilation is present.

Grade IV – intraventricular and parenchymal bleeding are present.

Grades I and II are graded as mild, and III and IV as severe.

Bleeding is usually asymmetrical and may occur on one or both sides of the brain.

Treatment

Mild haemorrhages (grades I and II) usually do not require treatment. Apnoeic spells can be terminated with aminophylline.

No specific therapy is available for severe bleeding. An attempt is made to control blood pressure, acidaemia, hypoxia, seizures, cerebral oedema and anaemia. Repeated lumbar punctures have been recommended to reduce intracranial pressure and prevent clot formation in the ventricles, but the efficacy of this measure is doubtful.

Outcome
Most mild cases resolve without complication. The severe variety has a high mortality rate (65%) and survivors are at risk for hydrocephalus, cerebral palsy and mental retardation.

Prevention
Antenatal steroid therapy (p. 62) reduces the risk of bleeding.

Septic meningitis
Meningeal infection is frequently associated with septicaemia and has the same predisposing factors. Causative organisms include the Group B streptococcus, listeriosis and enteric bacteria such as *E. coli*.

Meningitis tends to occur later than hypoxic-ischaemic encephalopathy and seldom presents before 24 hours of age. Group B streptococcus and listeria infections can occur earlier. Preterm infants are particularly susceptible, especially when there are preceding risk factors for sepsis (p. 73).

Pathology
Histology reveals a purulent exudate of meninges and ventricles in those who die, and there is an associated vasculitis. Other complications include hydrocephalus, subdural effusion and vessel occlusion from thrombophlebitis.

Clinical features
Early signs are non-specific and similar to those of septicaemia. They are:
- excessive lethargy
- exaggerated Moro reflex
- tachycardia
- abdominal distension
- vomiting
- labile temperature.

Local signs present later and include nystagmus or squinting, seizures, hypertonia and bulging fontanelle. Neck stiffness is unusual.

Diagnosis
A lumbar puncture should be done wherever there is a reasonable suspicion of meningitis. The CSF may be clear, hazy or frankly purulent. Polymorph white cell count and protein levels are usually raised. A Gram stain is done as the sample may contain many bacteria and relatively few white cells. This sometimes occurs in the early stages of a Group B streptococcus infection.

Confirmation is obtained from culture. The organism may also be grown from a blood culture.

Treatment
Specific: Start antibiotic therapy immediately. Ceftriaxone and ampicillin (p. 307) may be used until culture results are available. They are given intravenously for several days. Continue therapy for at least two weeks.

General: Complications such as seizures, apnoea and blood gas derangement require correction, and assisted ventilation may be needed during the acute phase.

Outcome
The following factors are associated with a poor prognosis:
- ventriculitis
- persistence of organisms in CSF

- high CSF cell count
- high CSF protein level.

The overall outlook remains poor as up to 50% of infants die and neurological abnormalities are found in 30–50% of survivors. They include seizures, and learning difficulties and disabilities.

Other brain insults
Metabolic brain insults (p. 272).
Kernicterus (p. 103).

SEIZURES

The causation, manifestations and significance of seizures in the newborn differ from those in older children or adults. Idiopathic epilepsy and febrile convulsions, for example, do not occur in the newborn period and typical grand mal seizures are most uncommon. Hypoxic-ischaemic encephalopathy accounts for more than 50% of cases.

Causes
Perinatal asphyxia and trauma: Intra-cranial haemorrhage; hypoxic-ischaemic encephalopathy.
Infection: Septic meningitis; viral meningoencephalitis; syphilis; tetanus; toxoplasmosis.
Metabolic: Hypoglycaemia; hypocalcaemia; hypomagnesaemia; pyridoxine deficiency, amino acid abnormalities.
Electrolyte imbalance: Hyponatraemia; hypernatraemia.
Drug-withdrawal syndrome.
Kernicterus (p. 103).
Congenital cerebral malformations.

Note
Hypoglycaemia and hypoxic-ischaemic encephalopathy are likely to cause seizures within two days of birth.
    The most common correctable causes are:
- hypoglycaemia
- hypomagnesaemia

- hypocalcaemia
- septic meningitis.

Clinical features
Five types of seizures are described, although there is some overlap.

Subtle convulsions
These are likely to occur in preterm babies and are characterised by one or several of the following signs:
- apnoea
- lateral deviation of the eyes or nystagmus
- repetitive flickering of eyelids
- exaggerated efforts of chewing, swallowing or sucking
- pedalling movements of limbs.

Multifocal clonic convulsions
Clonic movements may start in one limb and shift to another in a disorderly manner.

Focal clonic convulsions
Clonus may remain in a limb or involve one side of the face or body. This is a feature of metabolic disorders, for example hypocalcaemia. The infant is often conscious.

Tonic convulsions
The body stiffens, the legs extend, eyes deviate upwards and breathing may be impaired. This indicates severe brain disease.

Myoclonic convulsions
These flexor spasms rarely occur in the newborn and are associated with widespread brain damage.

Differential diagnosis
Seizures must be distinguished from:
- jerky movements which occur during REM sleep
- jitteriness
- spasticity.

Diagnosis and treatment
Prolonged seizures can cause damage owing to hypoxia and a decrease in adenosine triphosphate in neurons.

The primary objectives are to:
- arrest the convulsion
- identify and treat a correctable cause.

Treatment of seizures
Phenobarbitone, a drug of choice, is given intravenously in a dose of 20 mg/kg.

A maintenance dose of 3–5 mg/kg/day is then prescribed in divided amounts.

Other useful anticonvulsants include phenytoin sodium and diazepam.

Supportive treatment is essential to ensure:
- a clear airway
- adequate oxygenation
- normal body temperature.

Intractable seizures
Midazolam (p. 306) can be added to dextrose water and given continuously into a peripheral vein.

Identification of cause
Appropriate studies are done to identify treatable conditions such as:
- Metabolic derangements – a rapid estimation is made of blood sugar level.
- Serum sodium, sugar, calcium and magnesium levels are determined.
- Infection – a lumbar puncture is done to examine CSF for meningitis. Total and differential white cell counts are obtained.
- Onther investigations may include X-ray, EEG and ultrasound brain scan.
- In obscure cases a blood ammonia level is needed as well as urine organic and amino-acid patterns.

Treatment of cause
- Hypoglycaemia (p. 261).
- Hypocalcaemia (p. 263).
- Hypomagnesaemia (p. 264).

If a correctable cause cannot be identified, give pyridoxine 50 mg intravenously. This will correct a rare and rather unlikely vitamin B6 deficiency.

Perinatal hypoxia or trauma may be considered on the history, but is not accepted as a cause until treatable conditions have been excluded.

Outcome
Prognosis is influenced by the underlying cause and by EEG changes.

Hypocalcaemia has a good prognosis. The likelihood of neurological damage is increased by:
- hypoglycaemia
- hypoxic-ischaemic encephalopathy
- meningitis
- prolonged or severe seizures.

BIRTH TRAUMA
Intracranial bleeding (p. 142).

Cervical cord
Excessive traction or rotation of the neck or legs can injure the spinal cord. The damage usually occurs in a breech extraction and results from haemorrhage necrosis or transection of the cord.

Clinical signs
A loud snap is sometimes heard during traction and neurological signs depend on the site of injury. This is usually in the lower cervical or upper thoracic region. Baby cries weakly and has a scaphoid chest and a protuberant abdomen. The legs are flaccid and in a 'frog' position. The arms may also be weak or paralysed and urine will dribble constantly if the bladder is paralysed. Inadequate breathing can cause respiratory failure.

Investigations
Nuclear magnetic resonance scanning of the spinal cord reveals the type and site of damage. Nerve conduction studies

indicate the degree of peripheral nerve involvement.

Differential diagnosis
Spinal cord injury must be distinguished from other causes of floppiness (p. 148). It is most likely to be confused with intracranial damage. Alertness is an important differentiating feature.

Treatment
Immobilise the neck in a foam rubber collar and use physiotherapy for the limbs and chest.

Assisted ventilation, nasogastric tube feeding and expression of urine may also be required. Treat respiratory and urinary tract infections with antibiotics.

Outcome
The prognosis depends on the degree of cord damage. Many who survive the first week will die later of respiratory infections.

Survivors have varying degrees of spasticity and weakness of the limbs.

Note
Caesarean section is the preferred mode of delivery for breech presentations and in this event spinal cord injury is rare.

Peripheral nerves
Brachial plexus
This network of nerves incorporates the last four cervical roots from the spine and the first thoracic root. It supplies the arm muscles and extends from the lower neck to the axilla.

Excessive traction on the shoulder or neck can overstretch the nerves. They are rarely avulsed.

Clinical features
A large baby is at risk and the right arm is affected more frequently than the left one. The damage may involve:

- the upper plexus (Erb-Duchenne)
- the lower plexus (Klumpke)
- the whole plexus.

The upper plexus
The fifth and sixth cervical roots are damaged and the forearm hangs limply with the elbow extended. It is pronated, while the palm of the hand is flexed in a 'waiter's tip' position. A Moro reflex is absent, but the grasp reflex is good.

This is the most common injury.
Treatment: Within 24 hours the pain and swelling subside. Gently put the arm through all movements. Instruct the mother to repeat passive physiotherapy at feed times. During sleep flex the elbow to keep the hand above the head. A collar around the wrist is pinned to the sheet to maintain this position.

The lower plexus
This rare injury involves the seventh and eighth cervical roots and causes weakness or paralysis of the wrist and hand. The grasp reflex is absent and the hand is kept in a claw-like position. The eye on the side of the lesion may be partially closed and the pupil may be constricted. This is a Horner syndrome, which results from concurrent sympathetic nerve damage.
Treatment: Put the wrist and hand through all movements several times a day and splint them in extension during sleep.

The whole plexus
Paralysis or weakness affects the whole arm.

This injury is very rare.

Differential diagnosis
Intracranial injury with paralysis of an arm. In most cases the leg on the same side is also affected.

A fracture of the clavicle or humerus can also impair arm movements.

Outlook

Overstretched nerves recover within weeks or months.

Severed nerves have a poorer prognosis.

Suspect avulsion if no improvement has occurred within six weeks. Nerve conduction studies should be done to determine the site and severity of damage.

Microsurgical implantation of nerves may be needed to restore muscle function if roots in the brachial plexus have been severed.

Phrenic nerve

Neck traction in a breech can damage the phrenic nerve as well as the upper brachial plexus. This causes paralysis of the diaphragm and Erb palsy.

Tachypnoea and recurrent cyanosis are characteristic features. On the affected side the chest wall moves rather than the abdomen.

Fluoroscopy shows upward movement of the paralysed diaphragm on inspiration. Nasogastric tube feeding and oxygen may be needed and assisted ventilation is used if respiratory failure occurs.

Respiratory infections must be treated with antibiotics.

The diaphragm recovers in many cases.

Obturator nerve

This may be compressed because of the position of a leg *in utero*. At birth the leg is flaccid, externally rotated, abducted and flexed at the knee. It recovers within weeks.

Sciatic nerve

The blood supply to this nerve can be impaired if drugs or solutions are injected into an umbilical artery. Injection into the gluteus muscle can also damage the nerve.

Weakness, paralysis or wasting of the lower leg and foot may occur. This can be temporary or permanent.

Note

Never inject into the buttocks or into an umbilical artery.

Facial nerve

The extra-cranial part of this nerve may be compressed by forceps, a shoulder or the sacral promontory.

Clinical features

The upper and lower face is weak on the affected side.

The eye remains open during crying.

The forehead and angle of mouth are immobile.

The nasolabial fold is obliterated.

Sucking is impaired.

Outcome

Most cases recover within weeks or months.

Do not confuse facial palsy with Cayler syndrome (p. 288).

NEUROMUSCULAR DISORDERS
The floppy baby

Hypotonia of the skeletal muscles results in floppiness. The baby is inactive and has excessively mobile limbs so that a foot can be positioned behind an ear. The arms and legs hang limply when the baby is lifted and the head lags when the infant is pulled by the arms to a sitting position.

Sucking, swallowing and breathing may also be impaired.

Causes

Common:

Prematurity (particularly below 30 weeks' gestation).

Less common:
Hypoxic-ischaemic encephalopathy (p. 139).
> Down's syndrome (p. 117).
> Hypoglycaemia (p. 261).

Uncommon:
Neuromuscular disease, for example spinal muscular atrophy, myasthenia gravis.
> Connective tissue disorders, for example osteogenesis imperfecta (p. 283).
> Endocrine abnormalities, for example hypothyroidism (p. 276).
> Aminoacidurias.
> Hypotonia-obesity syndrome (Prader-Willi).
> Benign congenital hypotonia.
> Cervical cord injury (p. 146).

Diagnosis
A perinatal and family history together with the physical examination may be sufficient to establish a cause for floppiness.

Sometimes a muscle biopsy is required as histological and chemical analysis of this tissue may be the only way to determine the diagnosis.

Other investigations include the following:
- The level of blood sugar – hypoglycaemia.
- Test dose of Tensilon (see below) – myasthenia gravis.
- Creatine phosphokinase – muscle dystrophies.
- Urine amino acids – aminoaciduria.
- Chromosomes – Down's and Prader-Willi syndromes.
- DNA structure – gene defects.
- Electromyography – neuromuscular disorders.
- Nerve conduction pattern – peripheral neuropathy.

Spinal muscular atrophy
This is also known as Werdnig-Hoffman disease. Degeneration of the anterior horn cells in the spinal cord causes hypotonia and atrophy of the skeletal muscles. This autosomal disease is caused by mutations in the SMN gene on chromosome 5 and occurs in several varieties.

An acute form (type 1) is usually present from birth. The serum level of creatinine phosphokinase is normal.

Clinical signs
Fetal movements are sparse and hypotonicity is characteristic after birth. The tongue and limb muscles may fibrillate, reflexes are absent and cranial nerves, sensation, sphincter action and intelligence are normal.

Progressive weakness and respiratory infections result in death within 18 months.

Myasthenia gravis
Two types occur:

Transient
Nerve conduction is impaired at the neuromuscular junction by acetylcholine receptor antibodies which are transferred from the mother. Twelve per cent of infants whose mothers have myasthenia may manifest signs after birth.

Congenital
These are rare genetic diseases with recessive or dominant inheritance.

Clinical signs
The transient variety usually presents several days after birth, whereas signs associated with the congenital type can occur *in utero* or be delayed for several weeks.

Floppiness, a feeble cry, weak sucking and swallowing, inadequate breathing and cyanosis are important features.

Diagnosis
An intravenous injection of Tensilon (edrophonium chloride) 0,5–1 mg is

followed by immediate improvement which lasts for several minutes.

This distinguishes myasthenia gravis from other causes of floppiness. The response is variable in the congenital types.

Treatment
Prostigmine 0,5–1 mg intravenously or 1–5 mg orally every one to eight hours.

Piridostigmine (Mestinon) 0,1–0,4 mg subcutaneously or 1–2 mg orally every 4 to 12 hours.

Prognosis
Prompt diagnosis and treatment determine the outcome. The transient type usually lasts three to four weeks, but ventilatory support may be needed. The congenital type is less severe, but persists into childhood. The aminoglycosides kanamycin, gentamicin and neomycin interfere with function at the neuromuscular junction and can increase weakness. They must not be used.

The jittery baby

Jitteriness refers to repetitive tremors of the limbs or extremities. The movements are induced or exaggerated by crying and are absent during sleep. The baby is alert and the tremor can be halted by flexing an affected limb. This distinguishes it from a clonic seizure.

Jitteriness is likely to occur in a large- or small-for-gestation baby as a result of hypomagnesaemia (p. 264) or hypocalcaemia (p. 263).

Other causes are hypoglycaemia (p. 261), hypoxic-ischaemic encephalopathy (p. 139) and the drug withdrawal syndrome.

Seek and treat a cause.

Narcotic withdrawal syndrome
The infant of an addicted mother is likely to be small for gestation and is at risk for hypoglycaemia, septicaemia, syphilis, hepatitis B, HIV and withdrawal symptoms.

Signs of withdrawal
Irritability, jitteriness, high-pitched crying, excessive salivation, convulsions, pyrexia, vomiting and diarrhoea may occur in some infants.

Treatment
Fluid: Prevent hypoglycaemia by giving the baby 10% dextrose intravenously. An electrolyte fluid (Neonatalyte) is used for diarrhoea or vomiting.
Sedation: Phenobarbitone 5 mg/kg/day is given for two weeks if signs of withdrawal occur.
Antibiotics: Infections require the appropriate treatment.
Outlook: With adequate therapy the mortality rate is less than 10%.

PROCEDURES
Lumbar puncture

Indications
Meningitis
Subarachnoid bleeding.

Requirements
A sterile tray containing:
- disposable short lumbar puncture needles with stylets, sizes 22 or 23 gauge
- a towel with aperture
- a metal bowl with cotton wool swabs
- tubes for specimens.

Method
The flexed spine must be kept parallel to the surface by holding the baby in the lateral position at the edge of the incubator or table.

One hand supports the shoulders, the other flexes the knees onto the abdomen. The head should not be held as neck flexion can obstruct breathing.

Clean the skin over the lower spine with Hibitane in water. Drape the area and locate the site for puncture.

A vertical line through the anterior

iliac spines transects the spine at the level of the fourth lumbar vertebra (L4). The space above or below L4 is suitable. Insert the needle at right angles to the back and advance it 1–2 mm with the tip in the midline. Withdraw the stylet. If fluid does not drip from the needle, repeat the process. Proceed cautiously as the subarachnoid space is close to the skin in the preterm baby. If the needle is inserted too deeply it will perforate the venous plexus adjacent to the vertebral column and cause bleeding.

Note
The spinal cord extends the full length of the embryo until 12 weeks of gestation. Then the vertebral column grows rapidly and by 40 weeks the cord ends opposite the third lumbar vertebra. Do not insert a needle above this landmark as it may penetrate the spinal cord.

Normal values of cerebrospinal fluid
The cerebrospinal fluid is clear in a full-term baby and often xanthochromic in a preterm one. It contains a few red blood cells and up to 10 white blood cells per mm^3.

The protein content ranges from 45 to 100 mg/dl.

Ultrasonography

Intracranial structures can be visualised through the anterior fontanelle by grey-scale ultrasonography.

This indispensable and accurate technique has advantages over other scanning methods:

- It can be done at the bedside.
- No sedation is needed.
- Movement does not affect the quality of the picture.
- No radiation hazard is encountered.

The skull contents can be examined in many planes and the ventricles, blood vessels, cerebral cortex and thalamus are readily identified.

Ultrasonography is the method of choice to detect peri- or intraventricular haemorrhage and hydrocephalus.

CHAPTER 12

Special Sense Organ Disorders

EYE

The eye develops in the fourth week of gestation and is derived from several embryonic tissues. Vesicles appear on the forebrain and protrude to form optic cups from which the layers of the retina are derived. The lens, eyelids and lachrymal apparatus are formed from surface ectoderm, and the muscles (other than ciliary) from mesoderm.

At term, the eye is fully developed, except for the retinal cells of the fovea, which continue to differentiate for several months.

Sight

Vision is well established in the term baby, who is able to gaze at a face and follow its movements.

Methods of assessment

Response to light: When a bright light is shone into an infant's face, the following reactions occur: the pupils constrict and the baby immediately blinks and withdraws the head. Heart rate increases, and an evoked response can be demonstrated on an occipital EEG.

Testing vision: Eyesight can be assessed when the baby is awake, alert and not crying. Hold a bright red ball between the thumb and forefinger and bring it into the baby's line of vision. The infant's pupils will constrict and the eyes widen as they fix intently on the ball.

Move the ball slowly to one or other side. The infant's eyes follow the object and the head rotates in the same direction.

After several attempts, the baby can usually track the ball through an arc of 180°.

Movements

Conjugate eye movements are the norm, even in preterm babies who appear to survey their surroundings with interest. Persistent squinting, nystagmus or eye rolling is suspicious and requires further assessment.

During REM sleep the eyes flicker under the lids and may be seen to roll when the lids are open.

Congenital abnormalities

These are rare and usually associated with teratogenic or genetic factors.

Anophthalmia

Failure of the optic vesicle to form results in an absent eyeball and lens. Eyelids are present.

Cyclopia

The eyes are fused into a median structure usually covered by a tubular nose. This is associated with other craniocerebral malformations incompatible with life.

Microphthalmia

Abnormal development of the optic cup results in an excessively small eye. This can be inherited or caused by teratogens, such as alcohol, cytomegalovirus or *Toxoplasma*.

Coloboma

Gaps may occur in the eyelids or iris. The defect in the iris is usually inferior and gives the pupil a keyhole appearance.

Heterochromia

The eyes are of different colours. This usually affects only part of the iris.

Blue scleras

The dark choroid imparts a blue tinge to scleras, which are abnormally transparent, as in osteogenesis imperfecta. This feature may be normal in dark-skinned babies.

Cataract (Colour plate IX)

This is a greyish-white opacity of the lens which may be inherited or caused by:
- rubella
- toxoplasmosis
- galactosaemia.

Treatment
Small incomplete cataracts may not require treatment in the initial stages, whereas large ones, which impair vision, will need removal. The decision is left to an ophthalmologist.

Glaucoma

This implies a raised intraocular pressure owing to inadequate drainage of the aqueous. The obstruction may be in the sinus venosus sclerae or the canal of Schlemm, and is associated with genetic or environmental factors such as rubella.

Diagnosis
Early diagnosis and treatment is essential in order to preserve the function of the eye.

The following features are important:
- Excessively large cornea.
- Haziness of the cornea.
- Photophobia.

Untreated glaucoma will result in the enlargement of the eyeball and blindness.

Treatment
Early surgery, that is, goniopuncture and/or goniotomy, offers a good prognosis.

Strabismus

A temporary squint is fairly common, but one which persists for more than two months is abnormal and may be associated with developmental faults, cerebral trauma or hypoxia. This usually results in paralysis of an extraocular muscle group.

Treatment includes:
- correction of any refractive error
- covering the healthy eye to strengthen the muscles of the abnormal one
- surgical correction.

Hypertelorism

The distance between the eyes is excessive (p. 19) and can be associated with other abnormalities, for example deafness and white forelock in Waardenburg syndrome.

Ptosis

This dominant hereditary condition is characterised by an inability to raise one or both upper eyelids. It must be distinguished from a facial palsy in which there is difficulty in closing the eye tightly.

Blocked nasolachrymal duct

Incomplete canalisation of this duct prevents drainage of tears into the nose. The obstruction is characterised by persistent tearing and an accumulation of white matter in the eye. Secondary infection occasionally occurs in the conjunctival or lachrymal sac.

Treatment

At each feed empty the duct by finger massage from the nose towards the eye. Remove accumulated matter with moist swabs and use an antibiotic, for example chloramphenicol Applicap for secondary infection. The obstruction persists for weeks or months, but resolves spontaneously and seldom requires probing.

Epicanthus (Colour plate IX)

A fold of skin may overhang the medial portion of the eye and partially obscure the sclera to give the illusion of squinting. This may be a familial characteristic or be associated with malformations such as Down's syndrome. No treatment is required.

Infection

Conjunctivitis (Colour plate II)

This common infection is usually caused by one of the following agents:

- *Neisseria gonorrhoeae.*
- Chlamydia.
- Staphylococcus or streptococcus.
- Coliforms.

Gonococcal conjunctivitis

Ophthalmia neonatorum varies in frequency and is most likely to occur where ante- and postnatal care are inadequate. The disease is rarely seen when prophylaxis is employed (p. 26).

Clinical signs

A purulent discharge which may be profuse occurs on the second or third day and is associated with red, swollen conjunctivae.

Diagnosis

A swab of the discharge is taken for Gram stain and culture. A presumptive diagnosis is made of gonococcal infection if Gram-negative diplococci are seen. They may be present in leukocytes.

Treatment

Many strains of the organism have become resistant to penicillin and the recommended treatment is a single intramuscular or intravenous injection of ceftriaxone 75 mg/kg.

Irrigate the eyes with normal saline using a dropper every five minutes until the purulent discharge subsides.

Chlamydia

These intracellular organisms can be transmitted from the genital tract to an infant's eyes or respiratory system. They are probably responsible for many cases of non-gonococcal conjunctivitis.

The infection is characterised by mild or severe conjunctivitis, which occurs one to three weeks after birth. It may be associated with pneumonia.

Diagnosis

Numerous lymphocytes are present and characteristic inclusion bodies are seen in cells obtained from conjunctival scrapings. An immunofluorescent test is available for the rapid detection of the chlamydia antigen.

Treatment

Treatment
Erythromycin 10 mg/kg/oral dose. Give this three times a day for two weeks.

Topical tetracycline ointment 1%. Instil into eyes twice a day for two weeks.

Secondary bacterial conjunctivitis
Secondary infections may follow conjunctival damage caused by silver nitrate drops or meconium. A variety of organisms may be responsible. Culture is needed for identification. A broad-spectrum antibiotic, chloramphenicol ointment, is instilled into the eyes for five days.

Choroidoretinitis
The eyes of the fetus are susceptible to infective agents, such as *Treponema, Toxoplasma*, rubella, cytomegalovirus and herpes simplex.

Systemic infection is frequently associated with choroidoretinitis.

Retinopathy of prematurity
The retina of the fetus remains avascular until the 16th week of gestation. The optic artery then grows towards the anterior boundary of the retina, which becomes vascularised after 38 weeks' gestation. The incompletely vascularised retina is highly susceptible to damage.

Factors implicated in retinopathy include:
- very low birthweight (about 50% of infants < 1 200 g show some degree of retinopathy)
- oxygen toxicity
- severe illness.

Two phases are observed: constriction of the optic artery, followed by proliferation of capillaries into the vitreous.

Vasoconstrictive phase
A high arterial oxygen tension (PaO_2) can constrict the optic artery. In the preterm baby this constriction may obliterate the lumen of the vessel. Such an event can be permanent and is likely to occur in the preterm baby once PaO_2 exceeds 12 kPa. In the full-term baby this danger exists if the PaO_2 is higher than 18 kPa.

In a very low birthweight infant (< 1 500 g) the growth of retinal vessels may be arrested and then constrict without exposure to high concentrations of oxygen.

Proliferative phase
An overgrowth of retinal capillaries may then extend into the vitreous.

The disease is categorised into zones and stages. Zone 1 surrounds the macular, and zones 2 and 3 are concentric circles that extend beyond this to the periphery of the retina. Aggressive disease rarely occurs in the outermost zone.

Five clinical stages are described, ranging from extra vascular growth to retinal detachment.

The disease can regress at any stage and the ultimate damage varies from blindness to myopia owing to a distorted retina.

Retinopathy owing to excessive oxygen is preventable, and the following measures must be taken to ensure the safe use of the gas:
- Use oxygen only to correct hypoxaemia.
- Measure the concentration of the inhaled gas.
- Maintain oxygen saturation between 89 and 92%, and oxygen tension between 8 and 12 kPa. Never exceed the upper limit, particularly in a preterm baby.
- Oxygen is a toxic drug. Ensure that a primary care unit has the means, that is, oximeter, to measure the saturation in the blood.

An ophthalmologist should examine the eyes of all preterm infants, at frequent intervals, particularly those under 1 500 g.

EAR

The organ is comprised of internal, middle and external sections. The internal ear is derived from the otocyst, a thickened plate of surface ectoderm, whereas the middle portion arises from the first pharyngeal pouch and the first and second branchial arches. The auricle or external ear is formed from the first branchial groove. In the embryo it develops in the upper part of the future neck and progresses to the side of the head as the mandible develops. It finally ascends to the level of the eye.

Hearing

Auditory responses are well developed in the term baby, who responds to the soothing talk of the mother by turning the head towards her voice.

A high-pitched rattle usually evokes a response from the sleeping baby. This ranges from facial movements such as blinking or grimacing to a startle reflex. Repetitive auditory stimuli tend to reduce this reaction and the infant eventually sleeps through the noise.

The following are risk factors for impaired hearing:
■ A family history of deafness, which accounts for about half the cases.
■ Syndromes associated with deafness, for example Down's and Waardenburg.
■ Cranio-facial abnormalities, for example mandibulo-facial dysostosis and Pierre Robin syndrome.
■ Intra-uterine infections, for example rubella, cytomegalovirus, herpes, syphilis and toxoplasmosis.
■ Exposure to ototoxic drugs, for example aminoglycosides, streptomycin and isotretinoin.
■ Meningitis.
■ Hyperbilirubinaemia.
■ Very low birthweight (< 1 500 g).

Formal hearing tests suitable for this group include the otoacoustic emission (OAE) assessment, and brainstem auditory evoked responses (AER).

The former requires an ear probe and a microphone. It measures the OAE generated by the cochlea and is suitable for screening. Auditory evoked responses show characteristic brainstem EEG patterns, which demonstrate the intact pathways of hearing to the brain. This test is preferred for follow-up assessment.

Congenital abnormalities
Auricular defects
Low-set or malformed ears are often associated with chromosomal abnormalities. The low position may also be indicative of severe fetal compression as in renal agenesis (p. 238).

Appendages or skin tags may occur (Fig. 12.1) and sinuses can be observed on occasion.

Infection
Otitis media
Middle-ear infection is uncommon in the first week, but should be suspected when non-specific signs of sepsis are present.

Predisposing factors include:
■ amniotic fluid infection
■ cleft palate
■ prolonged nasotracheal intubation.

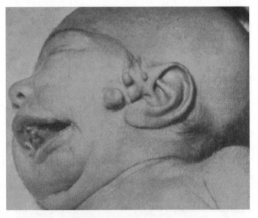

Fig. 12.1 *Auricular appendages. These will require surgical excision*

Diagnosis
The tympanic membrane is dull and inflamed and a purulent discharge may be present if the drum has ruptured.

Use systemic antibiotic therapy for 10 days.

NOSE

Primitive nasal sacs develop beneath the brain in the embryo and are separated from the mouth by an oronasal membrane. This regresses and is replaced by the hard and soft palate and a nasal septum.

Specialised olfactory cells develop in each nasal cavity and are connected by nerve fibres to the brain. Paranasal air sinuses develop during late fetal life and infancy.

Smell

Olfactory function is well established at birth and a term baby can distinguish its mother's milk from that of others.

Congenital abnormalities

Malformations of the nose may be caused by genetic or teratogenic factors. Important defects are associated with:

- cleft lip and palate (p. 206)
- warfarin toxicity (p. 113)
- achondroplasia (p. 282).

Atresia of the posterior nasal passages (Fig. 12.2)
Unilateral or bilateral choanal atresia is caused by a bony or membranous obstruction. The condition is twice as frequent in girls as in boys.

The newborn infant is an obligate nose breather and complete nasal obstruction can lead to cyanosis and death. Bilateral choanal atresia is characterised by sternal and rib recession and cyanosis. The infant may become pink during bouts of crying. This process is repeated and eventually results in death if not treated.

No air can be heard to leave the nostrils and a catheter cannot be passed beyond the back of the nose.

Treatment
Immediate: An oropharyngeal airway permits adequate mouth breathing by depressing the tongue from the soft palate to create a passage for air.

Give milk feeds through an orogastric tube that is removed after each feed.

Corrective: An adequate air passage should be established as soon as possible by laser surgery.

Infection
Congenital syphilis
Snuffles, an early sign, is characterised by a blocked nose, and a discharge which may be clear, purulent or sanguinous (Colour plate II).

Diagnosis
Spirochaetes may be identified in nasal secretions, or there may be characteristic clinical and radiological features of the disease (p. 88).

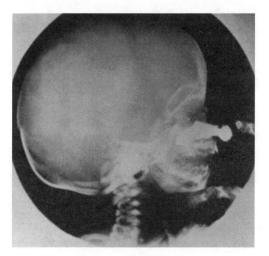

Fig. 12.2 *Choanal atresia: Radiopaque dye has been instilled into the nose and shows an obstruction posteriorly*

Bacterial infection

The nasal mucosa can be damaged by:

- vigorous suctioning of nostrils
- indwelling nasogastric catheter
- nasal tube for CPAP.

This can result in superimposed bacterial infection and a purulent discharge. The organism, usually a *Staphylococcus aureus*, can be identified on Gram stain and culture and relevant antibiotic therapy is used for a week.

Respiratory Disorders

PHYSIOLOGY OF BREATHING

The initiation of air breathing at birth is probably the most crucial physiological adjustment of any age and depends on many pre-existing factors, such as a functioning respiratory centre in the brain, intact nerve pathways, active carotid chemoreceptors and mature lungs.

Lung development

The lungs originate in the 24-day-old embryo from a pouch in the primitive gut, and dividing tubules grow from this endoderm into a mass of mesoderm. Subsequent development proceeds outwards from the trachea and includes:

- vascularisation of the tubular framework: 20th week
- development of alveolar air spaces: 13th–25th week
- formation of alveolar capillaries: 26th–40th week.

Adequate gas exchange is possible only after birth if sufficient alveoli and capillaries have been formed.

Breathing movements

Chest movements are detectable at 11 weeks *in utero*, when the lungs are grossly immature and unable to support life. They occur during REM sleep and involve the diaphragm. They are essential for normal lung development and can be supressed temporarily by smoking, alcohol or hypoglycaemia. The movements normally cease a day before labour, probably as a result of increased secretions of prostaglandin E2.

Lung fluid

The alveoli secrete a fluid which fills the respiratory tract and differs from amniotic fluid in that it has less protein and a lower pH. It is produced continuously and enters the pharynx intermittently to mix with liquor. Under normal circumstances amniotic fluid does not flow into the respiratory tract, but may do so during gasping in fetal hypoxaemia. (Fig. 13.3)

Surfactants

Alveolar cells (type II) secrete phospholipids, which are essential for lung stability after birth. These surfactants retain air in the alveoli during expiration by reducing surface tension. This volume of air is essential for normal gas exchange in the lungs and is known as the functional residual capacity. It is greatly reduced in immature lungs that lack surfactant.

The phospholipids are secreted into lung fluid before birth and can be detected in samples of amniotic fluid. Lecithin, the main constituent, is present from 26 weeks of gestation and rises sharply after 35 weeks. This contrasts with the level of sphingomyelin, which remains constant throughout pregnancy. A lecithin-sphingomyelin (L/S) ratio of more than 2,5 indicates lung maturity.

Phosphotidylglycerol appears after 35 weeks and also heralds lung maturity.

The presence of surfactants in amniotic fluid can be demonstrated by a simple 'bubble test'.

'Bubble test' method

Pipette 1 ml of amniotic fluid into a clean test tube containing 1 ml of absolute alcohol. Cover the top with parafilm and shake the tube vigorously for half a minute. Examine the surface 15 minutes later for foam. The absence of foam implies lung immaturity.

The onset of breathing

The initiation of breathing can be divided into two phases:
1. Deep crying to inflate the lungs – this occurs within half a minute of birth.

2. Quiet rhythmic breathing to maintain ventilation – this is established within a minute and a half. The amount of air inhaled with each breath is the tidal volume (TV).

Lung inflation at birth

During normal labour there is usually a progressive but small decrease in fetal arterial oxygen tension, oxygen saturation and pH, with a rise in carbon dioxide tension. This probably stimulates the carotid chemoreceptors to initiate the deep breaths that occur at birth.

Initially, a considerable transthoracic pressure may be needed to expand the fluid-filled alveoli. This negative pressure ranges from 2 to 3 kPa, but can be as high as 7 kPa. It is achieved by elastic recoil of the compressed chest wall at birth, downward movement of the diaphragm and contraction of the intercostal muscles. Subsequent breaths require less negative pressure (0,6 kPa) as surfactant now lines the alveoli and maintains a functional residual capacity (FRC).

Clearance of lung fluid

The air that is inhaled at birth forces lung fluid through alveoli into the interstitial spaces. This fluid averages 30 ml/kg.

Its absorption into the circulation is enhanced by labour and takes place through the interstitial capillaries and lymphatics.

The maintenance of breathing

After birth, this is probably regulated by a number of factors that on their own would not be essential for the maintenance of respiration.

Various chemical and non-chemical stimuli may act directly on the respiratory centre in the brain or indirectly through nerve receptors in the skin, muscles, lungs and large blood vessels. These stimuli include:

Chemical factors
- Rise in arterial carbon dioxide tension ($PaCO_2$).
- Acidaemia.

Non-chemical factors
- Change in skin temperature.
- Tactile stimuli.
- Auditory and visual stimuli.
- Taste bud stimuli.
- Lung reflexes, e.g. Hering–Breuer.

BLOOD GAS AND ACID-BASE FUNCTIONS

A lung alveolus and its capillary comprise the gas exchange unit (Fig. 13.2). Gases, like water, flow "downhill" i.e. from a high to a low pressure area so that oxygen diffuses rapidly across the alveolar membrane into the blood stream while carbon dioxide in returning venous blood swiftly enters the alveolus and is then exhaled from the lungs by breathing.

Oxygen carriage

Oxygen diffuses into the blood from the lungs and is transported in two ways:
1 In combination with the haemoglobin (98%) of red blood cells (oxyhaemoglobin).
2 As a dissolved gas in plasma (2%).

The partial pressure of dissolved oxygen in plasma (PaO_2) determines the amount of the gas that will combine with haemoglobin in the red blood cells oxygen saturation (SaO_2).

The association between oxygen saturation and the partial pressure of oxygen is illustrated in Fig. 13.1 (oxygen dissociation curve).

The flat portion of the S-shaped curve (right-hand side) represents the situation in the lungs. The PaO_2 in lung capillaries

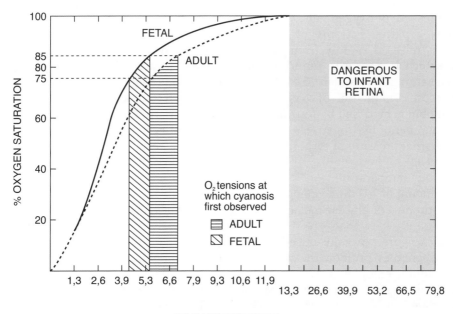

Fig. 13.1 *The oxygen dissociation curve for haemoglobin. The curve remains in the fetal position for several months after birth. (From Klaus and Fanaroff. 1975.* Care of the High-risk Neonate. *Philadelphia: WB Saunders)*

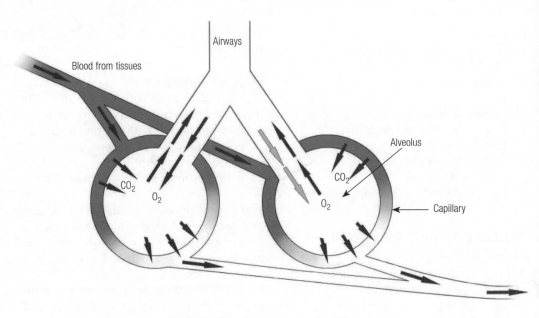

Fig 13.2 *The gas exchange unit of the lung*

is approximately 13 kPa and the hae-moglobin molecule is completely satu-rated with oxygen (over 98%). When oxygenated blood reaches the tissues (left hand side) the curve drops steeply as the partial pressure of oxygen falls.

Below a partial pressure of 5,3 kPa, oxygen is released rapidly from haemo-globin which is now in a reduced state (oxygen saturation less than 75%).

The loose combination of oxygen with haemoglobin is modified by four factors:
1. The number of hydrogen (H+) ions.
2. The partial pressure of carbon dioxide ($PaCO_2$).
3. The body temperature.
4. The amount of 2–3 diphosphoglycerate (a by-product of glucose metabolism).

These factors are normally raised in the tissues where they promote the release of oxygen from haemoglobin. They can also be raised throughout the body in patho-logical states such as hypoxaemia. This hinders the combination of oxygen with haemoglobin and shifts the dissociation curve (Fig. 13.1) to the right.

Oxygen–haemoglobin affinity also depends on the type of haemoglobin. It is enhanced by the fetal variety, which facilitates the transfer of oxygen from mother to fetus at a relatively low PaO_2. In fetal life the curve (Fig. 13.1) is shifted to the left.

Arterial oxygen tension

This is measured on a sample of arte-rial blood (technique p. 189). The normal range is 8 to 12 kPa.

The partial pressure of oxygen has direct effects on various organs. After birth the relatively high PO_2 dilates the pulmonary artery and constricts the ductus arteriosus.

Hazards of a high PaO_2

An excessive partial pressure of oxygen in plasma (over 12 kPa) is produced by inhaling high concentrations of oxy-gen. This contributes free oxygen radicals which may harm tissues.

Damage to the endothelium of the retinal capillaries results in a retinopathy (retrolental fibroplasia) (p. 155). Destruc-tion of lung alveolar cells impairs sur-factant production, induces oedema and possibly results in chronic lung disease (bronchopulmonary dysplasia) (p. 179).

Hazards of a low PaO$_2$
A fall in oxygen tension to 6,6 kPa can cause:
- pulmonary artery constriction.
- impairment of thermoregulation.

A PaO$_2$ of less than 5,5 kPa is associated with a low oxygen saturation, cyanosis and metabolic acidaemia owing to tissue hypoxia. This will result in death if not corrected.

Cyanosis
This literally means 'blue', from the Greek word *kyanos*. It is caused by reduced haemoglobin in the circulation and is obvious when the oxygen saturation is below 75%. Two types are described, peripheral and central.

Peripheral cyanosis
The extremities, that is hands, feet or tip of the nose, may be blue. Red blood cells containing reduced haemoglobin are trapped in capillaries where the circulation is sluggish. This may be due to hypothermia and is not significant.

Central cyanosis
The mucous membranes are blue because of excessive amounts of reduced haemoglobin in the systemic circulation. This is always ominous. Cyanosis is best detected on the tongue and inner lips. It must be differentiated from the blueness produced by bruising of the face and lips at birth. This commonly occurs in very small babies and is distinguished from cyanosis by a pink tongue.

Central cyanosis indicates pulmonary, cardiovascular or central nervous system disorders.

Arterial oxygen saturation (SaO$_2$)
This is measured by pulse oximetry. The safe range in an ill baby is 89 to 92%. When it exceeds 92% further increments are associated with large rises in the partial pressure of oxygen in blood. This occurs because the dissociation curve (right hand side) is relatively flat (Fig. 13.1).

When oxygen saturation falls below 89% it is associated with:
- low PaO2
- tissue hypoxia
- cyanosis.

Carbon dioxide carriage
Carbon dioxide (CO$_2$), a volatile acid, is formed continuously in the tissues and is excreted by the lungs.

The solubility in blood is far greater than that of oxygen and it is transported in various forms:
- In red blood cells (95%). Here it is converted to bicarbonate ions by carbonic anhydrase
- Attached to haemoglobin (5%)
- Dissolved in plasma (5%)

When blood reaches the lungs the partial pressure of carbon dioxide is higher in the pulmonary capillaries than in the alveoli and the gas diffuses rapidly from blood into the air sacs. Its final elimination depends on the adequacy of breathing.

The partial pressure of carbon dioxide in arterial blood (PaCO$_2$) reflects the state of breathing
It averages 5,3 kPa (40 mmHg) at birth and falls to 4,6 (35 mmHg) within 24 hours.

Hazards of a very high PaCO$_2$
Hypercapnoea causes acidaemia, lethargy, increased cerebral blood flow and coma. The latter may occur when PaCO$_2$ exceeds 10 kPa.

Hazards of a very low PaCO$_2$
Hypocapnoea suppresses breathing and diminishes the cerebral blood flow. The

$PaCO_2$ must therefore be controlled during mechanical ventilation, particularly when using oscillation.

Acid-base balance

pH

The acidity or alkalinity of a solution depends on the concentration of its hydrogen (H+) ions.

Pure water contains 10^{-7} moles of ionised hydrogen per litre. This is conveniently expressed as pH 7 where p stands for the negative power of 10 and H for the concentration of H+ ions.

The pH of blood is maintained within narrow limits to permit adequate metabolism. It averages 7,34 at birth and rises to 7,42 within 48 hours.

A reduction of pH (less than 7,30) implies an excess of H+ ions and is called acidaemia. The H+ ions may be due to an excessive accumulation of volatile acid (carbon dioxide) or non-volatile acids (mostly lactic) in the blood.

An increase in pH (more than 7,45) implies a deficiency of H+ ions and is termed alkalaemia. The lack of H+ ions can be caused by too little carbon dioxide or by an excessive amount of bicarbonate in the blood

Three mechanisms prevent fluctuations in blood pH:

1 Elimination of volatile acid by the lungs.
2 Excretion of non-volatile acid by the kidneys.
3 Buffers.

Excretion of non-volatile acid

The kidneys play a major role in acid-base regulation as they excrete non-volatile acids. Some, such as sulphuric acid, are the products of protein metabolism.

The acids are neutralised by bicarbonate and then the excess H+ ions are secreted into the renal tubules. They combine with acid phosphate and ammonia salts and pass into the urine.

The bicarbonate ions are reabsorbed to conserve the body's base.

The quantity of non-volatile acids can be determined indirectly by measuring the level of bicarbonate in the blood.

The actual bicarbonate ranges from 20 to 24 mmol/l.

Buffers

These chemicals prevent marked changes in H+ ion concentration when acids or alkalis are added to the blood.

Bicarbonate/carbonic acid buffer

This important system accounts for half of the plasma's buffering action. It

Respiratory disorders		
Gas exchange terminology		
Term	Symbol	Explanation
Partial pressure	P	Gas molecules are in constant motion. When they strike a surface they exert a pressure. In a mixture of gases such as air in the alveoli, the pressure exerted by each one is known as partial pressure.
Alveolar ventilation	VA	This is the volume of alveolar air that takes part in gas exchange with the blood. It cannot be measured directly.
Partial pressure Carbon dioxide	PCO_2	The pressure of carbon dioxide in the alveoli ($PACO_2$) is similar to that in arterial blood ($PaCO_2$). If ventilation is inadequate, $PACO_2$ rises and so does $PaCO_2$. Hence $PaCO_2$ is cardinal measurement of the adequacy of breathing.

consists of a weak acid H_2CO_3 (dissolved carbon dioxide) and a weak alkali HCO_3 (bicarbonate).

pH is proportional to $\dfrac{base}{acid}$, i.e. $pH\alpha \dfrac{HCO_3}{H_2CO_3} \dfrac{20}{1}$

Plasma bicarbonate and carbonic acid are in a ratio of 20 to 1 and the pH will not alter if the ratio remains constant. The plasma level of carbonic acid is dependent on the rate and adequacy of breathing and the concentration of bicarbonate is determined by kidney function.

Mechanism of buffering
A strong acid, for example lactic acid, combines with bicarbonate to form carbonic acid.

HLA + NaHCO$_3$ = NaLA + H$_2$CO$_3$ $\longrightarrow$ CO$_2$
lactic   sodium   sodium   carbonic   carbon
acid   bicarbonate lactate   acid   dioxide

This causes a temporary fall in the pH until sufficient carbonic acid has been blown off as CO_2 by the lungs.

A strong alkali, for example sodium hydroxide, combines with carbonic acid to form bicarbonate.

NaOH + H$_2$CO$_3$ = NaHCO$_3$ + H$_2$O
sodium   carbonic   sodium   water
hydroxide   acid   bicarbonate

The pH may rise until the excess bicarbonate has been excreted by the kidneys.

Rapidity of acid base-equilibration
Buffers act immediately to prevent alterations in the pH.

Lung control is achieved within minutes to hours.

Renal control is completed with in hours but may take several days.

Although the kidneys take considerably longer to regulate acid-base balance they can neutralise any excess acid or base completely.

Measurement of acid-base status
This is determined from the pH, PaCO$_2$ and HCO$_3$ values of arterial blood (technique p.189). The three measurements are necessary for accurate interpretation. The actual bicarbonate, for example, can be altered by respiratory and metabolic factors. A normal PaCO$_2$ would rule out a respiratory component.

Respiratory acidaemia
Inadequate ventilation causes the PaCO$_2$ to rise (over 6 kPa or 45 mmHg) and the pH to decrease.

Apnoea (p. 184) and respiratory distress (p. 172) are important causes.

Respiratory alkalaemia
Overventilation causes the PaCO$_2$ to fall and the pH to rise. This can occur during mechanical ventilation of the lungs, especially if they are normal.

Metabolic acidaemia
Hypoxaemia produces large amounts of lactic acid which can reduce the levels of pH and bicarbonate (below 20 mmol/l). Birth asphyxia is an important cause.

Metabolic alkalaemia
The use of citrated blood for exchange transfusion or large quantities of sodium bicarbonate can increase the pH and the bicarbonate. This is usually an iatrogenic problem.

Examples of common problems

	pH	PaCO$_2$ (kPa)	Bicarbonate (mmol/l)
Respiratory acidaemia	7,20	9,1	23
Metabolic acidaemia	7,20	4,9	16
Respiratory and metabolic acidaemia	7,20	9,1	16

Birth asphyxia and respiratory distress account for a significant number of

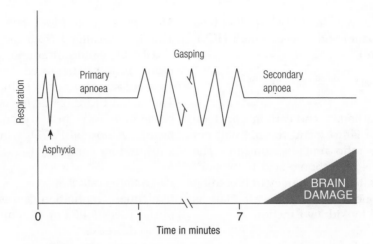

Fig. 13.3. *The pattern of respiration during experimental asphyxia*

deaths within the first 48 hours. They often occur during the transition from intra- to extrauterine life and are usually preventable.

ASPHYXIA NEONATORUM

Asphyxia literally means being born 'without a pulse'. In practice it implies a failure to initiate breathing at birth. This is commonly associated with fetal hypoxaemia which can result in death, respiratory depression, meconium aspiration or brain damage. These complications form the spectrum of the asphyxia syndrome.

Experimental asphyxia

When a fetal animal, like a monkey, is asphyxiated *in utero* by clamping the cord, a constant pattern of events occurs (Fig. 13.3). Brief efforts to breathe are followed by *primary apnoea,* which lasts for about one minute. Rhythmic gasping begins and then weakens over the next five to eight minutes, terminating in *secondary apnoea.* This is associated with a rapid fall in heart rate and blood pressure, and the animal dies.

Acidaemia occurs as a result of carbon dioxide retention and a fall in oxygen tension. In secondary apnoea the blood pH can be as low as 6,8, the PaO_2 0,26 kPa, and $PaCO_2$ can be as high as 16 kPa.

When animals are delivered at various stages of the experiment, a distinction can be made between primary and secondary apnoea. During primary apnoea a variety of stimuli, such as pain, cold and analeptic drugs, can initiate gasping and spontaneous breathing. Such stimuli are ineffective during secondary apnoea and breathing can only be induced by artificial ventilation of the lungs and correction of acidaemia.

Histological brain damage can only be demonstrated during secondary apnoea and its severity is related to the duration of asphyxia after the last gasp. The time interval to the last gasp is influenced by factors such as pre-existing acidaemia, which shortens it, whereas sedatives and anaesthetics tend to prolong primary apnoea and gasping.

The human baby probably manifests a similar pattern, but primary and secondary apnoea cannot be distinguished on clinical criteria alone.

Causes of asphyxia neonatorum
Respiratory depression can result from:
- fetal hypoxaemia
- maternal oversedation, for example pethidine
- gross immaturity

- lung pathology, for example diaphragmatic hernia.

Fetal hypoxaemia

The fetus may be deprived of oxygen as a result of:

- acute blood loss, for example early separation of the placenta or rupture of vasa praevia
- impairment of blood supply, for example cord prolapse, tetanic uterine contractions
- inability to compensate for stress, for example intrauterine growth retardation, prolonged labour.

The signs vary and include fetal heart-rate irregularities, meconium staining of the liquor and fetal acidaemia.

Fetal heart rate

Various patterns are described during labour. Listen to the fetal heart before, during and after contractions or use a cardiotocograph for continuous monitoring.

Normal pattern
The rate varies between 120 and 160 beats per minute with beat-to-beat variations and no slowing in the rate during uterine contractions.

Early deceleration
This is ascribed to vagal stimulation from pressure on the fetal skull during contractions. The heart rate slows with the onset of a contraction (type I dip), beat-to-beat variations persist and the basal rate is regained before or shortly after the contraction has ended. This is not considered to be a sign of fetal hypoxaemia.

Late deceleration
During a contraction there is a significant slowing of the heart rate (type II dip). The onset is delayed and the duration is prolonged in contrast to the type I dip. Deceleration often lasts for more than 30 seconds and the basal rate may be regained long after the contraction has ended. A significant bradycardia (below 100 beats/min) associated with loss of beat-to-beat variation is an ominous sign.

Varying deceleration
Compression of the umbilical cord can result in slowing of the heart rate, which varies in time of onset, duration and amplitude in relation to contractions.

Decrease in beat-to-beat variability
The heart rate normally varies slightly between one beat and the next. Hypoxia reduces this variability and in severe cases of the disorder can result in a flattened cardiotocograph tracing.

Basal tachycardia
Many factors alter the basal heart rate. Maternal anxiety, pyrexia, smoking and drugs such as atropine may cause a persistent fetal tachycardia (that is, over 160 beats per minute).

This is also a feature of fetal hypoxaemia, particularly when associated with decelerations and loss of beat-to-beat variability.

A change in the fetal heart rate is one of the earliest signs of acute fetal hypoxaemia. In some cases the abnormal pattern can be corrected by lying the mother on her left side.

An abnormal heart-rate pattern necessitates further assessment of the fetus with a view to early delivery.

Acid-base state of the fetus

The fetal pH declines slowly during a normal labour to between 7,35 and 7,25. Fetal hypoxaemia causes the pH to fall below 7,15 due to an accumulation of acid by-products from anaerobic metabolism.

Fetal blood can be obtained from the presenting part during labour, once the membranes have ruptured. An endoscope is used for this purpose and blood is obtained in a capillary tube from a small scalp incision.

A reasonable correlation exists between fetal pH and the state of an infant at birth. Consecutive pH readings of less than 7,15 in association with an abnormal heart-rate pattern are indicative of fetal hypoxia.

This procedure should not be done in regions with a high incidence of HIV infection.

Meconium staining of the liquor

The passage of meconium may be linked with fetal distress, but the mechanism is unclear. The hypoxaemic fetus who passes meconium *in utero* is likely to be a full-term baby or a growth-retarded baby of any gestation rather than one who has grown normally and is preterm.

Meconium can be seen in the liquor through an endoscope before the membranes have ruptured. It is significant when coupled with fetal heart irregularities or acidaemia in labour.

Assessment of infant at birth

A baby's ability to initiate and maintain breathing after birth can be determined by a clinical score devised by Virginia Apgar (Table 13.1). This consists of five physical signs, each scoring 0, 1 and 2 points. The total score indicates the clinical condition of the infant and the need for resuscitation.

This rapid assessment is done at one and five minutes after delivery.

An example of the clinical signs associated with birth asphyxia is as follows:

Heart rate below 100 per minute	1	point
No respiratory effort	0	
Limbs slightly flexed	1	point
No response to stimulation	0	
Body blue, mucosae blue	0	
TOTAL	2	points

Interpretation of Apgar score

Score	Respiratory depression
0–3	Severe
4–6	Mild to moderate
7–10	Absent

The Apgar rating cannot predict the neurological status of an infant, nor can it assess the immediate effects of preceding fetal hypoxaemia. A baby may suffer severe hypoxia *in utero* as reflected by cord blood acidaemia and yet have a high score at birth. An oversedated infant who has not been subjected to fetal hypoxia may have a low score.

The assessment offers a clinical guide to the immediate management of a baby at birth and methods of resuscitation are based on the score.

Resuscitation procedure

Place the baby onto a resuscitation table and rapidly dry the skin with a clean towel. Warmth is provided by an overhead infrared or a wall-panel heater.

Remove meconium, blood or froth from the nose and mouth to ensure a clear airway. Proceed cautiously, as vigorous suctioning of the pharynx can cause reflex apnoea or mucosal damage.

TABLE 13.1

Apgar score					
Score	Heart rate	Respiratory effort	Muscle tone	Response to stimulation	Colour
0	Absent	None	Flaccid	None	Pale or blue
1	Less than 100/min	Slow or irregular	Slight flexion	Grimace	Body pink, limbs blue
2	More than 100/min	Good, crying	Active, moves	Vigorous cry	Pink all over

The suction pressure should not exceed 2 kPa. Note the time and determine the Apgar score.

Apgar score 0–3

Place a neonatal resuscitator (Samson™, Ambu™, Laerdal™) firmly over the baby's nose and mouth and compress the bag as rapidly as possible, using fingers only. If oxygen is used in the circuit, do not exceed a rate of 1 l/min to ventilate the lungs.

An increase in the heart rate (over 100/min) and pink mucosae are the first signs of recovery. If they do not occur immediately, intubate the larynx (p. 170) and attach the endotracheal tube to the resuscitator. Even if you are unfamiliar with the procedure, do not panic, stay calm! Use face mask ventilation (p. 170). It is highly effective in the majority of cases. *Oxygen is not essential*. Lung expansion is the most important requirement for the initiation of breathing. Observe respiratory movements during ventilation and ensure that air entry is equal on both sides of the chest.

Use external cardiac massage (p. 171) to improve the circulation if a bradycardia (less than 100/min) persists.

Delay in spontaneous breathing

Breathing may not occur for several minutes despite the improvement in heart rate and colour. This could be due to oversedation or hypoglycaemia. These conditions cannot be distinguished by clinical signs so ask an assistant to inject the following substances into a peripheral or umbilical vein while you continue to expand the lungs:

Dextrose water 5%	– 2 ml
Naloxone	– 0,05 mg

These are the recommended dosages for a full term baby. The response is usually dramatic.

Failure to respond to resuscitation

Most depressed babies (99%) breathe adequately following these procedures. The remainder may have ominous signs such as:

- an absent heart beat or bradycardia (less than 60/min)
- apnoea or gasping
- cyanosis or pallor of mucosae
- hypotension or prolonged blanching of the skin after compression
- hypotonia
- fixed dilated pupils.

Treatment

Attempt to identify a correctable factor such as blood loss (p. 224) or pneumothorax (p. 180).

Use a blood volume expander, such as normal saline or stabilised human serum (10 ml/kg), to improve perfusion, and obtain an X-ray of the chest.

Discontinue resuscitation if these factors are not applicable and the clinical state has not improved.

The likelihood of hypoxic brain damage is high and the chance of recovery is negligible.

Apgar score 4–7

Hold a resuscitator mask firmly over the baby's nose and mouth and flow oxygen through the circuit (4 l/min).

Flick the feet with a finger.

If regular breathing is not established within 30 seconds then expand the lungs with face mask or endotracheal tube ventilation.

Outcome

Skilful resuscitation ensures the recovery of most depressed babies.

The following infants need to be observed after birth:

- Preterm babies – as they are liable to develop hyaline membrane disease.
- Meconium-stained babies – as they

may show symptoms of aspiration pneumonia.

- Babies with abnormal neurological signs and those with low five-minute Apgar scores. Preceding fetal hypoxaemia may have caused hypoxic-ischaemic encephalopathy (p. 140).

Other organs such as the kidneys and heart might also have been damaged. The long-term outlook depends on the degree of hypoxaemia and ischaemia which preceded resuscitation. Cerebral palsy, mental retardation and seizures are the result of these complications. Follow-up examinations are essential for those who were severely asphyxiated at birth.

Techniques

Face mask ventilation
A variety of resuscitators are used for the newborn. They must not generate pressures of more than 30 cmH$_2$O.

The Ambu resuscitator (Fig. 13.4)
This consists of a face mask, valve and bag that can be autoclaved. It can be attached to an endotracheal tube by removing the mask.

Method
- Lie the baby with the face up and the neck semi-extended.

- Attach an oxygen line to the resuscitator and let the gas flow at 4 l/min.
- Hold the mask firmly over the baby's nose and mouth and squeeze the bulb rapidly (60–120 times a minute).

Sufficient oxygen should enter the airways to inflate the lungs. Some gas will pass into the stomach. It can be expelled later through a nasogastric tube.

Endotracheal intubation
A size 2,5 mm endotracheal tube is suitable for infants over 1 500 g. A 2,0 mm tube can be used for the smaller ones.

Method
Lie the baby on a flat surface with the face up and the head fully extended. With the left hand insert a straight-bladed laryngoscope (appropriate size) (p. 171) along the surface of the tongue. Ensure that the tongue does not slip to the side.

When the blade tip reaches the angle between the epiglottis and the base of the tongue, lever up the epiglottis to expose the vocal cords.

A better view is obtained by asking an assistant to apply external pressure on the larynx.

Insert the endotracheal tube between the vocal cords. The narrow portion of a shouldered tube extends about 2 cm

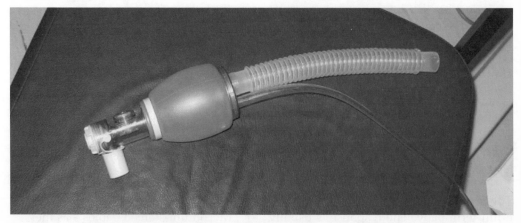

Fig. 13.4. *The Ambu resuscitator with a face mask attachment*

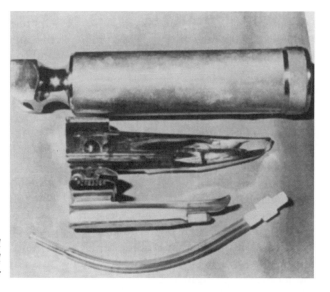

Fig. 13.5. *A suitable kit for laryngeal intubation. The tube attachment will fit a Samson resuscitator*

below the vocal cords. The broad portion rests lightly on the cords to provide an airtight fit.

Remove the blade and strap the tube to the chin. Apply intermittent positive pressure with a resuscitator or with a mechanical ventilator.

Complications
Trauma to the larynx or pneumothorax, passage of the tube into a bronchus or into the oesophagus.

External cardiac massage
Place a hand around the baby's chest and compress the mid sternum against the vertebral column with the thumb. Do this 100 to 120 times a minute. You should be able to feel a femoral pulse with each compression.

Complications
Fractures of ribs or sternum, rupture of the liver, haemopericardium, or pneumo- or haemothorax.

Resuscitation unit

A well-illuminated area is set aside in each delivery ward for the care of the baby. A wall clock with a second hand should be visible from here. The ideal unit incorporates a table with an over-head infrared heater, a mechanical suction apparatus, an oxygen supply and an infant ventilator.

In the absence of such a unit the following substitutes can be used:
- A table or trolley with a flat surface.
- Wall attachments or cylinders for oxygen and vacuum suction, infant resuscitator.
- Water bottles with a double layer of towelling to provide a warm surface.

A drawer on the resuscitation table should contain the following:

Equipment
- Stethoscope.
- Disposable endotracheal tubes with fittings – sizes 2,0, 2,5 and 3,0 mm.
- Infant laryngoscope with spare batteries and bulbs.
- Laryngoscope blades – Miller size 00 for infants under 1 500 g; size 0 for infants under 2 500 g; size 1 for term babies.
- Suction and nasogastric catheters – sizes 5, 8 and 10 French.
- Syringes, needles and IV cannulas (24 and 26 gauge).

Drugs
- Naloxone 0,2 mg/ml.
- Vitamin K$_1$ 1 mg.

Fluids
- Sodium bicarbonate 4% – 10 ml ampoules.
- Dextrose 5% – 10 ml ampoules.
- Dextrose water 10% – 200 ml vacolitres.

Miscellaneous
Test tubes, identification tags, scissors, forceps, umbilical clamps, sterile swabs.

Check all items daily and replace those that have been used. Ensure that the laryngoscope light is bright and that all endotracheal tubes, resuscitator and ventilator fittings are interchangeable.

RESPIRATORY DISTRESS

This accounts for up to 30% of neonatal deaths. The condition is caused by intra- or extrapulmonary factors, many of which are unique to this age group.

The following are common:

Pulmonary causes
- Hyaline membrane disease.
- Transient tachypnoea.
- Meconium aspiration pneumonia.
- Congenital bacterial pneumonia.
- Pneumothorax.

Extrapulmonary causes
- Patent ductus arteriosus (p. 194).
- Congenital heart disease (p. 192).

Diagnosis
The clinical presentation is often non-specific and is characterised by at least two of the following signs:
- Tachypnoea – a sustained respiratory rate over 60 per minute.
- Rib and sternal recession (Fig. 13.6).
- Expiratory grunting.
- Cyanosis.

Distressed babies other than those with the mildest signs should be investigated and treated in an intensive care unit.

Indications for referral to an ICU:
- Less than 1 500 g in weight.
- Oxygen requirements in excess of 40%.
- Cyanosis or apnoea.

Investigations
The following are important:

Chest X-ray
Obtain a radiograph in all cases. Often this is the only way to detect underlying pathology.

Gastric fluid
Collect a few millilitres for:
Bubble test: Mix equal quantities of fluid and absolute alcohol in a clean test tube. Cover the top with parafilm and shake for 30 seconds. The lungs are considered to be mature if foam collects at the surface of the mixture.
Microscopy: Smear a drop of fluid onto a glass slide for a Gram stain. This test is to detect meconium, polymorphs and bacteria.

Blood
Obtain capillary blood for a total white cell and band cell count (p. 232) to detect infection.

Urine
Send a specimen for a Group B streptococcal latex test to detect the streptococcal antigen.

Common pulmonary causes of respiratory distress can usually be identified by these preliminary tests (Table 13.2).

Specific diseases
Hyaline membrane disease
A normally grown preterm baby can

TABLE 13.2

	Diagnostic aids in respiratory distress.				
	Test	Hyaline membrane disease	Transient tachypnoea	Meconium aspiration pneumonia	Strep pneumonia
Gastric aspirate	Bubbles	Absent	Present	Present	Present
	Pus or bacteria	Absent	Absent	Absent	Present
Blood	Stab count	Normal	Normal	Normal	Raised
Urine	Strep latex	Negative	Negative	Negative	Positive
Chest X-ray		Diffuse granular pattern Air bronchograms	Hyperinflation Hilar streaking	Patchy atelectasis	Resembles HMD or patchy pneumonia

develop respiratory distress because of immature lungs. The likelihood is greatest under 34 weeks of gestation.

This syndrome is aptly called surfactant deficiency disease. The lung alveoli lacking surfactant collapse on expiration and considerable effort is needed for re-expansion.

Clinical signs

A significant number of babies are asphyxiated at birth and have to be resuscitated. The lungs offer resistance to inflation owing to their decreased compliance.

The course is progressive. Tachypnoea, sternal recession and expiratory grunting are prominent and cyanosis may occur if oxygen therapy is delayed. Very small babies may develop irregular breathing and bouts of apnoea.

Bowel sounds may be absent and the passage of meconium can be delayed for several days. Generalised oedema is usually noted within 24 hours.

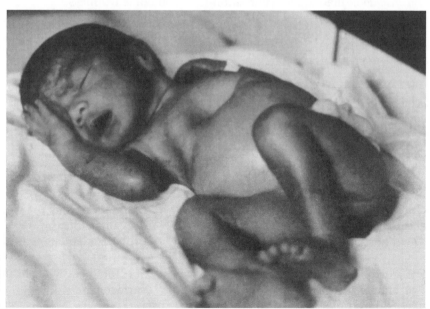

Fig. 13.6 *Rib retraction and sternal retraction*

Fig. 13.7 *Hyaline membrane disease*

Note the coarse granular pattern
and air bronchograms

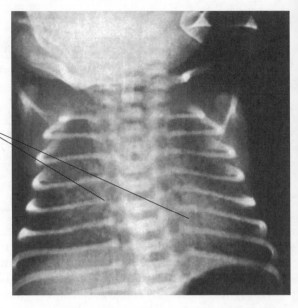

Metabolic derangements

If treatment is inadequate or delayed the following can occur:

Hypoxaemia: Imperfect matching of blood and air at alveolar level as well as right to left shunting of blood through the foramen ovale and ductus arteriosus lead to a reduced arterial oxygen tension (PaO_2).

Hypercapnoea: Inadequate ventilation results in retention of carbon dioxide and a fall in pH due to the accumulation of carbonic acid.

Metabolic acidaemia: Tissue hypoxia elevates the serum lactates which contributes up to 30% excess acid in the blood and lowers the pH.

Hypoglycaemia: The work of breathing is increased tenfold and may lower blood sugar by depleting liver glycogen.

Other abnormalities include azotaemia and hyperkalaemia due to the breakdown of tissue from hypoxia.

Special investigations

The bubble test on gastric fluid is negative and radiological signs are typical.

The size of the lung fields is diminished and there is a diffuse granular appearance due to alveolar collapse (Fig. 13.7). The conducting passages show prominent air bronchograms and the outline of the heart and thymus is often obscured.

Pathology features: The lungs are dark red and of liver-like consistency, and they sink in water. Any fluid expressed from them is frothless.

Histological examination shows intense alveolar collapse with dilated terminal bronchioles and alveolar ducts that are lined with hyaline material (the hyaline membrane).

Electron microscopy reveals the underlying alveolar surface to be disrupted in these regions.

Treatment

These are the principles for all causes of respiratory distress:

- Maintain normal oxygenation.
- Prevent acidosis.
- Provide adequate warmth, energy and fluid.
- Specific therapy for example surfactant

Oxygenation

At a primary care centre oxygen is essential even in the absence of cyanosis, which is a late clinical sign of hypoxaemia. Use a blender to regulate the concentration of oxygen and humidify the gas in a nebuliser. Flow it into a perspex hood that covers the baby's face and head.

Set the initial concentration at 40% and then measure oxygen saturation in baby's hand or foot (p. 187). Adjust the blender to maintain a saturation between 89 and 92%. This ensures a normal arterial oxygen tension (8–12 kPa).

Prevent excessive or inadequate oxygenation by:

- monitoring oxygen saturation continuously with a pulse oximeter
- maintaining a stable oxygen environment at all times.

A brief fall in oxygen concentration, from removal of the head box, for example, can result in cyanosis and apnoea.

In an intensive care unit oxygenation is best achieved by Continuous Positive Airway Pressure (CPAP) ventilation.

CPAP

A distressed baby attempts to expand lung alveoli by grunting. This Valsalva manoeuvre provides a functional residual capacity by keeping air in the lungs during expiration.

A similar effect can be produced or enhanced by breathing against a continuous positive airway pressure. This prevents collapse of the alveoli and infants who have signs of respiratory distress should receive CPAP as soon after birth as possible.

The most suitable device is a flow-driver. It has a specially designed nosepiece which fits snugly into the nostrils and ensures a constant and stable positive pressure to the lungs (nCPAP). This increases the functional residual capacity and reduces the work of breathing fourfold.

Indications: Use nCPAP as soon after birth as possible for all infants who are suspected of having hyaline membrane disease. Allow air to drain from the stomach through an oro- or nasogastric tube.

Intermittent positive pressure ventilation (IPPV)

Use ventilatory support for a baby who develops apnoea or who cannot maintain O_2 saturation above 89% despite being given CPAP. In most cases tracheal intubation is necessary.

Assisted ventilation has many hazards. Ensure safety by:

- keeping the mean airway pressure as low as possible
- allowing expiratory time to exceed inspiratory time
- transilluminating the chest frequently to detect a pneumothorax (p. 180).

Acid-base correction

Adequate oxygenation and ventilation prevents respiratory or metabolic acidaemia.

Respiratory acidaemia: Hypercapnoea is invariably present in hyaline membrane disease, but the side-effects of excessive carbon dioxide are usually preceded by those of hypoxaemia. Hypercapnoea is rarely the primary indication for IPPV unless $PaCO_2$ exceeds 9 kPa and the pH is less than 7,25.

Metabolic acidaemia: A severe acidaemia (pH below 7,25, HCO_3 below 18 mmol/l) needs correction. Sodium bicarbonate 4% is suitable. Give 0,25 mmol of this solution intravenously per minute for 30 minutes and recheck the acid-base status.

A mild or moderate acidaemia (pH 7,25–7,35, HCO_3 above 18 mmol/l) usually does not require correction with $NaHCO_3$.

Warmth, energy and fluid

Nurse a distressed baby in a closed

incubator or open crib to provide a neutrothermal environment.

Prevent hypoglycaemia by giving an intravenous solution of 10% dextrose water and introduce milk feeds after the acute phase (p. 68).

Contraindications to nasogastric feeding are:

- nCPAP, because of abdominal distension
- vomiting
- ileus.

Parenteral nutrition (p. 71) is needed if milk feeds cannot be commenced within three days of birth.

Specific therapy

Surfactant replacement is a major advance in the prevention and treatment of hyaline membrane disease. It has decreased the incidence and mortality significantly without major side-effects. Treatment necessitates intubation of the larynx and must be undertaken only by those familiar with the technique.

Prevention: Preterm babies, especially those under 34 weeks' gestation, may be given surfactant immediately after birth. About one-third have mature lungs and will receive it unnecessarily. As the product is very expensive many centres reserve treatment for established disease (see rescue therapy below).

Rescue: Respiratory distress should be severe enough to require an environmental oxygen concentration of at least 40% and a suitable recipient must not have obvious infection, intracranial haemorrhage or congenital abnormalities.

In centres with limited budgets weight will also be a consideration and treatment may be reserved for those over 750 g who have a good prognosis. Early treatment (within eight hours) is more effective than late treatment.

Advantages:

- The mortality rate is reduced.
- The duration of ventilatory support is shortened.
- Air leaks such as pneumothorax are infrequent.

Disadvantages:

- The product is expensive.

Surfactant is injected into the trachea in divided doses. This encourages dispersal of the substance into the alveoli.

Dose: 100–200 mg/kg.

Check oxygen saturation. Lung compliance improves rapidly and can result in overventilation in babies on IPPV. Adjust the oxygen concentration and respiratory pressure to maintain normal acid-base values.

Record blood pressure and pulse rate. A decrease in pulmonary vascular resistance can cause left to right shunting of blood through the ductus arteriosus. This may result in a fall in blood pressure and a decrease in cerebral blood flow. It rarely happens but needs treatment with a volume expander such as normal saline or stabilised human serum (p. 310).

About 30% of infants do not respond or relapse within 24 hours and require additional surfactant.

Nursing care

The staffing of a neonatal intensive care unit is costly and the recommended 1:1 nurse-to-baby ratio is unattainable in many underdeveloped countries. If this is so, ensure that at least a 1:3 ratio is applied. Constantly move among the infants on the alert for warning signs. The sight of a small infant 'smothered' by monitoring devices is alarming for parents and a nurse is pivotal in allaying their fears

Encourage parents to touch and hold their infant and permit visiting at all times. Explain the need for and the function of equipment. Provide parents with the relevant facts of an illness. Stress normal aspects such as alertness, colour and activity, and offer hope when there is a reasonable chance of recovery.

Encourage the mother to express her milk daily and impress upon her the essential role that she plays in promoting the nutrition and recovery of her baby. Allow her to kangaroo care her sick infant even for periods when assisted ventilation is necessary, and encourage breastfeeding.

Important complications
Cyanosis and apnoea: These may be caused by preventable factors such as inadequate oxygenation, aspiration of a feed, or hypoglycaemia.

Air leaks: Interstitial emphysema, pneumothorax or pneumomediastinum can occur at any stage, particularly during resuscitation, IPPV or CPAP.

Suspect a pneumothorax if the oxygen requirements increase unexpectedly or if apnoea occurs. Clinical signs may not be obvious so establish the diagnosis by transillumination or X-ray of the chest.
Unconjugated bilirubinaemia: Jaundice occurs in many babies and may require phototherapy.
Intraventricular haemorrhage: This is probably the commonest cause of death and morbidity. A pneumothorax or excessive crying increases the risk by raising the intracranial pressure.
Chronic lung disease (bronchopulmonary dysplasia): This taxing problem results from severe disease, oxygen toxicity and barotrauma. It is characterised by dependence on oxygen and mechanical ventilation and must be considered if these are needed for more than two weeks. Tachypnoea, sternal recession, diminished air entry and crepitations are typical signs.

Radiological features: Multiple areas of hyperinflation and atelectasis give the lungs a 'bubbly' appearance.

The chronic respiratory distress can be exacerbated by infections or heart failure. Appropriate therapy includes antibiotics, diuretics and digoxin. Dexamethasone is no longer favoured as it has been implicated in an increased risk for cerebral palsy. The outlook is variable. Survivors need oxygen for many months, but can improve to the extent of having normal lungs by four to six years of age. Recurrent chest infections occur in the early years.

The risk of chronic lung disease can be reduced by the early use of nCPAP breathing, low tidal volumes and sufficient positive end expiratory pressure (PEEP) during IPPV, the avoidance of hypocapnoea and the provision of adequate nutrition.
Pneumonia: The risk of infection is enhanced by intubation, tracheal suctioning and mechanical ventilation. Antibiotics are not ordinarily prescribed for hyaline membrane disease but may be needed during intubation.
Patent ductus arteriosus: Blood may shunt from right to left in the early stages of the disease when pulmonary artery pressure is high. Later the shunt may reverse as oxygenation improves. The overloaded pulmonary circulation can cause pulmonary oedema and heart failure. Suspect a patent ductus arteriosus if assisted ventilation is needed for more than 48 hours.

Course and outcome
The majority (over 95%) recover.

The early days are critical and improvement usually occurs within a week. This is heralded by diuresis, diminished oxygen requirements and a reduced dependence on assisted ventilation in severe cases.

Antenatal prevention

Cortisone increases the production of sur-factant in fetal lungs. Women in preterm labour ought to have an amniocentesis to determine the presence of surfactant. When absent or inadequate, a 48-hour course of betamethasone (12 mg daily) is advisable. During the therapy every attempt is made to arrest labour.

Transient tachypnoea ('wet lung' syndrome)

This condition may be indistinguishable from hyaline membrane disease in the early stage. It usually occurs in near- or full-term babies who are delivered by Caesarean section following excessive maternal analgesia.

The cause is unknown but is thought to be due to a delay in the absorption of lung fluid from interstitial spaces. This produces a temporary decrease in lung compliance.

Diagnosis

The signs of respiratory distress are present from birth and the chest is over-distended.

Radiographs show hyperinflation of the lungs and prominent bronchovascular streaking at the hilum. Lung fissures may be filled with fluid.

The bubble test on gastric aspirate is positive.

Course

Oxygen requirements are variable and improvement usually occurs after 24 to 48 hours. Assisted ventilation is unnecessary and the prognosis is excellent.

Meconium aspiration pneumonia

A fetus subjected to severe hypoxia *in utero* may expel meconium and inhale the substance into the lungs during gasping. This causes airway obstruction, mucosal damage, pulmonary vasoconstriction and impairment of surfactant production.

The resultant 'chemical' pneumonia occurs mainly in growth-retarded babies as a consequence of fetal hypoxaemia.

Clinical presentation

At birth, meconium is often seen in the pharynx and on the skin. The placenta, cord and fingernails are stained brown in longstanding cases.

Asphyxia is common and signs of respiratory distress are evident after resuscitation, such as the chest is overdistended and crepitations may be heard in the lungs.

Resultant hypoxic ischaemic brain damage may cause hypotonia and seizures.

Blood and protein may be detected in the urine as a result of hypoxic renal damage.

The gastric fluid contains meconium and the bubble test is positive.

Radiological signs show hyperinflation of the lungs and multiple areas of atelectasis and consolidation (Fig. 13.8). A pneumomediastinum or pneumothorax is present in up to 20% of cases.

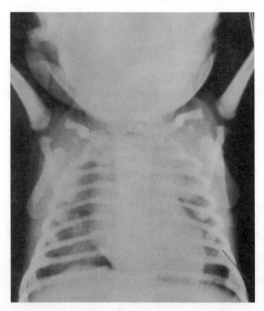

Fig. 13.8 *Meconium aspiration pneumonia*

Treatment

Meconium aspiration is preventable, as it is a consequence of intrauterine hypoxia. Fetal distress must be avoided especially in a pregnancy complicated by growth retardation. Signs of fetal distress, particularly meconium-stained liquor, indicate the possibility of aspiration and the need for resuscitation at birth.

Suction the nasopharynx after delivery to remove meconium. If crying and movements are vigorous transfer the baby to the ICU for further assessment. Oxygen therapy may be needed during transportation. If resuscitation is needed, inspect the larynx and intubate the trachea if thick meconium is seen beyond the vocal cords. This is rarely necessary and should be done only by one skilled in the procedure. Suction the material from the airway. Cease after five seconds if nothing is obtained.

Meconium should later be cleared from the stomach with a 2% sodium bicarbonate solution.

Treat the distressed baby similarly to one with hyaline membrane disease and constantly check for a pneumothorax.

In a severe case consider the following additional treatment:

- An antibiotic, such as ceftriaxone – to protect the denuded mucosal surfaces from infection.
- Dexamethasone – to reduce inflammation.
- Surfactant – to improve the lung compliance.

Specific therapy will be needed for hypoxic brain or renal damage.

Outcome

Approximately 50% of infants die, mainly from hypoxic-ischaemic encephalopathy. Survivors usually regain normal lung function within weeks, but some may have neurological sequelae from hypoxic brain damage.

Pneumonia

A fetus can develop pneumonia from bacteria that enter the uterine cavity through the cervix. The risk is enhanced by:

- premature labour
- prolonged rupture of membranes (over 18 hours)
- prolonged labour and obstetric manipulations.

Group B streptococcus is the most common cause in the first week. Later, cross-infection can occur from organisms such as *Klebsiella* and *Pseudomonas*. Prolonged endotracheal intubation increases the risk.

Rare causes include *Treponema*, *Listeria*, rubella and cytomegalovirus.

Diagnosis

Respiratory distress occurs soon after birth in streptococcal disease but later in cross-infection. The gastric contents contain polymorphs and bacteria and the bubble test is positive. The neutrophil stab count is frequently raised and streptococcal antigen may be detected in the urine.

X-ray signs vary from coarse mottling to diffuse granularity in streptococcal infection.

Treatment

An antibiotic, like ceftriaxone, is essential for a suspected or confirmed pneumonia and is given for 7 to 10 days.

The antibiotic may have to be changed depending on the results of bacteriological cultures.

Some infants will need oxygen and assisted ventilation depending on the severity of infection. The indications are similar to those for hyaline membrane disease.

Outcome

Pneumonia rarely causes death unless associated with streptococcal septicaemia.

Pneumothorax

A pneumothorax usually results from the rupture of an alveolar sac. Air tracks up the vascular sheath into the mediastinum and thence into the pleural cavity. This can be spontaneous but is more likely to result from:

- vigorous resuscitation
- abnormal lungs, such as hypoplasia, meconium aspiration
- ventilator therapy.

Clinical signs

Suspect a pneumothorax in a baby with respiratory distress who deteriorates unexpectedly, for example cyanosis, apnoea. The signs are not always obvious. They include:

- Abdominal distension.
- Apparent enlargement of the liver.
- Overdistension of one or both sides of the chest.
- Poor chest movement.
- Hyperresonance to percussion.
- Diminished air entry.
- Diminished heart sounds and a displaced apex beat.

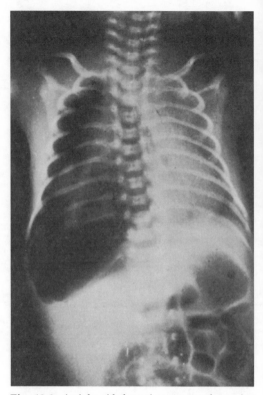

Fig. 13.9 *A right-sided tension pneumothorax in hyaline membrane disease. Note the right lung, which is too stiff to collapse*

Diagnosis

An X-ray of the chest (AP and lateral views) is imperative when a pneumothorax is suspected. The entrapped air contrasts with that in the lungs in that it is dark and has no lung markings (Fig. 13.9).

Transillumination of the chest with a fibroscope assists in the early diagnosis. This non-invasive technique is safe and is recommended for all babies with respiratory distress. When transilluminated in the dark, the chest lights up like a lantern on the side of the pneumothorax (Fig. 13.10).

Treatment

Normal lungs: Specific treatment is not necessary in most cases. Oxygen therapy hastens the reabsorption of trapped air.

Abnormal lungs: Intrathoracic pressure must be relieved as an underlying stiff lung cannot collapse to accommodate the trapped air. The compressed heart and large veins may cause tamponade and shock. A drain is inserted into the pleural space to remove air, thereby reducing pressure.

Drainage of a pneumothorax

Give the baby an analgesic (morphine 0,1 mg/kg IV) and clean the chest wall with Hibitane in spirit. The drainage site is located in the anterior axillary line at the second or third intercostal space.

Make a 2 mm incision in the skin and dissect the underlying tissue by reopening the tips of a mosquito forceps until the parietal layer of the pleura is reached.

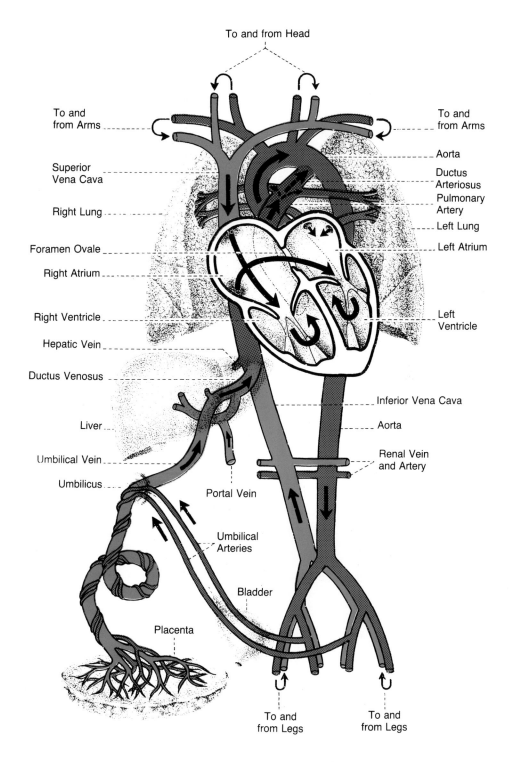

COLOUR PLATE I

The fetal circulation

Oxygenated blood (red) from the placenta flows through the ductus venosus into the inferior vena cava (stippled red). It is then pumped through the left atrium and ventricle into the aorta (stippled red)

Deoxygenated blood (blue) from organs is channelled through the right atrium and ventricle into the pulmonary artery (mauve). It bypasses the lungs through the ductus arteriosus (mauve) and mixes with blood in the aorta (stippled red) to be returned to the placenta

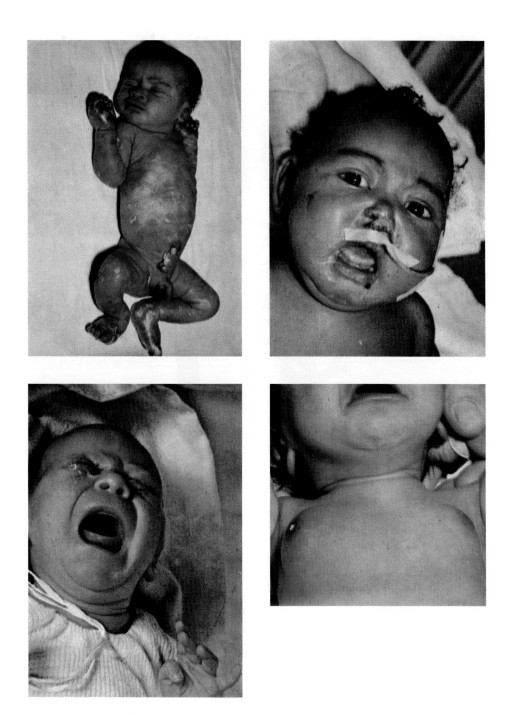

COLOUR PLATE II

Upper left: The bullous skin lesions of congenital syphilis
Upper right: The nasal discharge of congenital syphilis
Lower left: Gonococcal ophthalmia neonatorum
Lower right: Neonatal mastitis caused by the staphylococcus aureus

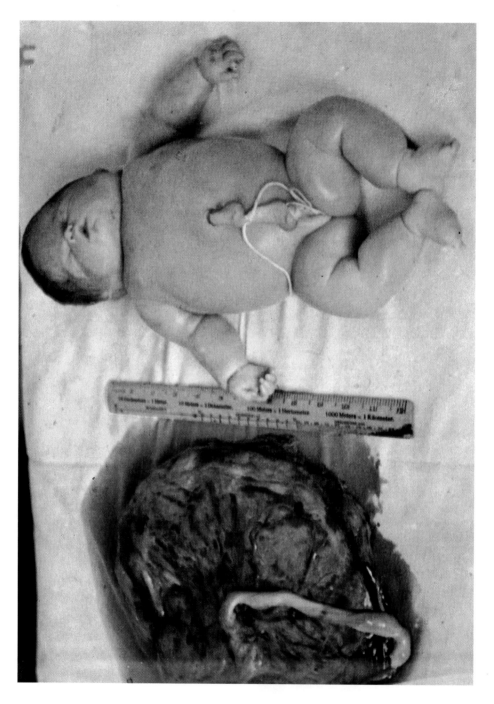

COLOUR PLATE III

Hydrops foetalis in severe rhesus disease
Infant: Grossly oedematous and pale
Placenta: Abnormally large

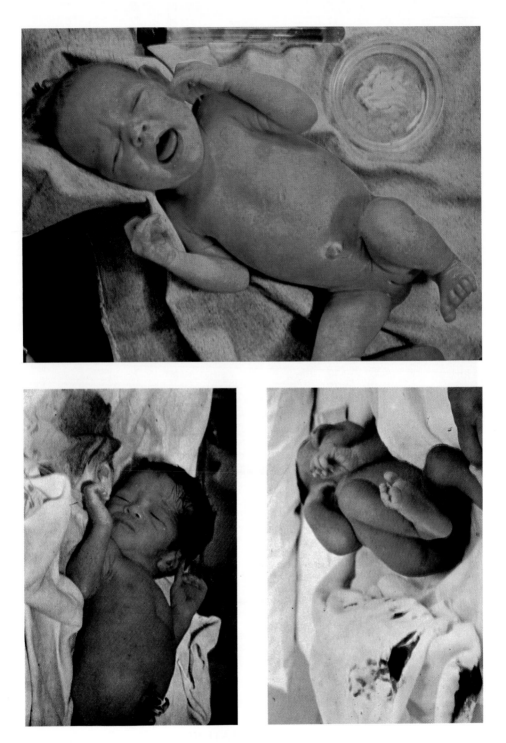

COLOUR PLATE IV

Upper: Atresia of the bile ducts. The infant, as a result of an obstructed flow to bile, has developed jaundice, pale stools and dark urine

Lower left: Intestinal obstruction: The infant shows marked abdominal distension and has vomited bile-stained material

Lower right: A melaena stool

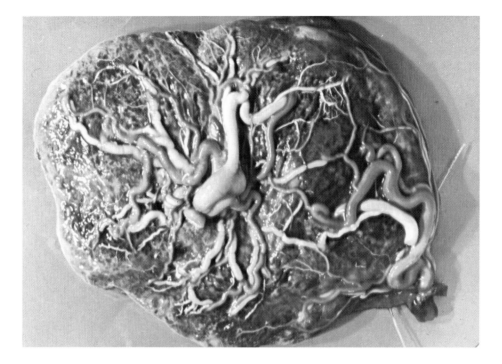

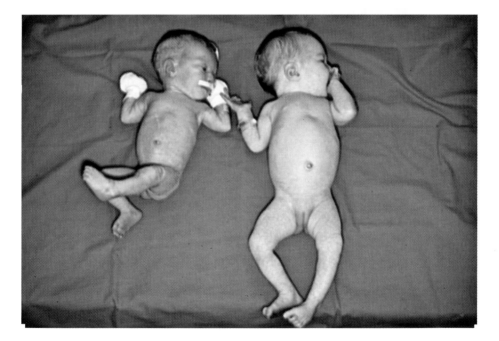

COLOUR PLATE V

A twin pregnancy

Upper: The blood vessels of this monochorionic, diamniotic placenta have been filled with dye. The two circulations show numerous vascular anastamoses

Lower: The twins from this placenta show characteristic features:

A. The transfusion syndrome: The large infant has lost blood to the small one who is plethoric

B. Intra-uterine growth retardation: The smaller twin was attached to the poorly developed portion of the placenta

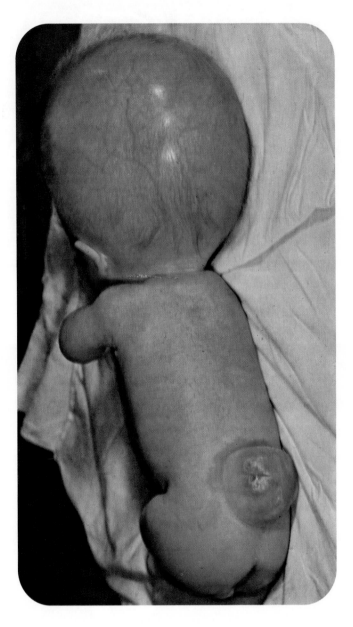

COLOUR PLATE VI

Hydrocephalus with a meningomyelocele: Posterior view

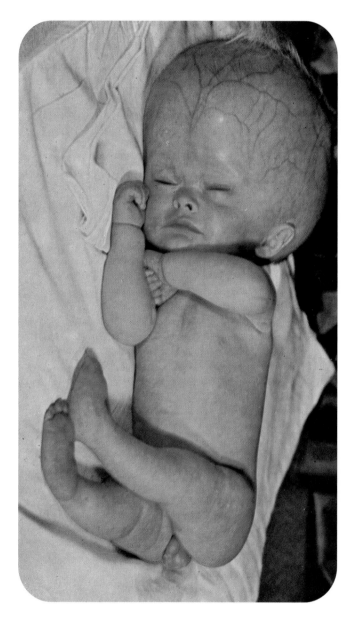

COLOUR PLATE VII

Hydrocephalus with a meningomyelocele: Frontal view of same infant. Note the paralysis of the lower limbs

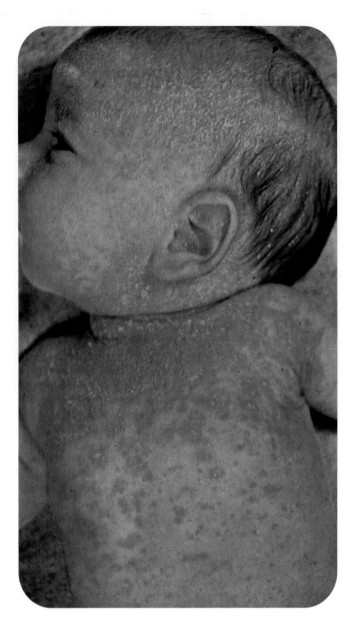

COLOUR PLATE VIII

Seborrhoeic dermatitis: The widespread form is termed `Leiner's disease'

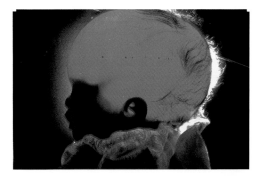
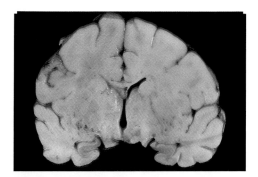
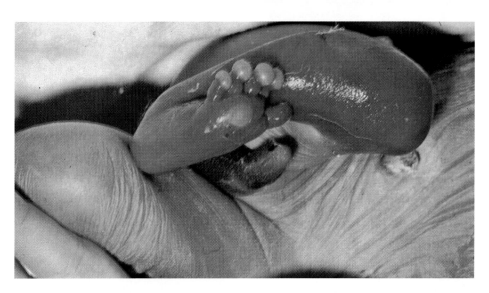
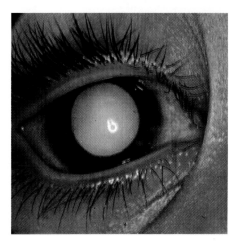
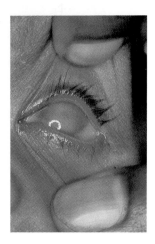

COLOUR PLATE IX

Uper left: Hydranencephaly. The head transilluminates like a lantern
Upper right: Kernicterus. The basal ganglia are stained yellow by unconjugated bilirubin
Middle: Epidermolysis bullosa. The loss of skin has been confined to one limb
Lower left: A congenital cataract of the lens. A prominent epicanthic skin fold is also present
Lower right: A thickened opaque cornea which is associated with absence of the anterior chamber of the eye

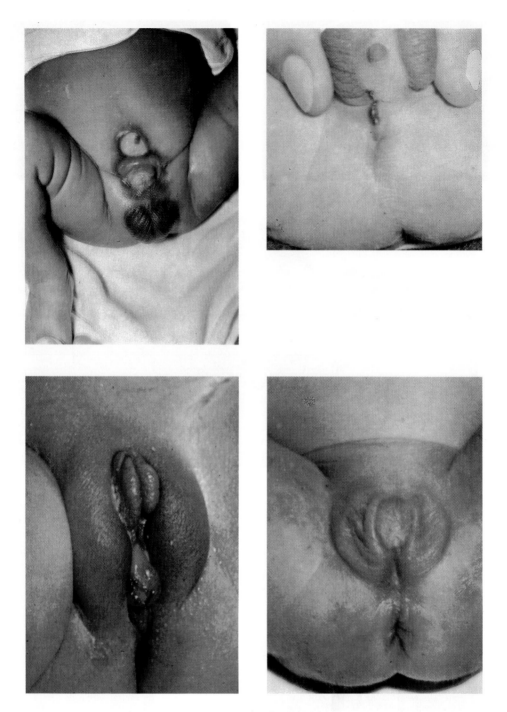

COLOUR PLATE X

Upper left: Extropia vesicae. The mucosal surface of the bladder is exposed on to the abdomen

Upper right: An ano-rectal malformation. The anus cannot be identified and meconium is seen tracking along a sinus to the scrotum

Lower left: A hymenal tag. This regresses spontaneously

Lower right: Ambiguous genitalia: The infant will need investigation for intersex

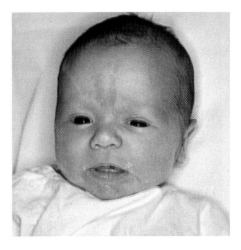

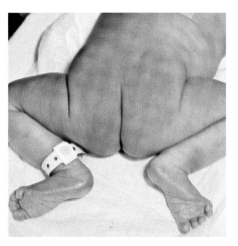

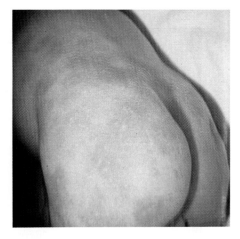

COLOUR PLATE XI

Upper left: A capillary haemangioma of the forehead

Upper right: Mongolian spots on the buttocks. These commonly occur in dark-skinned infants

Middle: Erythema toxicum. This common rash consists of yellow papules surrounded by a red base. It fades spontaneously

Lower left: The Harlequin colour change. Vasomotor activity has caused dilatation of blood vessels to produce a characteristic pink colour of the lowermost portion of the body

Lower right: Normal vaginal discharge after birth

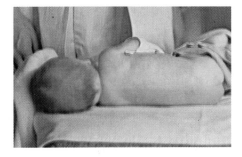

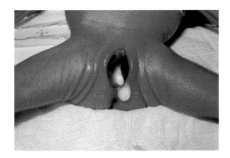

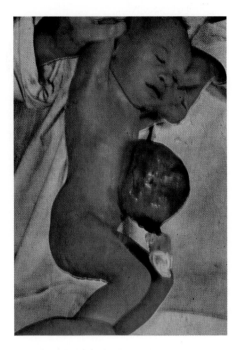
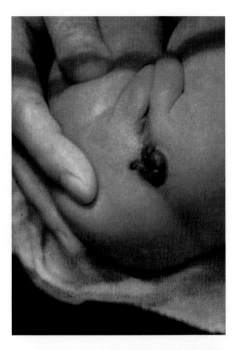
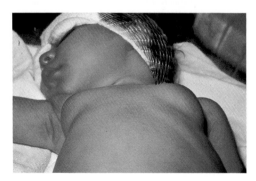
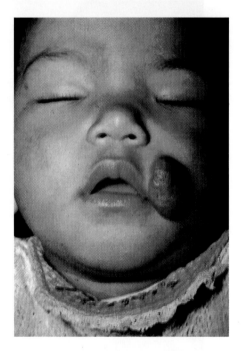

COLOUR PLATE XII

Upper left: Exomphalos. Portions of bowel and organs are contained in a sac outside the abdomen

Upper right: Haemorrhoids have prolapsed as a result of excessive rectal pressure in a breech delivery. They usually regress within a week

Lower left: Normal engorgement of breasts after birth

Lower right: A strawberry naevus. This increases in size and then gradually subsides without therapy

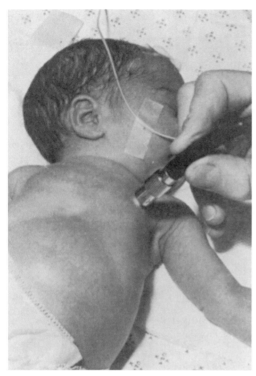

Fig. 13.10 *Transillumination of the chest. This is done hourly in cases of respiratory distress to detect a pneumothorax, which presents with an increased halo of light*

When this shiny membrane is pierced with the forceps air may gush out. Guide a plastic end-hole catheter (10 French) into the pleural cavity before removing the forceps.

Clamp the catheter and close the incision with a purse-string silk suture. Loop this around the catheter to prevent displacement.

Attach the catheter to an underwater drainage bottle and ensure that the water column moves on inspiration when the tube is unclamped.

Obtain an X-ray of the chest to check the position of the catheter and the amount of air in the pleural space.

When ventilator therapy is used it is necessary to suck off air from the chest. Attach a low-pressure pump to the drainage bottle and set the vacuum between 24 and 26 cmH_2O. The suction is continued for as long as air drains from the pleural space. The tube is then clamped for 48 hours. Remove the catheter if no more air accumulates in the chest cavity.

Pneumomediastinum
Aetiology
The predisposing factors are similar to those of a pneumothorax (p. 180).

Diagnosis
The chest bulges anteriorly and is hyper-resonant. On an AP X-ray the heart is bordered by a translucent area which lies between it and the sternum on the lateral view (Fig. 13.11).

Treatment
The trapped air rarely causes complications and is reabsorbed within days.

Less common causes of respiratory distress
- Cardiac failure (p. 190).
- Persistent pulmonary hypertension (p. 197).

Several congenital abnormalities also cause breathing difficulties. They include:

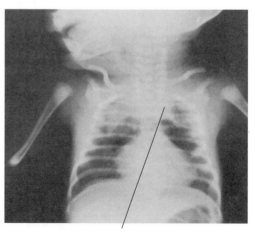

Note the clear outline of the thymus

Fig. 13.11 *A pneumomediastinum*

- Choanal atresia (p. 157).
- Congenital stridor.
- Diaphragmatic hernia.
- Tracheo-oesophageal fistula (p. 213).
- Lobar emphysema.

Congenital stridor
Common cause: Laryngomalacia.
Uncommon cause: Congenital abnormalities of surrounding structures, e.g. great vessels may compress the trachea.

Laryngomalacia
The following features are characteristic:
- Inspiratory 'crowing' is noted several weeks or months after birth.
- The stridor is exaggerated by excitement and usually disappears during sleep.
- Crying is usually normal and cyanosis is absent.
- The infant continues to thrive and is not bothered by the impediment.

Laryngoscopy
The larynx and surrounding tissues are soft and collapse during inspiration. The epiglottis is elongated.

Course
No treatment is needed and the stridor usually subsides within a year.

Note
Further investigations are required if the presentation or course is atypical, such as onset at birth, spells of cyanosis, hoarse cry, failure to thrive. Investigations include X-ray neck, bronchoscopy, CT scan and angiography.

Diaphragmatic hernia (Fig. 13.12 and 13.13)
Embryology
The diaphragm develops from pleuroperitoneal outgrowths of the lateral and posterior thoracic cavity. These fuse together by the eighth week of gestation to form the major portion of the diaphragm. Failure of fusion can result in a diaphragmatic hernia. This is five times more likely to occur on the left than on the right side. The aetiology is unknown. Various drugs have been implicated, like quinine and nitrofen, and vitamin A deficiency. A genetic defect involving chromosome 15q is also a possibility in some cases.

Classification
Important herniae include the following:
- Left posterolateral, i.e. foramen of Bochdalek. This is the most common type. The stomach, spleen and portion of the liver and intestine can enter the thoracic cavity to displace the heart and compress the developing lungs. This results in varying degrees of lung and pulmonary vascular hypoplasia, particularly on the left side. The arterioles show excessive amounts of muscle tissue.

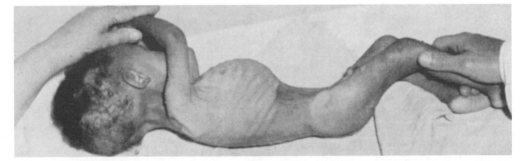

Fig. 13.12 *The small scaphoid abdomen with a diaphragmatic hernia*

- Anterior, i.e. foramen of Morgani. This is a rare form of hernia.

Before birth
The defect can be detected by ultrasound examination which is also prognostic. If the liver has not entered the chest, the chance of a livebirth is over 90%. About 50% are stillborn and most of these have additional abnormalities.

Clinical presentation
Signs depend on the extent of herniation and the degree of lung hypoplasia.

Severe lung hypoplasia and herniation: The infant is often asphyxiated at birth and may gasp, but cannot establish normal breathing. The lungs display marked resistance to inflation despite the use of tracheal intubation and artificial ventilation. Approximately 50% die soon after birth because of irreversable pulmonary failure.

Obtain an X-ray of the chest to exclude a tension pneumothorax before resuscitation is abandoned.

Moderate or mild lung hypoplasia: The infant may not require resuscitation or will respond well to lung ventilation.

Features include tachypnoea, rib recession, cyanotic episodes, small scaphoid abdomen (Fig. 13.13), right-sided heartbeats and sounds, and bowel sounds audible in left chest.

Note
Signs may be absent in mild cases and only present later in life.

Treatment
Intubate the trachea and ventilate the lungs with a bag resuscitator. Avoid face mask ventilation as the bowels in the chest may distend with air. Constantly deflate the stomach by aspirating air through a nasogastric tube. Elevate the head and chest and transfer the baby to a neonatal unit.

The outcome depends on the degree of lung hypoplasia. Persistent pulmonary

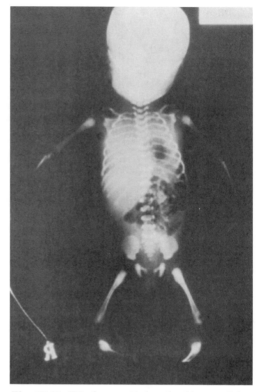

Fig. 13.13 *Diaphragmatic hernia. Air-containing bowel may be noted in the left chest*

hypertension is a significant problem that will need to be corrected (p. 199). Be careful not to overinflate the lungs during assisted ventilation. Use the lowest tidal volume that will maintain an arterial oxygen saturation above 85% and permit arterial carbon dioxide tension to rise to 6–7 kPa (45–55 mmHg) and the pH to fall to approximately 7.25. This is known as permissive hypercapnoea.

Surgery is undertaken only if ventilation is adequate. The postoperative survival rate is approximately 70%. Gastro-oesophageal reflux (p. 207) can be troublesome after surgery and must be addressed.

Eventration of the diaphragm
Part of the diaphragm may bulge into the chest because of muscle aplasia or nerve

paralysis. The signs resemble those of diaphragmatic hernia and the diagnosis is made by X-ray examination.

Treatment
The eventrated diaphragm is plicated.

Congenital lobar emphysema
Bronchial obstruction can cause lobar emphysema by a ball-valve effect. Air enters a lobe on inspiration but cannot be exhaled. Excessively compliant airways are thought to cause the obstruction.

Clinical signs
Emphysema must be distinguished from a pneumothorax. Respiratory distress is prolonged and becomes progressively worse. A radiological examination is needed to establish the diagnosis.

Treatment
The emphysematous lobe is excised.

APNOEIC ATTACKS

Periodic breathing
This occurs frequently in preterm babies in the first week. It consists of brief spells of apnoea (5 to 10 seconds). The mucosae remain pink and the heart rate and blood pH do not change significantly. Adverse effects are unlikely and the condition must be distinguished from true apnoea.

Recurrent apnoea
Babies under 1 500 g are prone to apnoeic attacks with cyanosis and bradycardia.

Characteristic features:
- A breathing pattern which becomes progressively more shallow and irregular and terminates in prolonged apnoea (more than 15 seconds).
- A fall in heart rate to below 100 beats per minute shortly before or during apnoea.
- Cyanosis of mucous membranes.

- A fall in blood pH.
- Absence of an underlying illness such as infection.

Initially breathing can be restarted by stimulation, e.g. flicking a foot, but eventually apnoea becomes refractory if not treated. Poor muscle control that causes obstruction to the upper airways, and unstable respiratory regulation in the brain, are reasons offered for the apnoea.

Treatment
Theophyline and caffeine can avert or prevent apnoea. The mode of action is uncertain, but is probably due to stimulation of the brain's respiratory centre.

Prophylactic treatment may be used for babies under 1 500 g, but must be tempered by the fact that long-term effects of these drugs are unknown.

Dosage: Theophyline – a loading dose of 4–6 mg/kg is followed by the maintenance amount of 1–3 mg/kg/day. Divided doses are given six-hourly for several weeks to maintain a blood level of 6–12 µg/ml.

Dosage: Caffeine – loading dose 10 mg/kg. Maintenance, 2,5–5 mg/kg once a day.

nCPAP: Nasal-prong treatment is recommended for an infant with established apnoea.

Discharge: An infant who has experienced recurrent apnoea of prematurity must be treated with caution.
- Provide parents with an apnoea mattress and resuscitation bag.
- Instruct them how to use face-mask ventilation should the baby develop apnoea.
- Continue aminophylline therapy for several months as the baby is at risk for sudden infant death.

Other causes
Apnoea can be precipitated by:
- a patent ductus arteriosus

- overheating
- aspiration of a feed
- hypoglycaemia
- infection.

Before labelling a baby as having apnoea of prematurity, check the temperature of the skin, inspect the pharynx for regurgitated milk, check the sugar level on heel blood, look for overt signs of sepsis and feel the pulses for evidence of patent ductus.

TECHNIQUES
Assisted ventilation
Mechanical ventilation can assist a distressed baby over critical periods by providing adequate gas exchange in the alveoli. The majority of infants who need assistance have stiff lungs as a result of hyaline membrane disease.

The therapy is hazardous if applied by inexperienced hands and must be confined to staff who are well versed in the procedure in intensive care units.

Numerous pressure or flow-controlled ventilators are available for the newborn, but no specific recommendation can be made. Successful management depends on the experience acquired from constant usage of a single model.

Basic requirements include:
- independent control of peak pressure, pump rate and inspiratory-to-expiratory ratio
- continuous positive airway pressure
- positive end-expiratory pressure
- a suitable humidifier
- a lightweight circuit with minimum dead space
- alarms – to indicate the failure of any system.

The device and its circuits must be easy to clean and sterilise after use.

Methods
Continuous positive pressure (CPAP) or intermittent positive pressure ventilation (IPPV) can be delivered through a nasal cannula or an endotracheal tube.

Nasal cannula
Flow-drivers have their own specially designed nasal connectors, which ensure stable and continuous positive pressure.

Insert the prongs into the nostrils and support the cannula upright by tying its flange to a cap fitted over the head. This avoids undue pressure on the nose, which must not be compressed or distorted during treatment. A constant check ensures that the cannula is in the correct position and that the prongs do not slip out of the nostrils. Turn the head to one side and keep it in that position for several hours.

Endotracheal tube
A suitable model is the Cole (Portex).

Sizes range from 2,0 to 3,0 mm internal diameter at the distal end.

Tubes are cut to lengths of 8–10 cm and then inserted through a flange (Portex). Very small babies require the narrowest and shortest tubes. The tip should lie halfway between the glottis and the bifurcation of the trachea after intubation. This position is checked on X-ray and adjusted if necessary.

Immobilise the tube by tying its flange to a cotton cap fitted over the head. Prevent displacement by encircling the tube with plaster strapping above the flange and fixing it to the chin.

CPAP
The majority of babies who will benefit from breathing against a constant positive pressure have reduced lung compliance as a result of hyaline membrane disease.

Set the ventilator to deliver a constant pressure of 5 cm H_2O and oxygen concentration at 40% through a gas blender. These values may need to be altered depending on blood gas results. Pressures rarely exceed 10 cm H_2O.

Weaning takes several days with an attempt to reduce the oxygen concentration. When this is below 50% decrease the pressure gradually.

A nasogastric tube is left open to ensure drainage of air from the stomach, especially when pressure is delivered through a nasal cannula.

IPPV

This treatment is used for severe hyaline membrane disease where CPAP has failed to maintain normal acid-base and blood gas values or where breathing efforts are too weak or absent.

Set the ventilator to deliver 50% oxygen at a peak pressure of 20 cmH$_2$O and a cycling rate of 50 to 60 per minute. Fix the inspiratory-to-expiratory ratio at 1:1,2 and the end expiratory pressure (PEEP) at 3 cm H$_2$O.

Measure oxygen saturation and adjust the concentration to give a saturation reading between 89 and 92%. Maintain these settings for 30 minutes, provided the infant remains pink. They may need adjustment when the results of blood gas analyses are available. Use the lowest tidal volume that will maintain normal oxygenation and acid-base balance.

Crying is to be avoided as it can increase the risk of complications such as pneumothorax.

During the recovery stage gradually wean the infant off the ventilator by reducing one factor at a time. Decrease oxygen concentration over several days and then reduce the peak pressure in increments.

The infant subsequently takes over the work of breathing, with occasional assistance from the ventilator and the use of CPAP.

Hyaline membrane disease is pressure-dependent and weaning is unlikely to be completed until peak pressures are below 15 cm H$_2$O.

A restless baby needs adequate analgesia. Morphine may be given continuously or intermittently, for example 0,1 mg/kg intravenous injection repeated every six hours.

Oscillation

In this form of ventilation the lungs are distended and very small volumes of air are introduced into them at rates of 500 to 2 000 oscillations min. This results in a rapid removal of carbon dioxide from the alveoli.

Indications

Oscillation is most effective for conditions that cause diffuse homogeneous lung disease such as:

- hyaline membrane disease
- pneumonia
- pulmonary haemorrhage.

It is also of use in very small infants (< 750 g) who have unstable lungs.

In non-homogeneous lung disease it may be tried when conventional ventilation has failed.

Important conditions in this category include:

- meconium aspiration pneumonia
- focal pneumonia
- interstitial emphysema (air leak syndrome).

An additional indication is lung hypoplasia. This is frequently associated with diaphragmatic hernia (p. 184).

Precautions

Oscillation is more exacting than conventional ventilation. The rapid removal of carbon dioxide can result in diminished blood flow to the brain and blood gas analysis has to be done frequently to ensure a safe level of PaCO$_2$.

Oscillation distends the lungs and repeat X-ray examination is advised to prevent overinflation.

Physiotherapy

An electric toothbrush provides gentle vibration and the covered head is applied to the chest several times a day. This enables mucus to be dislodged into the larger air passages.

Tracheobronchial toilet

Tracheal suctioning is done two or three times a day or when indicated.

Attach a sterile Argyle 5F polythene end-hole catheter to suction tubing and set the vacuum pressure at −1,0 kPa. Clean the attachment on the endotracheal tube with surgical spirits before it is opened. Use sterile gloves to guide the catheter down the endotracheal tube as far as it will go. This process should not exceed 15 seconds as the infant is liable to become hypoxic.

It may be repeated if secretions are not cleared at first attempt.

The nostrils and mouth are then cleared of mucus using a pressure of 2 kPa. Closed-circuit suctioning, for example Trach Care Mac may also be used. Oxygenation and assisted ventilation is maintained during the procedure and there is less chance of atelectasis. In addition, it can be used to introduce surfactant into the respiratory tract.

Measurement of oxygen saturation (SaO₂)

The continuous monitoring of oxygen saturation is desirable for ill babies.

A sensor that is attached to an extremity gauges the amount of oxygenated and reduced haemoglobin in the red cells during arterial pulsations. These measurements are displayed as oxygen saturation (SaO_2) and pulse rate. The correlation between SaO_2 and PaO_2 is illustrated in Fig. 13.1 (p. 161) and the safe range of SaO_2 is 89 to 92%.

Arterial blood – method of collection for PaO₂ and acid base analysis

Radial artery puncture (this is not recommended as a routine procedure) Ensure analgesia (p. 293)

Extend the infant's hand and locate the radial artery by dividing the wrist into thirds. The artery lies in the mid-portion of the radial third.

It can be identified as a dark band when the dorsum of the wrist is transilluminated with cold light.

Clean the site with an alcohol swab and insert a fine needle (26 gauge) through the skin at an angle of 60°. It usually transfixes the vessel and blood runs into the hub as the needle is slowly withdrawn. Collect this blood in a heparinised tube (100 μl).

Remove the needle and compress the site with a cotton swab for a minute. Cover the puncture mark with an adhesive dressing.

If blood is unobtainable or if the flow rate is inadequate reinsert the needle lateral or medial to the original site. Attempt the opposite radial artery should this fail.

This method is effective and safe, but can give inaccurate oxygen tension results if crying occurs. This usually subsides after the initial stab and blood can be collected while the infant is quiet.

When used with oxygen saturation monitoring, radial artery sampling is required once or twice a day if the infant's condition is stable.

Umbilical or peripheral artery catheterisation is advised if larger or frequent samples of blood are required.

Cardiovascular Disorders

THE FETAL CIRCULATION (Colour Plate I)

The fetal heart functions as a pump from the eighth week of gestation and circulates blood as follows:

Oxygenated blood from the placenta enters the fetus through the umbilical vein. The major portion bypasses the liver through the ductus venosus into the inferior vena cava (IVC). Here it mixes with deoxygenated blood, which has been returned from organs below the diaphragm.

Blood from the IVC is selectively channelled into the left atrium of the heart across the foramen ovale. From the left atrium it enters the left ventricle through the mitral valve and is pumped into the aorta to supply head, neck and arms. Venous blood from these regions is returned to the heart through the superior vena cava (SVC). It enters the right atrium and is streamed into the right ventricle through the tricuspid valve. It is pumped into the pulmonary artery and flows mainly into the aorta through the large ductus arteriosus. A smaller portion of blood supplies the fetal lungs.

Blood returns to the placenta through two umbilical arteries, which arise from the internal iliac vessels.

Note

The umbilical vein carries oxygenated blood (saturation 80%) from the placenta to the fetus.

The umbilical arteries carry deoxygenated blood (saturation 58%) from the fetus to the placenta.

Circulatory changes after birth
Arrest of umbilical circulation

The umbilical cord ceases to pulsate within minutes of birth and the vessels constrict. During the stage of pulsation 50 ml of blood may cross into the fetus through the umbilical vein.

Closure of foramen ovale

This valve-like structure closes as a result of:
- A drop in pressure in the IVC owing to cessation of umbilical circulation.
- An increase in pressure in the left atrium owing to improved venous return from the lungs.

Constriction of ductus arteriosus

This large vessel constricts within 4 to 12 hours after birth. This is probably as a result of the increase in arterial oxygen tension (PaO_2). It can reopen at this stage if PaO_2 falls or if pulmonary hypertension is present.

The intima of the vessel proliferates over the next two weeks and permanent closure is effected within three months.

Closure of ductus venosus

The ductus venosus constricts within several hours of birth and is subsequently obliterated to form the ligamentum venosum.

HEART RATE AND BLOOD PRESSURE

Heart rate

This is readily determined by placing a stethoscope over the praecordium and counting the beats.

It averages 120 per minute (range 80–150) on the first day and gradually rises to 140 per minute (range 100–180) by the end of the week. During crying the rate can exceed 180 per minute.

Blood pressure

Methods

- Cuff.
- Flush.
- Doppler.

Cuff

Place a small conventional cuff around the upper arm, covering two-thirds of its length.

Inflate the cuff to 100 mmHg and place a stethoscope over the brachial artery in the elbow. It may be possible to record blood pressure in this manner if the infant remains quiet.

Flush

Apply a small conventional cuff around the infant's forearm or lower leg. Lift the limb and wrap a crêpe elastic bandage firmly round the limb, starting at the baby's fingers or toes and working up to the cuff.

Inflate the bag to a pressure of 130 mmHg and remove the bandage. The hand or foot should look pale.

Lower the limb to the level of the heart.

Slowly release pressure in the cuff. The hand or foot will turn pink as the pressure falls.

Read the manometer at the point where the colour-change takes place. This indicates the systolic pressure.

Doppler

The apparatus consists of a sensing device and a cuff. Strap the cuff round the upper arm or leg.

This is the method of choice for long-term monitoring of blood pressure. A device such as Dinamap is most suitable and gives an intermittent read-out of systolic and diastolic blood pressure.

Note

Repeated measurements are needed to ensure accuracy.

The blood pressure rises with gestational age.

A full-term baby has a mean upper arm systolic pressure of 70 mmHg systolic and 45 mmHg diastolic. Little variation occurs during the neonatal period.

The preterm baby of 2 000 g has a mean systolic pressure of 60 mmHg systolic and 32 mmHg diastolic on the first day. A preterm baby weighing 1 000 g has a mean pressure of 50 mmHg systolic and 25 mmHg diastolic. These rise gradually during the neonatal period. Most blood pressure monitors used in an ICU measure the pressure throughout the cardiac cycle, i.e. during systole and diastole and express the average as Mean Blood Pressure. The value depends on the shape and size of the pressure-wave curve. Mean Blood Pressure represents the average perfusion of the body's organs. Most preterm infants over 24 weeks'gestation will have a value of 30 mmHg or more.

PRESENTATION OF CARDIOVASCULAR DISEASE

The following clinical features should alert you to the possibility of cardiovascular disease:

- A murmur.
- Abnormal heart rate.
- Cyanosis.
- Tachypnoea,
- Poor sucking.
- Signs of heart failure.

Murmur

After birth an ejection systolic murmur may be heard down the left sternal border or in the pulmonary area. It usually disappears within days and may be due to the flow of blood across the pulmonary valve or to a patent ductus arteriosus.

A murmur may be abnormal when:

- it persists beyond the first week
- a diastolic component is present
- a thrill is palpable.

Note

The absence of a murmur does not exclude cardiovascular disease.

Heart rate

A rate persistently more than 180 per minute is abnormal and may indicate:

- heart failure
- paroxysmal tachycardia (p. 201).

A rate persistently less than 60 per minute may be associated with heart block (p. 201).

Cyanosis

Congenital heart lesions with shunting of blood from the right to the left side or severe heart failure can cause cyanosis. This sign is always significant, but may be difficult to distinguish from cyanosis produced by respiratory failure.

Hyperoxia test

Give a cyanotic infant 100% oxygen to breathe for 10 minutes and then determine the oxygen saturation on the right hand radial artery. An SaO_2 of 95% or more rules out cyanotic heart disease. In defects such as transposition of the great vessels, the SaO_2 seldom exceeds 85% during hyperoxia. A low SaO_2 does not rule out lung disease such as hyaline membrane disease.

Heart failure

The signs differ from those in an older child.

Common features are:

- enlargement of the liver
- tachypnoea (over 60 breaths min)
- tachycardia (over 180 beats min)
- triple rhythm.

Hepatomegaly is a cardinal sign of heart failure. The normal liver does not extend more than 2 cm below the costal margin in the nipple line.

Other signs such as crepitations, cyanosis and oedema are variable.

Common causes of heart failure are:

- patent ductus arteriosus
- hypoplastic left-heart syndrome
- transposition of the great vessels.

Uncommon conditions include:

- polycythaemia
- cardiomyopathy
- hypoglycaemia
- arteriovenous fistula
- atrial tachycardia.

Specific investigations

Certain investigations are indicated when cardiovascular disease is suspected on clinical grounds.

Chest X-ray

Cardiomegaly is an important sign of heart disease, but can be difficult to detect on clinical examination.

Obtain an X-ray to assess the site, size and shape of the heart and the vascularity of the lungs.

Heart size: A cardiothoracic ratio greater than 0,6 is indicative of cardiomegaly, but must be interpreted with caution as:

- the phase of respiration cannot be controlled during the procedure
- the position of the infant can be altered by crying or movement
- the thymus can obscure the upper mediastinum.

Heart shape: Certain defects are associated with characteristic shapes of the heart, for example transposition of the great vessels is characterised by an egg-shaped heart with a narrow base.

Lung vascularity: The right pulmonary artery is usually visible at the hilum, but vascular markings disappear towards the periphery as the branches are too small to be seen. The prominence of pulmonary vessels depends on the blood flow to the lungs.

Increased pulmonary blood flow: This occurs in most defects associated with shunting of blood from the aorta to the pulmonary artery (Table 14.1). The pulmonary vessels:

- are prominent at the hilum
- can be seen at the periphery of the lung
- have an increased cross-sectional area when viewed 'end on'.

Decreased pulmonary blood flow: This is characterised by:

- dark lung field
- insignificant hilar vessels
- lack of vessels throughout the rest of the lung field.

Electrocardiography
The normal ECG pattern is characterised by right ventricular dominance in the praecordial leads.

R is greater than S in lead V1.
S is greater than R in lead V5.

The heart rate is variable, depending on the activity of the infant and sinus arrhythmia may be noted.

The following features indicate heart disease:

- Persistent left-axis deviation.
- Left ventricular dominance.
- Left or right ventricular hypertrophy.
- Arrhythmias and heart block.

Echocardiography
Two-dimensional ultrasonography has revolutionised the investigation of cardiovascular disease. This non-invasive technique can be used to detect most defects when heart disease is suspected. Doppler colour flow imaging is indispensable in the diagnosis and management of heart lesions, particularly those with shunts, but it should not be used as a screening procedure.

TABLE 14.1

Important congenital heart lesions		
	Cyanotic	*Acyanotic*
Overperfused lungs	Transposition of great vessels Total anomalous pulmonary venous drainage	Hypoplastic left-heart syndrome Septal defects Coarctation of aorta Patent ductus arteriosus
Underperfused lungs	Fallot tetralogy Tricuspid atresia Pulmonary atresia	

Cardiovascular disorders

Echocardiography
It determines the natural course of blood through the heart, as well as the situation of the various structures and their relationship to one another. Initially the positions of the atria are established together with blood flow from the superior and inferior vena cava into the right atrium and the pulmonary veins into the left atrium. Then the tricuspid and mitral valves as well as right and left ventricles are assessed. Finally blood enters the pulmonary artery and aorta. The former crosses the aorta and bifurcates to the lungs; the latter conveys arterial blood to the head and body.

Angiography
Cardiac catheterisation and angiography provide definitive evidence of the physiological and anatomical abnormalities and are utilised for most ill babies despite their risks.

CONGENITAL HEART DISEASE

Embryology
The cardiovascular system develops in the third week of gestation and is the first system to function in the embryo.

The heart is formed from paired tubes that fuse and bend into the recognisable cardiac shape. It becomes partitioned into four chambers between the fourth and seventh weeks. Most anomalies occur during this critical stage and often involve the ventricular septum.

At least 3 of every 1 000 liveborn babies will have a congenital heart lesion. The problem should be anticipated in the following circumstances:
- Down's syndrome – 50% have heart lesions.
- Arachnodactyly – 15% have mitral or aortic incompetence.
- Turner syndrome – coarctation of the aorta may occur.
- Rubella syndrome – various cardiovascular defects are common, especially patent ductus arteriosus.

Important congenital heart lesions are listed in Table 14.1. They can be categorised into groups, depending on the presence or absence of cyanosis and the vascularity of the lungs.

Cyanotic heart disease

Transposition of the great vessels
This defect should be suspected in every infant who has cyanotic heart disease. It occurs twice as frequently in boys as in girls.

The great vessels are transposed so that systemic venous blood enters the aorta from the right ventricle and oxygenated blood from the lungs enters the pulmonary artery via the left ventricle.

Life can only be sustained after birth if there is a communication between the two circulations. In the fetus this occurs through the foramen ovale and ductus arteriosus. When these channels close the infant develops severe cyanosis and cardiac failure. Heart murmurs may not be audible.

X-ray – the heart is enlarged and egg-shaped. Pulmonary vascularity is increased.

ECG – the pattern is usually normal, with right-sided dominance.

Echocardiography confirms the diagnosis and angiography provides the specific physiological and anatomical details.

Treatment
Palliative: A shunt is created between the atria by tearing the septum with a balloon catheter (Rashkind procedure).

Definitive: Blood can be directed into the correct channels by the Mustard operation, which is usually done later in infancy.

Fallot tetralogy
This is a relatively common abnormality characterised by pulmonary stenosis,

ventricular septal defect, overriding aorta and right ventricular hypertrophy.

The defect is difficult to diagnose in the newborn as cyanosis and heart failure are not prominent features at this stage.

A systolic murmur may be present and X-ray and ECG are variable. The suspicion of heart disease would prompt the use of echocardiography to establish a diagnosis.

Cyanosis develops after weeks or months and may occur in spells.

X-ray features may be characteristic at this stage and show a small pulmonary artery, oligaemic lung fields and a boot-shaped heart.

The ECG displays right atrial and ventricular hypertrophy. A palliative shunt may be needed (p. 196) and the defect can be corrected with cardiopulmonary bypass surgery before four years of age.

Pulmonary atresia

This rare anomaly is important to detect as it is amenable to surgery.

The pulmonary valve consists of an imperforate membrane and blood can only reach the pulmonary vessels through the ductus arteriosus. This circulation ceases when the ductus closes after birth.

Cyanosis is severe and is observed soon after birth. It can be followed by signs of heart failure. X-ray features consist of cardiomegaly and oligaemic lungs, and the ECG shows left-axis deviation and peaked P waves.

The diagnosis can be confirmed on echocardiography.

Death will occur unless the obstruction is relieved. The ductus can be kept patent by prostaglandin E and a pulmonary valvotomy is performed.

Acyanotic heart disease
Hypoplastic left-heart syndrome

This is a common cause of cardiac failure and death due to congenital heart disease. It is characterised by an underdeveloped left ventricle, which may be associated with atresia of the mitral and aortic valves and hypoplasia or atresia of the aortic arch.

In the fetus the left-sided obstruction causes most of the circulation to enter the right atrium and ventricle. The ductus arteriosus is widely patent and an atrial defect is present. After birth the cardiac output is reduced and the blood pressure is low.

X-ray – the heart is enlarged and the lung fields are congested.

ECG – right atrial and ventricular enlargement commonly occur.

The diagnosis can be confirmed on echocardiography and angiography.

Note

Severe heart failure, cyanosis and shock may occur early if the ductus arteriosus closes. If warning signs of heart disease (p. 190) have been overlooked this may result in a misdiagnosis of neonatal sepsis.

Ventricular septal defect

This is the most common heart anomaly. It varies in size and position and may occur as a single lesion or in association with other defects.

The clinical features of an isolated VSD vary with the size of the opening, the degree of shunting from left to right ventricle and the vascular resistance in the pulmonary circulation.

The usual presentation of a small defect is a harsh systolic murmur that is audible down the left sternal border. A systolic thrill may be palpable. X-ray and ECG features are normal and the infant is asymptomatic. Angiography is not necessary as the condition has an excellent prognosis.

Large lesions may cause heart failure within a week of birth. X-ray examination indicates cardiomegaly and accentuated vascular markings, and the ECG shows right ventricular hypertrophy. Diagnosis may be confirmed on echocardiography.

Outlook

Most small defects close spontaneously and even large ones can close or become significantly smaller. Spontaneous closure takes place in 75% of cases by the age of 10 years.

Surgery is recommended for the infant with a large defect who fails to respond to anti-heart failure measures.

Coarctation of the aorta

This vessel can be narrowed at any point beyond the innominate artery. Blood bypasses the obstruction and reaches the lower part of the body through collateral vessels. Patency of the ductus is the most common associated anomaly.

Signs of heart failure may be observed within days or weeks of birth. Murmurs are variable. The most striking finding is weak or absent femoral pulses and bounding arm pulses. The blood pressure in the arms is usually higher than that in the legs.

Cardiomegaly is noted on X-ray. Left ventricular hypertrophy is seen on ECG. Surgery is recommended for infants who develop symptoms in early life.

Patent ductus arteriosus (PDA)

The ductus is derived from the sixth aortic arch in the embryo and communicates with the left pulmonary artery. It plays a vital role in the fetus's survival by directing most of the circulation away from the lungs to the aorta.

The factors that control patency of the ductus before and after birth are poorly understood. Prostaglandin E is thought to keep the vessel open *in utero,* but there is uncertainty about its site of production and mode of action.

Oxygen plays a major role in constricting the ductus after birth. It appears to have a direct action on the muscular wall.

Failure of the ductus to close after birth can be associated with:

- prematurity
- cardiac defects
- congenital rubella syndrome.

Prematurity

The vessel may remain patent for days or weeks after birth and the physiological derangements can cause blood to shunt from the aorta to the pulmonary artery. This can overload the pulmonary circulation and result in heart failure.

The risks of symptomatic patent ductus arteriosus in a preterm infant are increased by the following factors:

- *Hyaline membrane disease (HMD):* A patent ductus may be an integral part of this illness as it seldom occurs in babies who do not develop respiratory distress.

  Symptomatic PDA is present in more than 70% of infants with HMD who are born at less than 30 weeks' gestation. It occurs during or after the acute phase of the illness.
- *Hypoxaemia and acidaemia:* Perinatal asphyxia is likely to be associated with transient patency of the ductus.
- *Fluid overload:* Symptomatic PDA can result from an excessive intake of fluid. This may occur when the daily volume exceeds 150 ml/kg.
- *Anaemia:* Anaemia of prematurity or acute blood loss, which results in hypovolaemia, can cause the ductus to open.
- *Drugs:* Theophylline, which is used to treat recurrent apnoea, has been associated with symptomatic PDA.

  Prolonged usage of furosemide in chronic lung disease is also considered to increase the chance of PDA.
- *Continual positive airway pressure (CPAP):* This, independent of other factors, appears to open the vessel on occasion.

Clinical features

These are easier to detect in a well baby than in one who has an underlying illness, such as hyaline membrane disease.

Characteristic signs in the preterm baby include:
- bounding peripheral pulses
- tachycardia
- systolic murmur along the upper left sternal border and also between the shoulder blades.

The murmur is the least significant sign and can be absent. A diastolic component may be heard, but is uncommon.

The signs of heart failure, particularly hepatomegaly, may be present in severe cases.

A patent ductus should be suspected in the infant with hyaline membrane disease when:
- oxygen requirements increase, or
- respirator support is needed for more than 24 hours.

Chest X-ray – signs may not be obvious in the early stages or they can be obscured by lung pathology such as severe hyaline membrane disease. Characteristic features include cardiomegaly and engorgement of the pulmonary vessels due to shunting of blood from the aorta to the pulmonary circulation.

ECG – the pattern is often normal and non-contributing. Left atrial and ventricular hypertrophy can occur.

Two-dimensional echocardiography can demonstrate the shunting, but may not be available at the bedside.

Clinical features remain a reasonable indicator of symptomatic PDA.

Management
Risk factors such as hypoxaemia, acidaemia, fluid overload and anaemia must be prevented or corrected.
Arterial oxygen tension: Keep the PaO_2 at 8–12 kPa.
Haematocrit: Maintain the PCV above 40%. This may necessitate transfusion with packed red cells.

Fluid: Restrict the daily amount to 100 ml/kg.
Heart failure: Digitalis may be needed in selected cases.
Closure of the ductus: This can be achieved by medical or surgical means.
Drug therapy: Indomethacin, an inhibitor of prostaglandin synthetase, can cause the ductus to constrict in approximately 66% of cases when given within the first two weeks of life. Give 0,1 mg/kg intravenously as a daily dose for up to five days.

Indomethacin can impair renal function and should not be used if the blood urea is raised or if oliguria is present. It can also impair the blood supply to the bowel to cause a perforation. Do not continue to give the drug beyond the stage of closure of the duct.

Surgical closure: The ductus can be ligated in symptomatic PDA when medical treatment has failed, particularly if an infant cannot be weaned off a ventilator.

Outlook for congenital heart disease
Great strides have been made in the investigation and correction of heart defects. An infant would require urgent admission to a cardiac centre should at least two of these signs be present:
- Cyanosis.
- Heart failure.
- Hypotension.
- Cardiomegaly.

Many infants with these features are dependent on a patent ductus arteriosus to maintain communication between right and left circulations. Closure of this vessel can result in hypotension, shock and death.

The baby who requires transferral also warrants a course of prostaglandin E to maintain patency of the ductus.
Dose: Prostin E 125 μg per dose by mouth every hour.

Surgery

Corrective or palliative surgery is available for a number of heart lesions. Corrective surgery has been performed successfully for:

- coarctation of the aorta
- patent ductus arteriosus
- pulmonary atresia or stenosis with an intact ventricular septum and normally developed right ventricle and pulmonary arteries
- total anomalous pulmonary venous drainage
- aortic vascular ring
- septal defects.

Palliative surgery

This is essentially a life-saving measure until complete correction can be undertaken when the infant is older.

This type of surgery has been performed successfully for:

- severe tetralogy of Fallot (a subclavian to pulmonary artery shunt to increase the pulmonary blood flow.)
- transposition of great vessels, immediate balloon septostomy of atria followed at one to two years of age by the Mustard operation for correction.
- ventricular septal defect with profuse left to right shunting,for example double outlet left ventricle and truncus arteriosus, pulmonary artery banding to restrict pulmonary blood flow.
- severe pulmonary stenosis in any potentially correctable lesion, shunt procedure.
- hypoplastic left heart. (In some cases this can be corrected in a three stage procedure).

  Initially the pulmonary venous return is redirected to the right atrium and the right ventricle ejects the systemic and pulmonary venous return into a reconstructed aorta.

  Between 4 to 6 months a superior cavo-pulmonary anastamosis is done.

Blood from the upper body now flows into the lungs. At 18 months to 2 years the inferior vena cava flow is channeled into the pulmonary circulation to complete the reconstruction.

Variations of the above procedures are used for tricuspid atresia and other single ventricle defects

OTHER CARDIAC PROBLEMS
Cardiomyopathy

The following factors can impair the muscular functions of the heart and cause cardiac failure:

- Transient myocardial ischaemia.
- Myocarditis.
- Endocardial fibroelastosis.
- Glycogen storage disease.

An infant with cardiomegaly and heart failure should be suspected of having one of these diseases if a specific defect cannot be demonstrated.

Transient myocardial ischaemia

This is associated with severe hypoxaemia and should be anticipated if signs of heart failure occur with HIE. Its responds to anti-failure therapy.

Myocarditis

This may be caused by the Coxsackie B infection or echoviruses.

Coxsackie B infection

In an adult, Coxsackie infection may present with pleurodynia, aseptic meningitis or a flu-like illness. A person with these features is a hazard to newborn babies, as the disease is highly infectious and often fatal.

Clinical features

The infection usually occurs within 10 days of birth and can cause myocarditis or meningoencephalitis. The onset is often acute and presents with pyrexia, diarrhoea, poor feeding, hepatomegaly, jaundice and a morbilliform rash.

Myocarditis is characterised by cardiomegaly, heart failure and pallor.

The virus may be cultured from the throat, stool, blood or cerebrospinal fluid.

Treatment
The infant is isolated and treatment is symptomatic, for example digitalis is prescribed for heart failure.

The outlook is grave, as 50% of infants die.

Endocardial fibroelastosis
The cause of this disease is unknown, but thought to be a Coxsackie virus infection *in utero.*

The illness may be acute, but usually presents in a chronic form, which can be difficult to diagnose in the newborn. Wheezy breathing, failure to thrive and difficulty with feeding may be noted in the early stages. Signs of cardiac failure occur and arrhythmias may be present.

Consider this diagnosis if the heart is grossly enlarged and there is left ventricular hypertrophy. Confirmation is obtained on echocardiography. Treatment is symptomatic. Infants with the acute form usually die, but recovery is possible in the chronic variety.

Glycogen storage disease
This rare autosomal recessive condition results from the accumulation of glycogen in heart muscles. The sugar cannot be degraded as the lysosomes lack the enzyme alpha-1 6-glucosidase.

The diagnosis is rarely made in the newborn unless there is a family history of the disease. It should be suspected in the presence of massive cardiomegaly, muscle weakness and macroglossia. Treatment is unsatisfactory and death usually occurs within a year.

Persistent pulmonary hypertension

Fetal lungs have a high pulmonary vascular resistance. After birth this falls rapidly when the alveoli fill with air. Functional or physical abnormalities of the pulmonary arteries can cause the pressure to remain high. The vessels may be inadequately dilated or diminished in number or have thick muscular walls. This results in cyanosis from right to left shunting of blood through the foramen ovale and the ductus arteriosus. It can mimic cyanotic heart disease and is associated with:

- birth asphyxia
- meconium aspiration
- lung hypoplasia
- prostaglandin inhibitors, for example aspirin, ibuprofen, naproxen during pregnancy
- polycythaemia.

Cyanosis and tachypnoea are evident after birth, and unexplained cyanosis may be the most significant clinical feature. The praecordial impulse is prominent and a soft systolic murmur may be audible on auscultation. There may be signs of an underlying cause, such as diaphragmatic hernia, aspiration pneumonia.

The most important differential diagnosis is cyanotic heart disease. The clinical findings that would favour a structural heart defect include cardiomegaly, weak pulses, oedema, a loud murmur, arrhythmias and a SaO_2 persistently below 87%.

Chest X-ray – the heart and lungs may appear normal or there may be signs of overinflated lungs, consolidation or atelectasis.

Echocardiography – this should be done in every case of unexplained cyanosis to exclude structural defects of the heart. It also indicates right-sided vascular pressure.

Treatment
The main objective is to provide adequate oxygenation. This can be difficult and

hypoxaemia may persist despite the use of high concentrations of oxygen and assisted ventilation either by intermittent positive pressure or high frequency oscillation. The latter provides small tidal volumes that promote uniform lung expansion. Infants are often restless and may require sedation while ventilated. Morphine, 0.05 mg to 0.2 mg/kg/dose may be given intravenously every four hours.

Address the following factors:
▪ Correct acidaemia (p. 175).
▪ Correct polycythaemia (p. 227).
▪ Provide an adequate fluid volume.
▪ Maintain a normal blood pressure.

Attempts have been made to dilate the pulmonary vessels with pharmacological agents.

The most useful drugs are:

Nitric oxide: The gas has a potent and sustained vasodilator effect on pulmonary vessels without decreasing the systemic vascular tone. It promotes the flow of blood to the lungs. Dose: 20 parts/million (ppm). After six hours a lower dose may be tried, 6 ppm. Duration: up to five days. Treatment can usually be stopped when inhaled oxygen requirements are less than 60%.

There is a risk of methaemoglobinuria (p. 227) at doses higher than 20 ppm and the level of blood methaemoglobin should be checked after four hours and daily thereafter.

To date the most successful therapy has been a combination of high frequency ventilation (p. 186) and nitric oxide inhalation. This optimises lung inflation and minimises lung damage.

Magnesium sulphate: this can be used if nitric oxide therapy is unavailable, 200 mg/kg and then 20–50 mg/kg/hour intravenously.

Hypotension: Bolus amounts of normal saline (10 ml/kg) may be given intravenously to increase fluid volume and raise blood pressure. If this is unsuccessful then use:

Dopamine 2 μg/kg/min by intravenous infusion. If necessary, this may be increased gradually to 20 μg/kg/min.

Other problems that may have to be addressed are:
▪ Meconium pneumonitis
▪ Bacterial pneumonia
▪ Surfactant dysfunction

Prognosis
The outlook is variable. Acid-base derangements, if uncorrected, lead to death in 30% of cases. Long term assessment is necessary to detect neurological abnormalities as well as the state of hearing.

CARDIAC ARRHYTHMIAS
Numerous tachy- and brachy-arrhythmias are described. They occur as isolated abnormalities or with heart defects or cardiomyopathy.

Tachyarrhythmias
These present with a narrow or a wide QRS complex. The former is more common and includes sinus tachycardia, atrial flutter and Wolff-Parkinson-White syndrome (a short P-R interval and a slurred upstroke of the QRS complex).

The latter includes ventricular tachycardia and fibrillation.

Treatment
Adenosine is used for many of the atrial tachyarrhythmias and where possible, all arrhythmias should be assessed and treated by a cardiologist.

Other effective drugs include digitalis, propranolol and amiodarone.

Brachyarrhythmias
These range from sinus arrhythmia to complete atrioventricular block. The latter is characterised by persistent bradycardia (heart rate <80) which may be detected before or after birth. It can be associated with maternal lupus erythematosis. In

general, the slower the heart rate the more severe the condition.

Diagnosis is made on ECG which shows a dissociation between P waves and the QRS complex.

Treatment is unnecessary for the asymptomatic infant – a pacemaker may be indicated later for the child who develops syncopy.

TREATMENT OF HEART FAILURE

Digitalisation
Digoxin is the drug of choice and the oral route is preferable. A response occurs within minutes and the maximum effect is attained within six to eight hours.

Lanoxin® elixir: This substance contains 0,05 mg/ml of digoxin. It is given in a calibrated dropper.

Dose: 0,01 mg/kg/day. Give this twice a day (0,005 mg/kg/dose) and check the serum level of digoxin weekly (normal range 1–2 ng/ml). Infants under 1 500 g can be given one dose a day (0.005 mg). A level in excess of 3 ng/ml can be toxic.

Precautions: **The prescribed dose should be confirmed by two doctors**. A nurse may not give Lanoxin unless a senior colleague has checked the amount. These steps are essential, as a mistake of a decimal point can be lethal.

Toxic effects
Preterm babies are more susceptible than term ones. The side-effects are relatively short-lasting and rarely persist for more than two days. Vomiting, diarrhoea and lethargy may occur. Arrhythmias are common, such as extra systoles, coupling and paroxysmal atrial tachycardia.

Treatment of toxicity
- Stop the digoxin.

- Wash out the stomach with 2% sodium bicarbonate if the drug has been given recently.
- Monitor the ECG continuously.
- Ensure an adequate intake of fluid to promote excretion of the drug.
- Potassium chloride (0,1 g/kg/day) may be given orally in divided doses.
- Treatment may also be needed for arrhythmias. Propranolol® 0,05 mg per kg will suppress ventricular arrhythmias.
- In life-threatening toxicity Digibind®, a digoxin-immune FAB, has been used successfully.

Oxygenation
An oxygen-enriched environment is recommended, particularly if the infant is anaemic.

Diuretic
Furosemide is suitable.

Dose: 1 mg/kg given intravenously, intramuscularly or orally. A maintenance amount of 1 mg/kg/day may be given to the infant orally. In long-term medication potassium chloride may be added and the level of serum electrolytes should be checked weekly.

Correction of anaemia
A low haemoglobin level can aggravate heart failure. Transfuse the infant with packed red blood cells (5 ml/kg) if the haematocrit is less than 35%.

Feeding
Avoid abdominal distension by giving small amounts of milk frequently.

Daily weighing
This is an important procedure, as excessive weight gain reflects retention of fluid and inadequate therapy.

CHAPTER 15

Gastrointestinal Disorders

PHYSIOLOGY

Before birth

From approximately 17 weeks of gestation the fetus swallows liquor and is capable of ingesting 500 ml daily in late pregnancy. The amount of swallowed liquor, as well as urine output, regulates the volume of amniotic fluid. Impaired swallowing results in polyhydramnios (excessive liquor). The role of amniotic fluid in gut development is unknown. It contributes to meconium, which is also derived from mucosal cells and secretions. At term the bowel contains approximately 200 g of meconium, which is rich in gut enzymes, bile pigments, urea, mucopolysaccharide, hair and epithelial cells.

Bowel motility depends on an intact autonomic nervous system and gut hormones such as motilin. Peristaltic movements are present in the colon at 14 to 16 weeks, and white stools have been detected in amniotic fluid at an early stage.

Green meconium is rarely ejected into the amniotic cavity except under adverse circumstances such as hypoxaemia.

At 12 weeks the anal membrane perforates and digestive enzymes can be detected in amniotic fluid. These decrease progressively and cease after 22 weeks, when the anal sphincter has developed. All enzymes except pancreatic amylase are sufficient for digestion at term.

After birth

Sucking and swallowing are vigorous and co-ordinated in the term infant. Air enters the stomach at birth and reaches the small bowel within two hours and the large bowel within 24 hours.

The pH of stomach contents averages 6,0 at birth and falls to 3 within hours due to the secretion of hydrochloric acid.

Meconium is usually passed within 24 hours of birth.

Feeding enhances bowel motility and

digestion. It stimulates the production of gut hormones and enzymes, promotes bacterial colonisation and is probably necessary for the growth of the bowel.

Fat absorption is impaired in the preterm infant, but is adequate for growth in the term baby. It shows a progressive increase in the first year. Carbohydrate absorption increases three-fold after birth.

Gut permeability
The small intestine of mammals including the human is permeable to globulin and other macromolecules. These substances are engulfed by the epithelial cells of the ileum and jejunum and transported by the lymphatics into the systemic circulation. This process is selective in some animals as it is the only route for the transmission of maternal antibodies to the newborn.

In the human, gut permeability exists before birth and subsequently decreases with age. It is of practical significance in that foreign proteins, like cow milk protein, may be absorbed in sufficient quantities to evoke a systemic immune response. This is more likely to occur in preterm babies and can result in allergy (p. 295).

STOOLS

Most babies (94%) pass meconium within 24 hours of birth. The initial stool is often cylindrical and shiny grey (meconium plug). It is followed by sticky black meconium, which becomes soft and brown when milk is introduced.

Yellow stools appear on the third or fourth day and their composition depends on the type of milk (Table 15.1).

Delay in passing stools

Preterm babies, particularly those with hyaline membrane disease, may not pass meconium for several days. This is associated with a lack of bowel sounds. In all others, a delay of more than 24 hours may be due to intestinal obstruction. Check the following clinical features:
- The anus –to establish patency.
- The abdomen – to exclude distension.
- Bowel sounds – to ensure that they are audible.
- Lack of vomiting.

Further investigations can be postponed if all these features are normal. At this stage (48 hours) 99,8% of normal babies should have passed a stool.

Abnormal stooling may be due to diarrhoea or constipation. If either of these occur, consider the causes under two categories
1. Those in babies who are entirely breast-fed.
2. Those in babies who receive other milks.

Diarrhoea

Breast-fed infant
A breast-fed infant may pass 10 or more stools a day. This is normal when linked with a gain in weight.

TABLE 15.1

Stool characteristics								
	Colour	Consistency	Odour	Frequency	Fat	Bacteria	pH	
Breast-fed	Bright yellow	Watery, little residue	None or sour	Variable	5%	Many bifido-bacteria Few E. coli	5,0	
Bottle-fed	Pale yellow	Bulky	Malodorous	3–4 a day	10–20%	Few bifido-bacteria Many E. coli	6,0	

The frequent passage of watery stools in the first week is abnormal when an infant fails to gain weight despite drinking an adequate amount of milk. This may be caused by transient 'lactose intolerance', or laxatives in breast milk. Infective gastroenteritis associated with viruses or bacteria, for practical purposes, does not occur in a baby who is entirely breast-fed.

Laxatives
Many substances are secreted into breast milk and can act on the infant's bowel to cause diarrhoea. Caution must be observed when these products are prescribed for a lactating mother. Senna preparations are considered to be relatively safe, as the amount that crosses into breast milk is usually insufficient to cause diarrhoea.

Lactose intolerance
This transient problem occurs in less than 1% of breast-fed infants and is characterised by diarrhoea, weight loss, excoriated buttocks and excessive lactose in stool water. A specimen is obtained in a urine bag that is fixed to the anus. It shows more than 0,5% reducing substances on Clinitest.

Treatment
Breast milk contains a large amount of lactose and the dietary load can be reduced by omitting one breast-feed a day. A milk that does not contain lactose, for example Alimentum can be substituted for the evening feed.

This usually reduces the output of stools and enables the infant to gain weight. Complete breast-feeding can often be re-established within months.

Bottle-fed infant
The stools of a baby who is fed cow milk do not vary much each day in number or consistency (Table 15.1). Diarrhoea is a cause for concern as it is likely to be due to infective gastroenteritis and should be treated accordingly (p. 222) even if the diagnosis cannot be confirmed.

Adequate fluids are provided and kanamycin (p. 222) is given orally to cover a possible *E. coli* infection.

Uncommon causes
These include necrotising enterocolitis, cystic fibrosis, congenital adrenal hyperplasia and sensitivity to cow milk protein.

Constipation

This refers to the infrequent passage of stools, which are hard and dry. Constipation does not occur in a baby who is entirely breast-fed. Stools may be passed infrequently, e.g. after several days or weeks, but they are always soft.

Bottle-fed infant
Constipation is a common problem in babies who are fed cow milk. It can occur as early as two weeks of age and is characterised by crying and straining when an infant attempts to defecate. Several days may lapse before a stool is passed. If neglected, the condition can result in fissuring of the anus and retention of stools in the colon.

Treatment
Constipation can become a chronic problem if not treated adequately. It is one of the few conditions that may benefit from a change in milk. A modified formula can be substituted for a non-modified one or a liquid preparation can replace a powder product.

Lactose is effective for softening stools as it retains water in the gut. Add a teaspoonful (5 g) to each feed for several weeks.

The combination of lactose and a change in formula is usually effective for most cases of mild constipation.

A glycerine suppository (paediatric)

lubricates faeces in the rectum and is often effective in the acute stage.

A laxative is rarely prescribed except for retained stools. Many products are unsuitable for infants because of side-effects. Lactulose, a synthetic disaccharide of fructose and galactose, retains water in the colon by a local osmotic action. This laxative is recommended for severe constipation in a dose of 1,5 g daily (2,5 ml) until the colon has been cleared of faecal masses and the stool consistency is normal.

An anaesthetic gel, Bonjela®, which contains choline salicylate, is applied to a fissure several times a day to relieve pain. This is essential in breaking the vicious cycle of fear of passing stools, pain and retention. If the above measures are unsuccessful, consider the possibility of Hirschsprung disease (p. 214) particularly if there is associated abdominal distension and failure to thrive.

Uncommon causes

Constipation may be associated with oral iron medication, over-concentrated feeds, pyrexia and pyloric stenosis.

VOMITING

Vomiting is usually benign, yet it may indicate serious illness when associated with signs listed in Table 15.2. Important causes of vomiting at different stagesof the neonatal period are presented in Table 15.3.

Vomiting in the first 24 hours

Gastric irritants

A fetus may swallow liquor contaminated with meconium, blood or pus. These products can cause vomiting shortly after birth. They should be removed from the stomach by gastric lavage.

Gastric lavage

Method: Introduce a nasogastric tube into the stomach (p. 71) and remove the contents with a 10 ml syringe.

Fill the syringe with a 2% solution of sodium bicarbonate, inject this into the stomach and then aspirate. Allow the residue to drain by gravity if aspiration

TABLE 15.2

Signs associated with serious causes of vomiting	
Sign	*Cause*
Polyhydramnios	Oesophageal atresia
Constant drooling of saliva	
Coughing spells or cyanosis	Tracheo-oesophageal fistula
Abdominal distension	Bowel obstruction
	Necrotising enterocolitis
	Sepsis
Diarrhoea	Necrotising enterocolitis
	Infective gastroenteritis
Down's syndrome	Duodenal atresia
Excessive lethargy	Sepsis
Bile-stained vomitus	Bowel obstruction
Projectile vomiting	Pyloric stenosis

TABLE 15.3

Important causes of vomiting		
Age	*Common*	*Uncommon*
First 24 hours	Swallowed blood or meconium Too much milk Incorrect food, e.g. dextrose water Prematurity	Oesophageal atresia
First week	Gastro-oesophageal reflux Infection	Hiatus hernia Necrotising enterocolitis Small or large bowel obstruction Inherited metabolic disorder, e.g. adrenal hyperplasia
Several weeks	Pyloric stenosis Gastroenteritis	

is difficult. Repeat the process until the returning fluid is clear.

Excessive volume of milk

The amount of colostrum ingested by a breast-fed baby probably does not exceed 20–30 ml per feed on the first day. Larger quantities of milk will be eagerly sucked from a bottle, but are likely to be vomited. A total amount of 30–40 ml per feed is sufficient for most bottle-fed babies in the first 24 hours.

Incorrect fluid

Sterile water may be offered to babies in the early hours of life, but dextrose water is unsuitable. It can disturb the normal rhythm of sucking and swallowing, irritate gastric mucosa and damage the respiratory tract if aspirated into the trachea. This solution is used only when there is a significant risk of hypoglycaemia (p. 261).

Note: Breast milk is the first choice after birth and rarely is any other fluid necessary even to prevent hypoglycaemia.

Prematurity

The stomach of a preterm baby is quite small and the gastro-oesophageal junction may fail to remain closed after feeds. This causes regurgitation and vomiting, particularly if large amounts of milk are ingested. The problem can be avoided or minimised by cautious feeding (p. 68).

Vomiting in the first week

Gastro-oesophageal reflux

The junction between the oesophagus and stomach is normally compressed by muscles in the cardia and by the diaphragm, which acts as an external sphincter. The opening pressure of this region is low and small amounts of milk may be posited especially during winding. This is considered to be normal and subsides within months.

The gastro-oesophageal junction may be sufficiently flaccid to cause regurgitation and vomiting. This is termed lax oesophagus or chalasia.

Vomiting occurs after a feed when the infant is placed flat in a cot. It is usually not forceful, but can be projectile on occasion. The infant has no physical abnormalities and gains weight in spite of vomiting mouthfuls of milk.

Diagnosis

Fluoroscopy shows the lower portion of the oesophagus to be dilated and flaccid, and dye may enter the oesophagus from the stomach during expiration.

Treatment

Add a thickening agent, Nestargel™, to milk (0,5–1,0 g per 100 ml). In the case of a breast-fed baby it is mixed in 20 ml of sterile water and offered before a feed.

An alternative thickener is Gaviscon™ which contains alginic acid, magnesium trisilicate, aluminium hydroxide and sodium bicarbonate. Add half a sachet to each feed.

Elevate the head of the cot on blocks or prop up the infant on a pillow in the cot. Do not disturb the baby.

These measures are usually successful and can be discontinued after several months as the problem is self-limiting.

Infants who continue to vomit may be kept upright in a small chair.

Hiatus hernia

A congenitally short oesophagus with an intrathoracic stomach may cause regurgitation and vomiting. The clinical presentation, course and treatment are similar to those of a lax oesophagus. The defect can be identified by fluoroscopy.

The condition reverts to normal with medical care in the majority of cases and no signs of organic dysfunction can be detected after 12 to 18 months. Surgery is seldom required.

Complications include bleeding from

TABLE 15.4

	Vomitus	Stool
Causes of blood in vomitus or stool		
Common	Swallowed maternal blood	Swallowed maternal blood
Uncommon	Oesophagitis in hiatus hernia Haemorrhagic disease	Trauma, e.g. thermometer Fissure, e.g. constipation Gastroenteritis Necrotising enterocolitis Haemorrhagic disease Sensitivity to cow milk protein

oesophagitis and recurrent lung infections from inhalation of milk.

Infection

Persistent vomiting may be a sign of sepsis, particularly when associated with lethargy or jaundice. Look for evidence of infection (p. 93) and remember hidden sources, such as the urinary tract or the ear.

Vomiting after several weeks

Persistent vomiting that starts at three to six weeks of age in a healthy baby is due to pyloric stenosis (p. 211) until disproved.

Infection is also important. Again remember occult sources, like urine, ears.

Vomiting associated with diarrhoea is probably caused by gastroenteritis (p. 221), particularly if the infant is bottle-fed.

Blood in vomitus or stool

Fresh or altered blood may be detected in the vomitus or stool (Colour plate IV). It can originate from the infant or the mother and a distinction is made by the Apt test. This is based on the fact that fetal haemoglobin resists denaturation by an alkali.

Apt test

Method: Shake equal amounts of the blood-stained specimen and tap water in a test tube and then centrifuge. Add one part of sodium hydroxide (0,25%) to five parts of the pink supernatant fluid. A sample containing maternal blood turns greenish-yellow while that with infant's blood remains pink.

In most cases blood is of maternal origin. It can be swallowed from the liquor following a haemorrhage, such as separation of placenta, or from a cracked nipple during feeding.

CONGENITAL ABNORMALITIES
Branchial disorders

The face, lips, tongue, jaws, palate, pharynx and neck are derived mostly from the branchial arches, grooves and pouches. The transformation starts during the fourth and fifth weeks of gestation and ends at 12 weeks. It can be impaired at any stage.

Lips and palate
Aetiology

Genetic and environmental factors play a role in cleft lip and palate, and chromosome defects may be associated with some cases.

The occurrence rate of cleft lip with or without cleft palate differs from that of an isolated cleft palate. A sibling of an affected infant has the following chance of a similar lesion:

	Cleft lip plus/ minus cleft palate	Cleft palate only
Parents normal, no affected relative	4%	2%
Parents normal, one affected relative	4%	7%
One parent affected	17%	15%

Cleft lip

This is the commonest abnormality of the face, with an incidence of 1 in 1 000. It is caused by failure of the nasal and maxillary processes (Fig. 15.1) to fuse and may be uni- or bilateral. The defect can vary from a tiny notch in the upper lip to a complete split that extends into the nasal cavity (Fig. 15.2).

A cleft lip is often left-sided and is more common in boys than in girls.

Cleft palate

This results from a failure of the palatine processes to fuse with one another or with the nasal septum. The lesion varies from a bifid uvula to a complete cleft of the hard and soft palate, which extends into the nasal cavity. Severe lesions may be associated with a cleft lip (Fig. 15.3).

Cleft palate is more common in girls than in boys and has an incidence of 1 in 2 500 births.

Treatment

A cleft lip is disfiguring, but the effect of a cleft palate is more serious in terms of eating and speaking.

Reassure parents that a pleasing result can be achieved by plastic surgery and orthodontic treatment. Photographs of similar defects before and after treatment will reinforce this advice.

Obtain orthodontic help for a cleft palate as soon after birth as possible. A plastic prosthesis is fitted in the upper jaw after an impression has been made. It covers the cleft and enables the infant to suck from a bottle or breast. The device is cleaned after feeds, but otherwise remains in the mouth

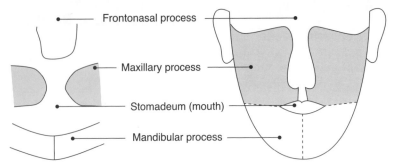

Fig. 15.1 *Embryological development of the face*

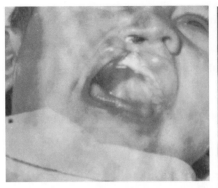

Fig. 15.2 *Cleft lip*

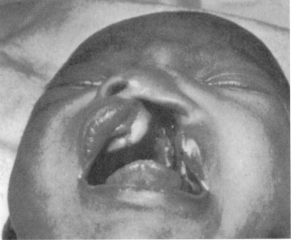

Fig. 15.3 *Cleft lip and palate*

at all times. This promotes alignment of the displaced jaw segments and prevents milk from entering the nasal passages. The prosthesis needs to be trimmed occasionally and has to be replaced after several months to allow for growth.

The deformity of the palate is repaired before 12 months of age. An isolated cleft lip is corrected at three months, but the complicated variety may be repaired later depending on the need for orthodontic procedures.

The treatment of severe lesions extends over many years. Speech training is essential for cleft palate, and teeth may need to be correctly spaced and aligned. Progress is supervised by a plastic surgeon, an orthodontist and a speech therapist.

Tongue
Ankyloglossia (tongue-tie)
Cells at the tip of the primitive tongue grow into the underlying mesenchyme and later degenerate to release the tongue. Failure of this development can result in the tip being anchored to the floor of the mouth by a fold of mucosa known as the frenulum (Fig. 15.4). Treatment is usually unnecessary as tongue-tie rarely impairs sucking or speech. The anterior portion of the tongue grows forward during infancy and the frenulum recedes and lengthens.

Macroglossia (enlarged tongue)
Moderate enlargement of the tongue may be associated with hypothyroidism (Fig. 15.5), Down's syndrome and glycogen storage disease.

Severe enlargement is seen in lymphangioma and Beckwith syndrome (Fig. 15.6). The latter condition is characterised by conditions such as macroglossia, omphalocele and hypoglycaemia.

Microglossia (small tongue)
This defect occurs in the Pierre Robin syndrome, which is characterised by severe

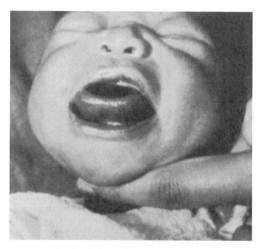

Fig. 15.5 *The enlarged tongue of hypothyroidism*

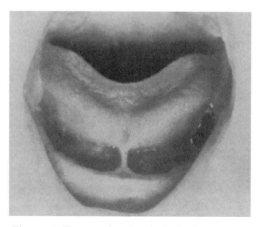

Fig. 15.4 *Tongue-tie – in which the frenulum is attached to the floor of the mouth*

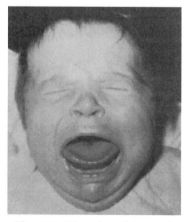

Fig. 15.6 *The enlarged tongue in Beckwith syndrome*

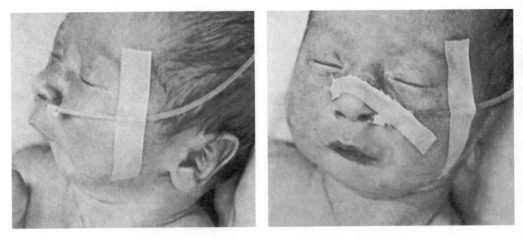

Fig. 15.7 *Recessed chin in Pierre Robin syndrome*

recession of the lower jaw (micrognathia), a small tongue and a U-shaped cleft palate (Fig. 15.7). Posterior displacement of the tongue can obstruct the airway and cause cyanosis.

Treatment
Orthodontic treatment is essential and a prosthesis is fitted into the upper jaw to cover the cleft. It has a posterior extension that elevates the uvula and maintains patency of the airways. The jaw and tongue grow to normal proportions in infancy and the palate lesion is repaired before 12 months.

Teeth
These develop from the ectoderm and mesoderm of the oral cavity. Calcification can be detected at 16 weeks in deciduous teeth and during the last month of pregnancy in permanent teeth. The lower central incisors erupt at about six months of age and the remaining deciduous teeth have appeared by two and a half years.

Natal teeth
Two lower incisors may be present at birth. Initially they may be covered by a thin layer of gum mucosa. Loose teeth with poorly developed roots can become dislodged and ought to be extracted to prevent inhalation.

Delay in eruption
This can be related to:
■ a family tendency
■ a faulty diet during pregnancy
■ rickets
■ cretinism.

Discoloration of teeth
■ Tetracycline can stain the teeth yellow.
■ Hyperbilirubinaemia can give them a green tinge.

Absent or deformed teeth
Genetic factors, like ectodermal dysplasia (p. 255), play an important role.

Defective formation of dentine
This can be associated with:
■ prematurity
■ prenatal infections.

Caries prophylaxis
Fluoride supplementation, such as Zyma-fluor® drops, is recommended during pregnancy and infancy in areas where the water content of fluoride is less than 0,7 parts per million.

Mouth
Ranula
This is a retention cyst of the sublingual

salivary gland. It is filled with fluid and is situated under the tongue, which may be displaced upwards. Small cysts usually subside, but larger ones need resection.

Epignathus
Various tumours may arise from the upper jaw or palate and protrude from the mouth (Fig. 15.8). They are thought to originate from remnants of embryonic tissue and are mostly benign. The lesion is excised to prevent respiratory difficulties.

First arch syndrome
Recognisable syndromes are caused by the defective formation of structures from the first branchial arch.

Treacher Collins syndrome (Mandibulofacial dysostosis)
This is characterised by micrognathia, flattened cheekbones, slanted lateral angles of the eyes, notched lower eyelids, ear deformities and deafness.

Pierre Robin syndrome (Fig. 15.7)
This has been described on page 207.

Neck
Branchial cysts (Fig. 15.9)
Cysts or sinuses are relatively uncommon and result from defective development of the second branchial cleft or groove. They are situated in the neck and require surgical resection.

Disorders of the gut
The gastrointestinal tract is formed during the fourth week of gestation. The head and tail sections of the embryo fold to enclose the primitive yolk sac (Fig. 15.10) and this invagination produces a fore-, mid- and hindgut. The structures that arise from these regions are listed in Table 15.5, and major defects in development are also shown.

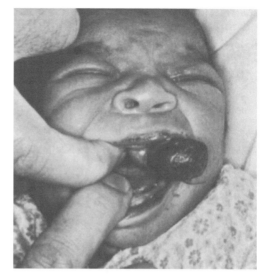

Fig. 15.8 *Epignathus protruding from the mouth*

Oesophageal atresia
Embryological background
Differentiation of the oesophagus and trachea occurs between the third and sixth week of gestation. These structures originate from a solid core of tissue that later becomes canalised. The trachea is divided from the oesophagus by a septum.

For reasons not yet established this tracheo-oesophageal septum can become deviated from its normal course to cause the various anomalies.

Classification
Five varieties are illustrated (Fig. 15.11). Atresia with a fistula between the lower oesophagus and trachea (C) occurs in more than 50% of cases. The two segments of the oesophagus are usually widely separated in this form.

Incidence
Oesophageal atresia is found in 1 in 3 000 live births and occurs in preterm infants more frequently than in the full-term.

Associated abnormalities
About 50% of infants show other malformations. These can involve the

intestine, cardiovascular system or anorectal region.

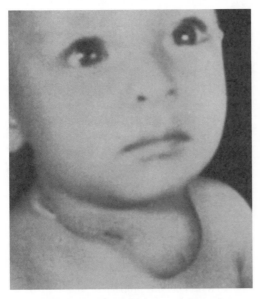

Fig. 15.9 *A branchial cyst of the neck*

Clinical presentation
Polyhydramnios is usually present during pregnancy. This must alert you to the possibility of an associated fetal abnormality such as oesophageal atresia. The affected infant is often preterm.

Mucus accumulates in the mouth and drools from the lips.

Choking spells occur during a feed, and can cause cyanosis and apnoea.

Signs of pneumonia may be present. In cases of persistent or recurrent pneumonia, an H-type fistula (Fig. 15.11E) without atresia should be suspected.

Diagnosis
Insert a nasogastric catheter in every infant suspected of having oesophageal atresia. This cannot be advanced more than 10 to 13 cm from the anterior nares. An AP X-ray of the chest will reveal the situation of the catheter.

The specific type of lesion can be confirmed by fluoroscopy (Fig. 15.12).

Complications
The aspiration of gastric juices or milk can cause pneumonia or death from obstructed airways.

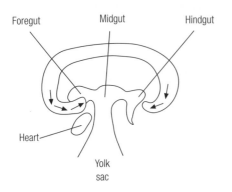

Fig. 15.10 *Formation of the primitive gut from the yolk sac*

Treatment
Oesophageal atresia is a surgical emergency. Immediate care is directed at constant drainage of the oesophageal

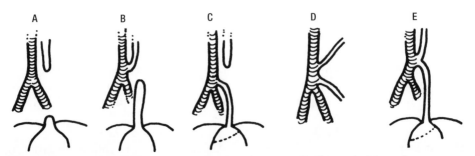

Fig. 15.11 *Tracheo-oesophageal fistula and atresia. The five varieties are shown*

TABLE 15.5

Development of the gut		
Primitive structure	*Organ*	*Important defects*
Foregut	Oesophagus and pharynx Stomach Part of duodenum Liver, bile ducts Pancreas	Oesophageal atresia Pyloric stenosis Duodenal atresia Bile duct atresia Annular pancreas
Midgut	Part of duodenum Jejenum and ileum and appendix Ascending and part of transverse colon	Atresia, malrotation Malrotation
Hindgut	Part of transverse colon Descending and sigmoid colon Rectum and part of anal canal	Hirschsprung disease Anorectal malformation
Yolk stalk, allantois, urachus	Umbilical contents	Exomphalos Gastroschisis Hernia Single umbilical artery Patent urachus Patent vitello-intestinal canal Meckel diverticulum

pouch, adequate hydration and transfer to a neonatal surgical centre. Insert a nasopharyngeal catheter and aspirate it repeatedly to keep the pouch empty. Set up an intravenous drip of 10% dextrose and transfer the baby in a portable incubator.

Prognosis
The type of surgery depends on the size and condition of the baby as well as on the nature of the lesion. Outcome is related to these factors and the overall survival rate is over 60%.

Oesophageal stenosis
Severe stenosis may present signs similar to atresia.

Infants with milder grades show:
- regurgitation of milk – this may occur during a feed
- persistent hunger
- weight loss.

Treatment
The oesophagus will require periodic dilation.

Hypertrophic pyloric stenosis
Incidence
- 1 per 1 500 births.
- Four times more common in boys than in girls.
- The first-born is more likely to be affected.

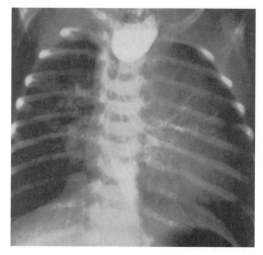

Fig. 15.12 *Lipidol swallow in oesophageal atresia. Although a small quantity of dye was used, it entered the bronchi and stomach through a tracheo-oesophageal fistula*

- It can occur in successive generations of a family.

Pathology

The pyloric muscles, particularly the circular layers, show marked hypertrophy. This extends into the gastric region, but ends abruptly on the duodenal side. The lumen of the pyloric canal is narrowed.

Signs

Clinical features seldom occur before the second week of life, but may occasionally be present from birth. They include:
- vomiting
- visible peristalsis
- palpable tumour
- constipation
- weight loss.

Vomiting: Initially vomiting may be intermittent, but soon it occurs after each feed and becomes projectile. Milk can shoot out immediately after a feed, or just before the next feed.

Vomitus consists of fresh or curdled milk. Bloodstained mucus may be found if there is an associated gastritis. Bile is never present in the vomitus. Appetite remains good and the infant is eager to drink again.

Visible peristalsis: Observe the abdomen in a good light during a feed. Peristaltic waves start below the left costal margin and move across to the midline. The direction is reversed just prior to vomiting.

Palpable tumour: Technique: During a feed a nurse supports the baby with the abdomen exposed. The doctor sits on the left side of the infant and gently palpates the abdomen with the left hand. A tumour is usually felt with the middle or forefinger just lateral to the right rectus muscle and about 4 cm below the costal margin. It feels firm and may measure 2,5 × 1 cm in size.

Constipation: Pellet-like stools are passed infrequently as a result of the decreased food intake.

Weight loss: Repeated vomiting causes weight loss with a reduction in subcutaneous fat.

Diagnosis

The clinical features that have been described are usually characteristic enough to make a diagnosis, particularly when a tumour is palpable.

In doubtful cases ultrasonography can demonstrate the tumour. Fluoroscopy shows narrowing and elongation of the pylorus and indentation of the duodenal cap.

Complications
- Dehydration (p. 265).
- Loss of chloride ions.
- Hypokalaemia.
- Metabolic alkalaemia.
- Tetany.

Differential diagnosis

Duodenal obstruction: Vomiting occurs much earlier and is usually bile-stained.

Hiatus hernia: Onset of vomiting is early. No tumour is palpable. Radiological signs are characteristic.

Treatment

Ramstedt operation: The hypertrophied muscles are split longitudinally down to the submucosa.

Correction of complications: Metabolic derangements must be corrected before surgery is undertaken.

Prognosis

Operative mortality is less than 1% and the complication rate is negligible.

Small and large bowel intestinal obstruction

Congenital malformations of the bowel often present with signs of intestinal obstruction and the ultimate prognosis depends on the stage at which the obstruction is detected and relieved. Often a precise diagnosis of the underlying pathology cannot be made prior to operation.

The clinical presentation of intestinal obstruction depends on the site and degree of blockage. In general, the higher and more complete the obstruction, the earlier and more severe the presentation.

The most important signs are:

- vomiting
- abdominal distension
- delay in passage of stools.

Vomiting (Colour plate IV)
High obstruction: Vomiting is often forceful and may occur shortly after birth. In lesions proximal to the ampulla of Vater it is colourless, whereas in obstructions distal to this site it is usually bile-stained.

Low obstruction: Vomiting may not be a prominent early feature as it is often intermittent and slight.

Note: Vomiting, however slight, must be reported. Notification is critical should the vomitus contain bile. Retain a sample of vomitus for microscopic examination.

The baby's stomach contains very little amniotic fluid after birth (usually less than 5 ml). In a high obstruction large quantities (over 50 ml) may be aspirated through a nasogastric tube.

Abdominal distension
High obstruction: Distension may not be a prominent early feature, in cases of duodenal atresia or stenosis only, for example, the duodenum and stomach can distend.

Low obstruction: Abdomen distension is prominent. The abdomen can become stretched and large veins may be obvious beneath the skin. Severe distension can impair respiratory function.

Delay in stooling
High obstruction: The excretion of meconium may be delayed, and in incomplete blockage the output of stools may be reduced. The excretion of meconium does not exclude the possibility of complete obstruction.

Low obstruction: In a case of complete obstruction, like colon atresia, the passage of meconium is unusual. In partial obstruction, stools may be infrequent and reduced in amount.

Other signs of intestinal obstruction include visible peristalsis and diminished or absent bowel sounds.

Diagnostic aids include an X-ray of the abdomen. This is taken with the infant in the erect position (Fig 15.13).

Characteristic fluid levels and air patterns may be seen. For example, in duodenal atresia two air bubbles with fluid levels are noted in the upper bowel ('the double bubble'), one situated in the stomach, the other in the duodenum. No air is present in the rest of the abdomen (Fig. 15.14).

Lower obstructions show distended loops of bowel with multiple fluid lev-

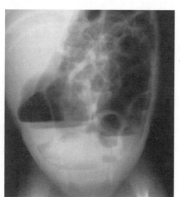

Fig. 15.13
Low intestinal obstruction with distended bowels and fluid levels

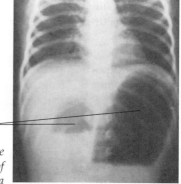

Double bubble

Fig. 15.14 *The 'double bubble' of duodenal atresia*

els. The size and number of fluid levels together with the situation of air gives an indication of the site of obstruction.

Meconium ileus: A characteristic granular appearance may be produced by the admixture of gas bubbles and sticky meconium. Intraperitoneal calcification may be present and in cases of perforation air will be seen under the diaphragm.

Barium enema: This study is important in the diagnosis of Hirschsprung disease. The enema shows a narrow rectum and sigmoid, and a dilated proximal colon in typical cases.

Treatment
Intestinal obstruction is considered a surgical emergency.

Prognosis
Most babies will die without treatment, but overall survival rates exceed 60% with surgery.

Specific abnormalities (Fig. 15.15)
Intestinal atresia or stenosis
Any part of the gut may be narrowed or atretic at birth. Atresia can involve a single portion or multiple sections of bowel and may extend over varying lengths.

Atresia below the duodenum is considered to have been caused by impaired blood supply to the gut during the development of the embryo.

Common sites of atresia: Ileum, duodenum. *Common sites of stenosis:* Duodenum, ileum. Atresia or stenosis of the duodenum can occur in Down's syndrome.

Annular pancreas
The second portion of the duodenum can be obstructed by a ring of pancreatic tissue. This may cause narrowing or even obliteration of the lumen.

Malrotation
Embryological background
From the sixth to the tenth week of gestation the primitive bowel grows more rapidly than the coelomic cavity and a portion of it is forced into the umbilical cord. This section, termed the midgut, extends from the second part of the duodenum to the middle of the transverse colon. While in this position, the midgut starts to rotate around the axis of the superior mesenteric artery in an anticlockwise direction (as you view the baby).

After the 10th week, the coelomic cavity has grown sufficiently to contain the midgut, which returns and continues its rotation. At this stage the terminal ileum and the colon lie on the left side, while the jejunum and rest of the small bowel are situated on the right side.

Rotation continues and the caecum, which is the last portion to return to the abdomen, passes the epigastrium and then the right upper abdominal cavity to fix finally in the right iliac fossa. The small bowel becomes attached to the posterior abdominal wall by mesenteric bands.

Rotation can be arrested at any stage. The most common variety of malrotation results in the duodenum lying to the right of the midline with the caecum anteriorly. Adhesions from peritoneum to caecum can cause obstructions to the second part of the duodenum.

Hirschsprung disease (Fig. 15.15)
Embryology
Ganglion cells enter the muscle layers of the upper alimentary canal at about the sixth week. They then migrate caudally through the canal. In Hirschsprung disease the course of migration is considered to have been interrupted, with the result that distal sections of bowel are devoid of these nerve cells.

Pathology
In most cases the rectum and lower sigmoid colon are affected, but the cells may be absent as high up as the ileum.

The abnormal sections are incapable of peristalsis and remain narrow, while the normal proximal bowel dilates and hypertrophies.

Hirschsprung disease occurs more frequently in boys than in girls and tends to recur in families.

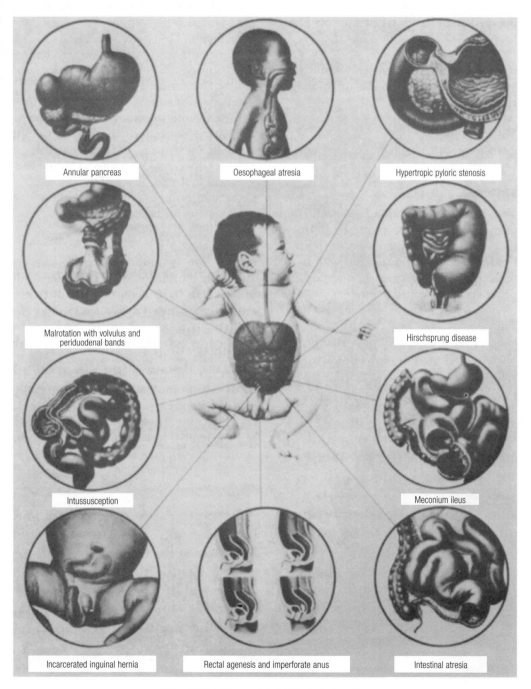

Fig. 15.15 *Neonatal intestinal obstruction*

Clinical signs

Features are those of an incomplete low intestinal obstruction and include constipation, vomiting and abdominal distension.

The passage of meconium may be delayed and vomiting often occurs early.

Diagnosis

Barium enema shows characteristic X-ray signs and confirmation is obtained on rectal biopsy.

Treatment

Colostomy and excision of aganglionic segment.

Meconium ileus

This, the earliest and most severe form of cystic fibrosis, occurs in about 10% of cases. Sticky meconium blocks the bowel to produce abdominal distension with partial or complete obstruction. Perforation may occur *in utero* to cause peritonitis.

Treatment

Gastrografin enemas may remove the meconium to produce temporary relief, but most infants require an enterostomy.

Supportive measures include:
- antibiotics
- pancreatic enzymes
- water-miscible vitamins
- intralipid infusions.

Complications

Bacterial peritonitis and pulmonary infection. About 50% of babies suffering this die in the neonatal period.

Cystic fibrosis is a generalised disease and all body secretions are thick and tenacious.

Other organs that may be affected by the disorder are as follows:

Lungs: Thick mucus obstructs the airways, resulting in chronic lung disease and infection.

Pancreas: (85% of cases) The enzyme output is diminished and steatorrhoea occurs.

Liver: (5% of cases) Fibrosis and failure can occur in the late stage of the disease.

Gonads: Infertility may result in those who survive beyond puberty.

Diagnosis

Cystic fibrosis is transmitted by a recessive gene (chromosome 7) and is a result of a lack of transmembrane conductance regulator protein (CFTR).

In many cases the mutated gene can be detected by the polymerase chain reaction. The amino acid, phenylalanine, is lost at codon 508 (mutation delta F 508).

The sodium content of sweat usually exceeds 60 mmol/l.

These investigations, in association with a family history and clinical signs, confirm the diagnosis.

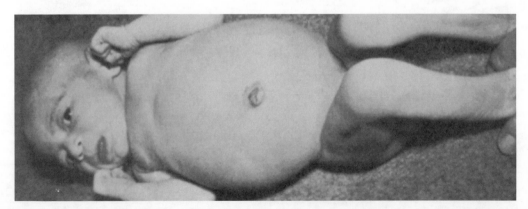

Fig. 15.16 *Abdominal distension due to Hirschsprung disease*

Other causes of intestinal obstruction
- Various hernias.
- Intussusception.

Ileus caused by:
- peritonitis
- chloramphenicol overdose
- hexamethonium overdose in mother.

The rectum and anus

Rectum

Embryology
The hindgut opens into a large cavity termed the cloaca. This becomes divided into a ventral portion, which forms the bladder and urethra, and a dorsal part, which develops into the rectum. The two sections remain joined by a narrow cloacal duct, which closes after the seventh week of gestation.

Anus

Embryology
An invagination of perineal skin grows towards the rectum to form the anus. This remains separated from the rectum by an anal membrane until the fifth week of gestation.

Malformations of the rectum and anus may be divided into 'high' and 'low' groups, ranging from rectal agenesis to imperforate anus, depending on the stage at which development was arrested. A fistula may be present if the cloacal duct fails to close.

In rectal lesions the puborectalis muscle is often poorly developed and can cause faecal incontinence. In anal lesions this muscle usually functions normally.

The simple 'imperforate anus', in which the anal opening is obstructed by a membrane, is rare (less than 3% of cases) and unfortunately most defects are extremely complicated. This implies that surgical correction should be undertaken only by skilled staff in a special neonatal centre.

Clinical features
A careful inspection of the perineum and anus after the baby's birth should detect most abnormalities. The anus may be covered with a membrane (Fig. 15.17). This membrane may be absent, narrowed, patulous or displaced anteriorly.

Fistula: Signs of this abnormality include:
- meconium-stained or green-coloured urine
- meconium passed per vagina
- visible tract extending from covered anus to frenulum in midline – this may contain meconium (Colour plate X).

Intestinal obstruction: See signs for lower obstruction, page 213.

Associated abnormalities: Genito-urinary malformation, abnormal vertebrae cardiac defects. Ultrasound or MR imaging of the sacrum and distal cord may be indicated to detect abnormalities.

X-ray features
A lateral film of the abdomen is taken with the infant inverted.

A marker, such as a forceps, is placed at the site of the anus. The distance between this marker and the gas bubble in the rectum indicates the site of the

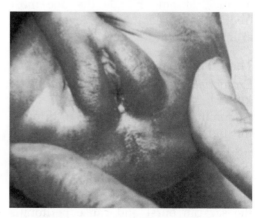

Fig. 15.17 *Anal membrane*

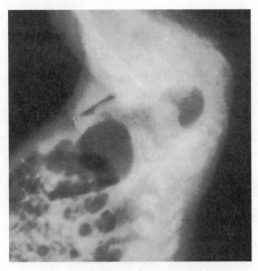

Fig. 15.18 *X-ray of rectal agenesis.*
Air cannot be seen in the rectum

lesion. In rectal agenesis this distance usually exceeds 1,5 cm (Fig. 15.18).

Radiological features of intestinal obstruction may be present.

Treatment
Refer the infant to a neonatal surgical unit for therapy.

Outcome
Outlook for survival is good. Faecal incontinence, however, can be a problem in later years, especially in high lesions.

Note: Of all major congenital abnormalities, absent anus is the one most frequently missed at birth. Never omit to examine the buttock area.

The umbilicus

Exomphalos (omphalocele) (Colour plate XII)
Abdominal contents may herniate through the umbilical ring into the base of the cord. The wall of the cord consists only of a layer of amniotic membrane so that the loops of intestine and other organs are clearly visible. If the defect is not treated, the sac can burst and cause peritonitis and death.

If the bowel herniates through a paraumbilical defect in the abdominal wall, the condition is termed gastroschisis. The lesion is usually situated to the right of the umbilicus.

Incidence of exomphalos
The incidence is 1 in 5 000 births.

Associated defects
About 30% of cases will have associated malformations, such as Meckel diverticulum, macroglossia (Beckwith syndrome).

Treatment
Exomphalos: At birth clamp the umbilical cord well beyond the sac to ensure that loops of intestine are not trapped.

Surgical repair is advocated for small defects.

For large defects conservative treatment is used. If the bowel cannot be accommodated within the abdomen, the sac containing the abdominal contents is painted with 1% mercurochrome in alcohol to encourage the formation of a fibrotic cover. This is continued for 24 hours, and most of the contents should have retracted into the abdomen by five to eight weeks.

Gastroschisis: A silastic bag is placed over the intestine and stitched to the abdominal wall. The bag is gradually reduced in size until the intestines have been returned to the abdomen.

Prognosis
About 40% of infants with a severe form of exomphalos die from associated malformations or infection.

Umbilical hernia (Fig. 15.19)
This is a soft, reducible swelling at the umbilicus, covered with peritoneum and skin. The swelling enlarges when the baby cries. The size of opening in the abdominal wall varies from a few millimetres to 5 or 6 cm. Evans found this

condition at birth in 31,8% of black and in 4,1% of white babies.

Prognosis
The hernia regresses spontaneously. Strangulation is very rare.

Treatment
Advise parents of the natural course of the hernia. Surgical repair is recommended after only two to three years of age if the hernia has not decreased in size and if the opening is larger than 1,5 cm.

Application of adhesive plaster to reduce swelling is not recommended.

Single umbilical artery
Faierman observed an absent artery in 2,7% of stillbirths and those who died within eight weeks of birth. Other sources quote a single umbilical artery in 1% of all births. The majority of infants are normal, but an accompanying defect should be sought in each case, particularly in a growth-retarded baby. Any system may be involved.

Examine the infant intermittently in the early years to exclude an occult lesion, such as a heart defect.

Patent urachus
The urachus connects the bladder to the umbilicus in the embryo. This canal may remain partially or completely open. A patent urachus causes urine to leak at the umbilicus. A partially closed canal may present as a mass below the umbilicus.

Treatment
Surgical removal.

Prognosis
Good.

Patent vitello-intestinal canal
The embryonic connection between the yolk sac and the small intestine normally atrophies in the embryo. If the whole of the connection remains patent, it is called a vitello-intestinal canal. This leads to the passage of meconium or faeces at the umbilicus.

Treatment
Surgical removal.

Prognosis
Good.

Meckel diverticulum
Only the distal portion of the embryonic connection between the yolk sac and the small intestine may atrophy, leaving a patent proximal canal in communication with the intestine. This is called a Meckel diverticulum. It is usually about 5 cm long.

The diverticulum is observed in about 2–3% of autopsies. It is situated on the ileum and usually does not cause any symptoms.

Complications
Infection: Diverticulitis can give signs similar to acute or chronic appendicitis.

Bleeding: Ulceration can cause bleeding, which may be profuse. This is the most common complication.

Intussusception: The diverticulum may be the starting point of this disorder.

Intestinal obstruction: Bands or an intussusception can cause obstruction of the bowel.

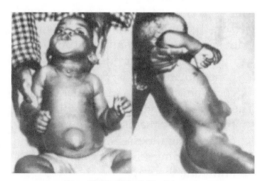
Fig. 15.19 *Umbilical hernia*

Treatment
A Meckel diverticulum is excised in complicated cases.

NECROTISING ENTEROCOLITIS

The incidence varies from one nursery to another and is highest in infants who weigh less than 1 500 g. The cause is unknown and predisposing factors are thought to be birth asphyxia, shock, catheterisation of umbilical vessels, hyperosmolar feeds or colonisation of the bowel with pathogenic bacteria, like *Klebsiella* and *Clostridium*.

The insult results in ischaemic necrosis of the gut, particularly the terminal ileum and colon. These portions are distended and lesions are infiltrated with organisms such as *Klebsiella*.

Bubbles of gas, formed by bacteria, may infiltrate the wall of the bowel. Perforation results in peritonitis.

Clinical features
Abdominal distension is usually noted three to five days after oral feeding has been started. Bowel sounds are diminished or inaudible and the outline of distended loops of gut may be seen under the abdominal wall.

Bile-stained vomitus and bloody stools are common and the abdominal skin may be red and oedematous. Non-specific clinical features include lethargy, hypothermia and shock.

The early triad of vomiting, abdominal distension and ileus is very suspicious in a preterm baby and warrants discontinuation of oral feeding, antibiotic therapy (see below) and an abdominal X-ray.

Radiological signs (Fig. 15.20)
Distended loops of bowel are noted and intramural air, pneumatosis intestinalis, may be seen. Air is present in the peritoneal cavity when perforation has occurred.

Laboratory findings
Leukopenia and thrombocytopenia are common in severe disease and organisms such as *Klebsiella* may be cultured from stools and blood.

Treatment
Feeds: Discontinue oral feeding and use intravenous alimentation (p. 72) until all signs of disease have subsided. Several weeks may lapse before milk feeds can be re-established.

Antibiotics: If the bowel sounds are present give a non-absorbable antibiotic, such as kanamycin, orally for five days.

Dose 80 mg/kg/day.

An aminoglycoside, such as gentamicin, and ceftriaxone are used in severe disease.

Gut decompression: Insert a Reprogle tube into the stomach and apply constant suction at a low negative pressure to remove air and secretions from the bowel.

Surgery: A laparotomy is performed in cases of perforation and the ischaemic segment of bowel is resected.

Outcome
Prompt diagnosis and early treatment have reduced the mortality rate to less than 20%. The mortality rate of perforation with peritonitis can exceed 50% with or without surgical intervention.

INFECTIONS

Thrush (Fig. 15.21)
This is produced by the fungus *Candida albicans*. It commonly infects the mouth or skin and may be transmitted from:
- mother's vagina or nipples
- contaminated hands, e.g. staff
- contaminated items, e.g. unsterile teat.

The disease is likely to occur with:
- prematurity, that is poor immunity
- debilitating illness
- bottle-feeding
- antibiotic therapy.

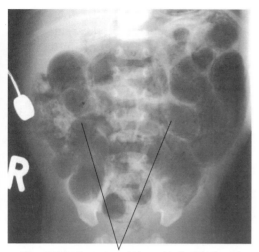

Fig. 15.20 *Pneumatosis intestinalis: The bowel walls are outlined by dark bubbles of intramural gas*

Antibiotics alter the normal microflora of the gut and encourage the overgrowth of *Candida albicans*.

Clinical features
Mouth: Small white patches appear on the dorsum and sides of the tongue and may spread to the inner cheeks and lips. The papillae of the tongue are prominent and mucous membranes are red and inflamed. In severe cases the whole mouth is white.

The infant sucks poorly or refuses feeds. The infection occasionally spreads to the gut and may produce diarrhoea and vomiting.

Milk curds may be mistaken for thrush and can be distinguished by the following features:

- Milk curds are found on the dorsum of the tongue and not on the sides or under the surface.
- They are not present in the mouth before feeds.
- They are easily scraped off and leave a normal pink underlying mucosa.

Treatment
Oral thrush: Nystatin drops, such as

Mycostatin®. Instill one drop into the mouth each hour up to 12 times a day. Continue treatment for a week.

Gentian violet 1% aqueous solution. Place two drops on the tongue after feeds for seven days.

Gastrointestinal thrush: Nystatin drops, 100 000 units orally four times a day after feeds for a week.

Note
The disease may recur if the source of infection is not eliminated. This applies to untreated vaginal thrush and to contaminated items such as gripe-water, sodium hypochlorite solution or dummies.

Gastroenteritis
This is highly infectious and can cause dehydration and death within hours. Outbreaks usually result from cross-infection and involve artificially fed babies, particularly preterm ones.

Aetiology
Most cases are associated with pathogenic

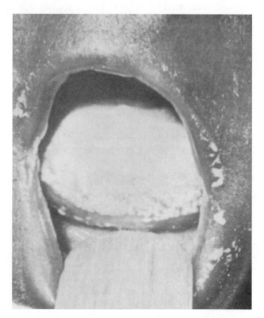

Fig. 15.21 *Thrush infection of the tongue*

E. coli, such as 011, 055. Other agents include:

- bacteria: salmonellae, shigellae
- fungus: *Candida albicans*
- virus: rotavirus.

Clinical signs

The onset may be insidious or explosive with:

- diarrhoea
- weight loss
- vomiting
- dehydration
- shock.

The loose, watery stools may be pale white, yellow or green and contain slime. Specks of blood are rare and indicate a possible shigella infection.

Signs of dehydration appear if the infant loses more than 5% of body weight. The features are described on page 265.

Obtain a stool specimen for the detection of bacteria and viruses.

Treatment

Isolation: The infant must be removed from the nursery and handled only by staff who have no contact with other babies.

Correction of dehydration (p. 266).

Antibiotics: Kanamycin is used orally (p. 306).

Prevention: Gastroenteritis rarely occurs in well-run nurseries and can be avoided through:

- prevention of cross-infection (p. 73)
- promotion of breast-feeding.

Omphalitis (Colour Plate II)

The umbilicus is a potential portal of entry for infection after birth. Care must be taken to keep the cord dry (p. 33) as moisture favours the growth of pathogenic micro-organisms.

Omphalitis is usually caused by coliforms, Group B streptococci or staphylococci and is always serious as the organisms can be transmitted into the bloodstream.

Clinical features

The skin at the base of the cord may be red and oedematous.

A red flare may extend onto the abdominal wall. A purulent or bloody discharge may be noted. The cord may have an offensive odour.

Complications

Infection can spread to produce:

- cellulitis of the abdominal wall
- umbilical vein phlebitis
- hepatitis and jaundice
- peritonitis
- septicaemia
- bleeding from the cord.

Late complications include a cord granuloma and portal vein thrombosis.

Treatment

Take a swab for Gram stain and culture. Dry the cord using alcohol every three hours. Give systemic antibiotic therapy for 7 to 10 days.

The choice of antibiotic will ultimately depend on the type of organism and its sensitivity.

Cord granuloma

Following separation of the cord a fleshy lump may develop at the base of the umbilicus. This moist granuloma probably results from a chronic low-grade infection.

Treatment

Protect the surrounding skin with a layer of Vaseline and cauterise the lesion with a silver nitrate stick. This results in resolution of the granuloma within days.

CHAPTER 16

Blood Disorders

This chapter in outline:

RED BLOOD CELLS

The erythrocyte values (Table 16.1) in a full-term infant depend on factors such as the site of sampling and age after birth. Figures obtained from a venepuncture are more accurate than those from a heel stab as they are not influenced by a poor peripheral circulation due to acute blood loss or hypothermia. This can be partly overcome by warming the heel to obtain arterialised blood (p. 232).

The blood volume, haematocrit and haemoglobin at birth depend on the time of cord clamping. The benefits of late vs early clamping are uncertain as those factors do not influence the level of haemoglobin at 12 weeks.

The haemoglobin concentration remains steady during the first week and a value below 14 g/dl is indicative of anaemia in a full-term baby.

Anaemia

Important causes of anaemia in the first week are listed in Table 16.2. Anaemia at birth is usually due to haemolytic disease or blood loss. After birth it is likely to be caused by haemorrhage or infection.

TABLE 16.1

Normal values of red blood cells (heel blood)			
Age	*Haemoglobin* g/dl	*Total cells* $\times 10^{12}$/l	*Haematocrit* %	*Reticulocytes* %
1 day	19 ± 2,2	5,1 ± 0,7	61 ± 7,4	3,2 ± 1,4
7 days	17,9 ± 2,5	4,8 ± 0,6	56 ± 9,4	0,5 ± 0,4
12 weeks	11,3 ± 0,9	3,7 ± 0,3	33 ± 3,3	0,7 ± 0,3

(From Maroth, Y; Zaizov, P, and Varsano I. 1971. Postnatal changes in some red cell parameters. Acta Paediat Scand 60: 317–23.)

TABLE 16.2

Important causes of anaemia	
At birth	*After birth*
Haemolytic disease	Blood loss
	Cord haemorrhage
Acute blood loss	*Repeated sampling of blood*
Placenta praevia	*Trauma, e.g. subaponeurotic bleeding, rupture of liver*
Abruptio placentae	
Incision of placenta	Haemorrhagic disease
Rupture of cord, e.g. velamentous insertion	Haemolytic disease
	Infection, e.g. septicaemia
Fetomaternal bleed	Physiological anaemia
Twin transfusion syndrome	Anaemia of prematurity
Antenatal infection, e.g. syphilis	
Congenital hypoplastic anaemia	

Investigations and diagnosis

The cause of anaemia can usually be established if adequate attention is given to the history, clinical examination and laboratory studies in each case.

History

The following antenatal details should be sought:

- Rh and ABO sensitisation
- bleeding during pregnancy
- drug ingestion, e.g. anticoagulants
- maternal infection, e.g. syphilis.

Clinical examination

Examine for:

- site of bleeding, e.g. cord
- jaundice, hepatosplenomegaly.

Laboratory investigations

Take a sample of the infant's blood for:

- haemoglobin
- reticulocyte count
- blood smear
- bilirubin
- Coombs test.

Characteristic features of major disorders are shown in Table 16.3.

Acute haemorrhage

Onset before or during birth

Severe bleeding, as in abruptio placentae, can result in fetal death.

Liveborn infants may not show any symptoms or show the following signs of acute blood loss:

TABLE 16.3

Laboratory tests for anaemia at birth.

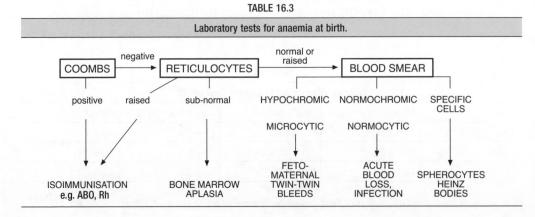

- Pallor of mucosae.
- Weakly palpable pulses.
- Tachycardia.
- Hypotension.
- Irregular or gasping breathing.

Note: These signs must be distinguished from those associated with asphyxia, which include pallor, hypotension, brady-cardia and absent respiratory efforts.

Treatment
Severe case (above clinical signs):
- Hold an oxygen mask over the face.
- Pass a catheter into the umbilical vein (p. 109).
- Take blood for cross-matching and for anaemia investigations. Leave the catheter in place.
- The circulating plasma volume can be enhanced by an infusion of normal saline.
  Inject 20 ml/kg into the vein.
- Reassess the clinical condition and PCV level. If there is no improvement in the clinical state give additional fluid (10 ml/kg).
- Unmatched Group O negative blood can be used, but should be reserved for dire circumstances. Initial expansion of the plasma volume usually tides an infant over the critical period.
- A transfusion of cross-matched blood may be needed later if clinical signs persist, such as tachypnoea, tachycardia and the Hb being below 10 g/dl.

Moderate case:
- Give a plasma volume expander to the infant who is not shocked at birth but has clinical and laboratory signs of blood loss, e.g. tachycardia, a PCV below 50%, an Hb below 14 g/dl. A total of 20 ml/kg is usually adequate.

Mild case:
- An asymptomatic infant with an Hb above 12 g/dl does not require a

plasma volume expander or blood. Administer iron (p. 304).

Note
Determine the source of bleeding. Examine the placenta carefully for abnormalities, like ruptured vasa praevia. An endoscopic examination of the abdomen may be indicated if rupture of a viscus, such as liver or spleen, is suspected.

Fetomaternal haemorrhage
Bleeding commonly occurs into the maternal circulation from the fetus and occasionally may be severe enough to produce anaemia.

Diagnosis
The clinical and laboratory signs are those of acute blood loss, but no site of bleeding can be detected.

The diagnosis is established by demonstrating fetal red cells in the maternal circulation (Kleihauer technique).

This depends on the fact that adult haemoglobin can be eluted from red cells at a low pH, whereas fetal haemoglobin is unaffected. Red cells containing fetal haemoglobin can be demonstrated on a slide by adding a citric-phosphate buffer solution to the smear. Adult cells appear as ghosts and fetal cells as dark refractile bodies.

Twin transfusion (Colour Plate V)
Vascular anastomoses are common in monochorionic placentae and bleeding may occur from one twin into the other via an artery-to-vein communication.

Clinical presentation
At birth one twin is strikingly pale, whereas the other appears plethoric.

Treatment
The anaemic twin usually does not require immediate treatment, whereas the plethoric infant is often distressed

and may die from fluid overload if not treated (p. 227).

Congenital hypoplastic anaemia

This uncommon disease presents with anaemia from birth. The reticulocyte count is low (less than 2%) and confirmation of diagnosis is obtained from bone marrow examination. The aetiology is unknown. Steroid therapy can sometimes stimulate the production of red cells.

Physiological anaemia

The production of red blood cells in the fetus is partly controlled by erythropoietin, a hormone secreted by the kidney. It has a maximum effect on the bone marrow in the last trimester of pregnancy and disappears from the circulation within days of birth. This is accompanied by a decrease in haemoglobin, haematocrit and red cell count, and the level of haemoglobin may reach 11–9,5 g/dl between 6 and 12 weeks (Table 16.1).

Erythropoietin is reactivated at this stage and there is a progressive increase in the formation of red cells and in haemoglobin concentration.

The iron stores of the body together with the iron in milk are sufficient to maintain a normal level of haemoglobin until approximately six months of age. Thereafter extra iron is required to prevent anaemia. This is obtained from a well-balanced diet.

The decrease in haemoglobin after birth is a physiological event that does not require treatment in a healthy full-term infant.

Anaemia of prematurity

Most preterm babies are born before their bone marrow has benefited from erythropoietin stimulation in late pregnancy. The values for haemoglobin, haematocrit and red cell count are lower than those of full-term infants at birth. There is a shortfall of iron transmitted from the mother in the last trimester of pregnancy.

Anaemia may present in two phases:

1 *Early anaemia*
   The haemoglobin level declines rapidly after birth and may reach 6,5 g/dl within four to eight weeks.
   This can be hastened by repeated vene-sections and by haemolysis owing to vitamin E deficiency.

2 *Late anaemia*
   An iron deficiency anaemia can occur after 12 weeks as a result of inadequate iron stores. This coincides with the stage of active erythropoiesis after birth.

Treatment

- Preterm babies require adequate amounts of iron to prevent anaemia (p. 304).
- The need for vitamin E prophylaxis is uncertain and supplementation is recommended if a haemolytic anaemia occurs.
- Early anaemia may be unavoidable in babies of less than 1 500 g.
- Erythropoietin has been used successfully in conjunction with iron to prevent anaemia.
- Indications: Haematocrit less than 35%.
- Dose: 200 units/kg once a week for six weeks.

A transfusion of packed red cells may be required if the haematocrit is less than 25% and there are signs or symptoms. These usually result from a patent ductus arteriosus and include tachypnoea, tachycardia and bounding pulses (p. 194).

Polycythaemia

This is defined as a haemoglobin of more than 22 g/dl or a haematocrit greater than 65%. It results from an absolute or relative increase in the mass of red cells due to overproduction or transfusion.

Important associations include:

- 'milking' of the cord at birth
- twin transfusion syndrome
- exchange transfusion
- intrauterine growth retardation
- maternal diabetes mellitus.

Blood viscosity increases when the haematocrit reaches 60%, and the following complications are likely to occur at a haematocrit above 70%: reduced blood flow, sludging of red cells and venous thrombosis.

Clinical features
Most infants are asymptomatic.
Some may show:

- heart failure (p. 190), or
- persistent pulmonary hypertension (p. 197).

Heart failure is more likely to occur when there has been a sudden increase in blood volume from overtransfusion.

Other complications include:

- hyperbilirubinaemia
- hypoglycaemia
- renal vein thrombosis
- thrombocytopenia.

Treatment
Asymptomatic infants with a haematocrit below 70% do not need to be treated.

Infants with a higher haematocrit or with signs such as tachypnoea and tachycardia require a partial exchange transfusion.

Blood is withdrawn (10 ml/kg) and replaced with an equal volume of stabilised human serum. Complications such as hypoglycaemia and hyperbilirubinaemia will need to be treated.

Haemoglobin

A haemoglobin molecule consists of four haem groups (iron-containing porphyrins), combined with globin polypeptide chains.

Its character is dependent on the types of globin chains. Haemoglobin F is the major form in the fetus and haemoglobin A the main type produced after birth.

Inherited structural disorders of haemoglobin can cause a variety of diseases, such as haemolytic anaemia and methaemoglobinaemia.

Haemolytic anaemias
Sickle cell disease is associated with abnormal polypeptide chains, whereas thalassaemia is caused by inadequate amounts of normal chains.

Methaemoglobinaemia
The iron in haemoglobin is in the ferrous (Fe++) state, which enables it to combine loosely with oxygen. This property is lost if iron is oxidised to the ferric state (Fe+++). The molecule is then known as methaemoglobin.

It can result from inherited abnormalities of the polypeptide chains or from chemicals such as nitric oxide, nitrates and aniline dyes, which oxidise iron.

Diagnosis
With methaemoglobinaemia, the mucous membranes have a slate-grey colour, which differs from the cyanosis caused by respiratory or cardiac abnormalities.

The cardiac and pulmonary systems are normal and in a mild case there is usually no evidence of distress. Blood is brown and does not turn pink on shaking.

The diagnosis may be confirmed on spectroscopic examination of blood, which shows an absorption peak of 634 mμ.

Treatment
Preventive measures include avoiding water that might contain nitrates, for example well water, the thorough washing of nappies that have been labelled with marking ink, and the monitoring of methaemoglobin levels during nitric oxide inhalation therapy.

TABLE 16.4

	Total count × 10⁹/l	Range × 10⁹/l	Neutrophil %	Lymphocyte %	Eosinophil %	Monocyte %
Cord blood	18	9–30	61	31	2	6
14 days	12	5–21	40	48	3	9
12 weeks	12	6–18	30	63	2	5

(From Behrman, R and Vaughan, VC, 1983. Nelson Textbook of Pediatrics. 12th ed. 1207.)

Specific measures:
- Methylene blue 1% (2 mg/kg) – single injection IV.
- Ascorbic acid – large doses can be given daily in the congenital type.

WHITE BLOOD CELLS

The values for white cells vary with age and are listed in Table 16.4. Neutrophils predominate at birth, whereas lymphocytes are more numerous at 12 weeks.

Most white cell disorders are secondary to other conditions. Specific changes occur in bacterial infection.

Bacterial infection

Clinical features of infection are preceded by changes in the white blood cells.

Bacterial invasion is associated with a movement of white cells to the site of the infection. The numbers of primitive neutrophils, which are called 'stab' or 'band' cells, increase and then the total white cell count rises.

White cell count
Method
- Collect a few drops of heel blood in an EDTA tube for analysis.
- A blood smear is stained and a differential count is done under x 40 oil immersion lens.
- Mature and immature neutrophils are counted separately.

Mature neutrophils contain two or more nuclei connected by thin filaments. Band (immature) neutrophils have nuclei that show no distinct lobulation or connecting strands (Fig. 16.1).

Absolute neutrophil and band counts are obtained by multiplying the numbers of mature and immature neutrophils by the total white cell count.

The values for full-term babies are shown in Fig. 16.2. Maximum counts are reached at 24 hours and there is a steady decline thereafter.

Preterm babies usually have lower counts and the absolute neutrophil count rarely exceeds 15 x 10⁹/l.

The following features are indicative of bacterial infections:
- Absolute neutrophil count – above or below normal range (Fig. 16.2)
- Absolute band count – above normal range for age (Fig. 16.2).

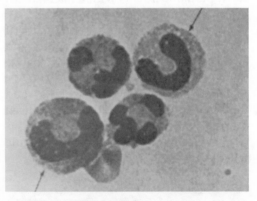

Fig. 16.1 *The 'band' forms of neutrophils are indicated by arrows. (From Akenzua, G. et al. 1974) Pediatrics 54:38–41*

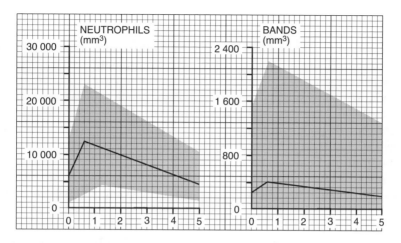

Fig. 16.2 *Absolute neutrophil and band counts in normal full-term infants. (From Akenzua, G et al. 1974. Pediatrics **54**: 38–41)*

- Band-to-total-neutrophil ratio – more than 0,2.
- Band cells as a percentage of total white cells – more than 10%.

Other haematological signs include:
- Döhle bodies, vacuoles and toxic granulation of neutrophils
- thrombocytopenia.

Other disorders of white cells

Eosinophilia may be associated with prematurity.

Lymphopenia may be a feature of defective immunity, e.g. Di George syndrome.

Rare conditions include neonatal leukaemia and the Chédiak-Higashi syndrome. This is an autosomal recessive disease characterised by albinism and recurrent infections. It is a disorder of neutrophils and lymphocytes that contain large granules and function poorly.

BLEEDING DISORDERS

Haemostasis

This depends on an adequate response to injury by capillaries, platelets and clotting factors.

Capillaries
Vasoconstriction reduces the risk of bleeding when a vessel has been severed.

Platelets
These release haemostatic factors and aggregate into a loose plug when they come into contact with the collagen in damaged capillaries.

In the laboratory the adequacy of this function can be assessed by the platelet count and the bleeding time:
- Normal platelet count: 150–$170 \times 10^9/l$.
- Normal bleeding time: 4–7 minutes.

Clotting factors (Fig. 16.3)
A firm clot of fibrin is formed by the sequential action of clotting proteins. One of these, factor X, is activated via two routes. An intrinsic pathway is stimulated when factor XII reacts with collagen in the injured vessel. An extrinsic pathway is activated when factor VII comes into contact with thromboplastin in damaged tissue.

The activated factor X is needed to convert prothrombin into thrombin and this proteolytic enzyme changes fibrinogen to fibrin.

The efficacy of the clotting process can be determined by various tests:

- *Prothrombin time (PT)*: This measures the activity of the extrinsic pathway. It is expressed as the international normalised ratio (INR).
- *Partial thromboplastin time (PTT)*: This provides an assessment of the intrinsic pathway.
- *Fibrinogen*: An adequate amount of fibrinogen is required for the formation of fibrin. Deficiencies may indicate liver disease or disseminated intravascular coagulation (DIC).

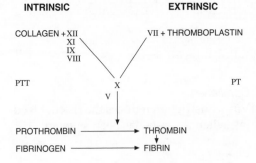

INTRINSIC   **EXTRINSIC**

COLLAGEN + XII   VII + THROMBOPLASTIN
XI
IX
VIII

PTT   X   PT
V

PROTHROMBIN ⟶ THROMBIN
FIBRINOGEN ⟶ FIBRIN

Fig. 16.3 *Factors involved in blood clotting (see text)*

Investigation of a bleeding disorder

The infant with a bleeding disorder may be asymptomatic at birth or present with petechiae, bruising, mucosal bleeding or severe haemorrhage. These may occur spontaneously or as a result of mild trauma or surgical procedure such as circumcision.

A history is important and includes:
- family – evidence of a bleeding tendency
- mother – infections, e.g. rubella; drugs, e.g. tolbutamide; illness, e.g. idiopathic thrombocytopenic purpura (ITP)
- infant – vitamin K_1 not given at birth.

Perform a clinical examination to detect signs of illness, such as septicaemia, jaundice or hepatosplenomegaly.

Laboratory tests include platelet count, bleeding time, INR and PTT.

Platelet abnormalities

Thrombocytopenia

This is the main cause of bleeding. It can be asymptomatic and is characteristically associated with petechiae or mucosal bleeding when the platelet count is less than $60 \times 10^9/l$.

Various types of thrombocytopenia are described.

Immune thrombocytopenia

Antiplatelet antibodies can be formed in the mother and then transferred to the fetus to produce a transient thrombocytopenia.

Platelets: Antibodies may be produced against fetal platelets that enter the maternal circulation. This is similar to ABO or Rhesus sensitisation.

Drugs: Various drugs can induce antibody formation and the drug-antibody complex may become attached to platelets and destroy them.

Maternal disease: Antiplatelet antibodies occur in diseases such as idiopathic thrombocytopenic purpura and systemic lupus erythematosus.

In most of these conditions only platelet function is altered (Table 16.5) and infants remain well apart from the effects of thrombocytopenia. Treatment is often unnecessary.

A platelet transfusion is recommended when the count is less than $20 \times 10^9/l$ as haemorrhage is a risk below this level. Steroids may also be used at this stage.

Thrombocytopenia and infection

Congenital infections such as rubella, cytomegalovirus, syphilis and herpes can cause thrombocytopenia.

After birth, thrombocytopenia may be associated with bacterial sepsis or disseminated intravascular coagulation.

Infants are ill and have general signs of infection, such as jaundice and hepatosplenomegaly.

Clotting defects are frequently present.

Treatment is directed at the underlying disease.

Clotting defects

The bleeding that occurs in clotting defects is usually more severe than that associated with thrombocytopenia. Mild trauma can produce excessive bruising, enclosed haemorrhage or constant oozing of blood from puncture sites.

Haemorrhagic disease

The condition is characterised by bleeding owing to inadequate coagulation factors dependent on vitamin K_1. They include factors II, VII, IX and X. The incidence varies widely throughout the world.

Note

Haemorrhagic disease is preventable and vitamin K_1 should be given to all infants after birth (p. 26).

Clinical signs

Spontaneous bleeding occurs from a variety of external or internal sites after the second day of life. The infant may develop epistaxis, haematemesis, melaena, haematuria or ecchymosis, depending on the organ involved.

Laboratory tests: The INR and PTT are abnormal (see Table 16.5).

Treatment

Vitamin K_1 1 mg is given intravenously and should correct defective coagulation within a few hours.

A transfusion of fresh blood will be required in cases of severe blood loss.

Haemophilia

Male infants who are deficient in factors VIII or IX may develop a haemorrhagic tendency in early life, for example after circumcision. Defective coagulation is detected on screening tests (Table 16.5). Specific investigations are required to identify the missing factor.

Treatment

Factor concentrates are used, as well as plasma cryoprecipitate.

Disseminated intravascular coagulation

This condition is characterised by the intravascular consumption of platelets and coagulation factors with deposition of fibrin thrombi. It occurs secondarily to a number of antenatal and postnatal diseases.

Causes

Antenatal: Thromboplastic material may enter the fetal circulation as the result of:
- abruptio placentae
- dead twin
- amniotic fluid embolism.

Postnatal:
- severe infections, such as Gram-negative septicaemia
- severe hypoxaemia, for example hyaline membrane disease.

TABLE 16.5

Laboratory screening tests for bleeding disorders				
Test	Vitamin K deficiency	Haemophilia	Disseminated intravascular coagulation	Thrombocytopenia
PTT	Prolonged	Prolonged	Prolonged	Normal
INR	Prolonged	Normal	Prolonged	Normal
Platelet count	Normal	Normal	Decreased	Decreased
Fibrinogen	Normal	Normal	Decreased	Normal

Clinical presentations
Most infants are extremely ill owing to their underlying disease. They may develop bruising and purpura and tend to bleed from injection sites.

Diagnosis
Laboratory tests show signs of abnormal coagulation (Table 16.15), thrombocytopenia, red cell fragmentation and hypofibrinogenaemia.

Treatment
In mild cases the process may revert to normal following treatment of the underlying disease. Severe cases may require an exchange transfusion with fresh blood.

Prognosis
Severely affected infants often die despite therapy.

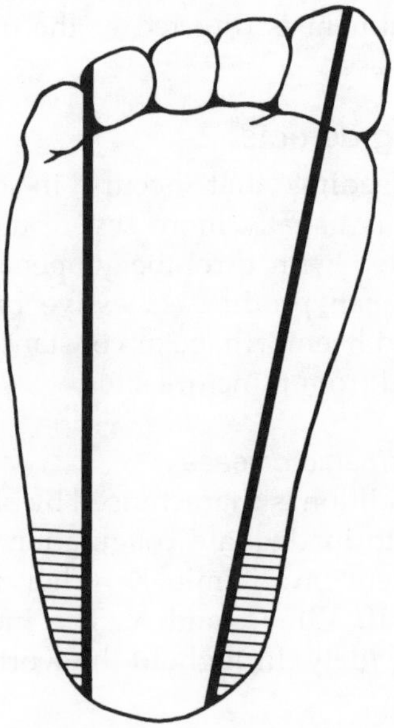

COLLECTION OF BLOOD SAMPLES

Heel stab
Heat a foot by placing it in a clean carton of warm water for five minutes (temperature 38° C).

Dry the heel and then clean it with an alcohol swab.

Encircle the heel between a thumb and forefinger and stab the dorsum on the medial side with a disposable metal blood lancet (Fig. 16.4).

The heel is held down, preferably below the level of the body, and drops of blood are collected in the required capillary or microtubes.

Note
Failure to warm the foot is the most likely explanation for a poor flow of blood.

Venepuncture
This may be necessary if larger amounts (2–5 ml) of blood are required.

No venepuncture is totally safe and

Fig. 16.4 *The warmed heel is held between a thumb and forefinger and a stab is made within the shaded areas*

certain sites are preferably avoided because of potential complications.

Avoid	Complications
Femoral vein	Arterial spasm Penetration of peritoneal cavity Osteitis of femur
Umbilical vein	Sepsis Thrombosis
Posterior fontanelle	Intracranial bleeding
Internal jugular	Occult bleeding, pneumothorax

Site of choice
- Cubital vein.
- Veins on dorsum of hand – difficult to obtain more than 1–2 ml blood.
- Scalp veins.

Requirements
- A good light source.
- Disposable 10 ml syringe.
- Scalp vein set, needle size 25.
- Cotton and alcohol swabs.

Method

Cubital vein: The infant is wrapped in a clean towel and placed on a flat surface with one arm exposed and extended.

A nurse compresses the upper arm above the elbow. The baby's lower arm is extended and 'milked' towards the elbow to distend veins. A distended cubital vein may be more readily palpated than seen, especially in a fat baby.

Clean and dry the skin. Insert the needle directly into the vein.

Occasionally the vein is transfixed, but blood is obtained as the needle is slowly withdrawn while aspirating all the time.

The lower arm may require intermittent 'milking' in order for the required amount of blood to be obtained.

Urogenital Disorders

RENAL PHYSIOLOGY

Before birth

Three sets of excretory organs are formed in the embryo at different stages: the pronephros (forekidney), mesophros (midkidney) and metanephros (hindkidney). The last develops into permanent kidneys, whereas the others degenerate and disappear.

Nephrons have formed by eight weeks and urine is excreted at nine weeks. This function regulates the volume of amniotic fluid that is diminished (oligohydramnios) in the absence of kidneys or when there is a urethral obstruction. The renal system is not essential for intrauterine life as products of metabolism are transferred to the maternal circulation through the placenta.

After birth

Homeostasis is regulated by the kidneys, which have to function near maximum capacity for several months. They have little reserve for additional loads such as drugs.

Glucose, bicarbonate, phosphate and amino acids are not completely retained by the tubules and sodium is poorly conserved in the preterm baby.

The kidneys have a limited ability to conserve water when fluid has been restricted or lost and cannot concentrate urine beyond a specific gravity of 1 025.

Urine output is thus an important reflection of the state of hydration in a newborn baby.

URINE

Output

The bladder contains 5–40 ml urine at birth, which is voided within 24 hours by 90% of babies.

The daily output gradually increases to 1–2 ml/kg/hour and by the end of the first week up to 10 wet nappies are changed each day.

Delay in micturition

Micturition can be delayed for 36 hours,

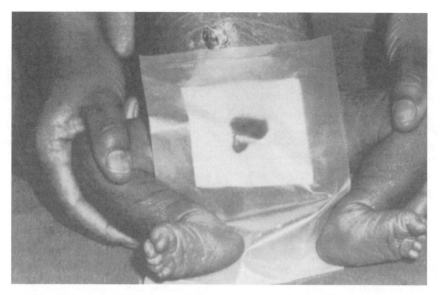

Fig. 17.1 *A plastic bag is attached to the perineum for the collection of urine*

particularly if the first voiding occurred at birth and was not observed. A further delay is unusual and may be associated with:

- asphyxia
- respiratory distress
- inadequate intake
- excessive evaporation from photo-therapy or radiant heating.

Rare causes include renal agenesis and urethral obstruction from valves.

An infant who fails to void can be offered a feed of sterile water (30 ml/kg). The bladder should be palpable within 30–60 minutes. If it is manually compressed, urine may be voided. Males should produce a good stream and not a dribble.

A full bladder can also be detected by ultrasonography, which may be used to demonstrate kidneys and the absence of urethral valves.

Collection (Fig. 17.1)
Method of obtaining urine specimen
A 'clean catch' specimen of urine may be collected as follows:

- Palpate infant's abdomen to feel the bladder. A full bladder is palpable above the pelvis.
- Apply an alcohol swab to the anterior abdominal wall and at the same time hold a sterile test tube in front of the genitalia to collect urine.

If this method is unsuccessful, collect urine in a plastic urine-collecting bag.

Method
- Wash the genitalia with an antiseptic solution, such as chlorhexidine 0,5% in water.
- Dry with a sterile towel.
- Use a neonatal urine-collecting plastic bag.
- Remove the paper strip to expose the adhesive surface.
- *Boys:* Place the opening of the bag over the penis and scrotum and fix it to the surrounding skin.
- *Girls:* Fix the adhesive section around the vulva, starting posteriorly.
- Remove the bag as soon as it contains urine and transfer a specimen to a sterile test tube.

Suprapubic puncture

Invasive techniques are avoided as far as possible, but occasionally the need may arise to collect a perfectly sterile specimen of urine. This situation usually occurs in cases of doubtful urinary tract infections.

The urine may be obtained by a suprapubic puncture:

- Wash hands.
- Palpate the abdomen and percuss it to detect a full bladder.
- Clean the lower abdomen with chlor-hexidine 0,5% in water, using sterile swabs.
- Insert a 22-gauge needle fitted to a syringe through the skin in the mid-line 1–2 cm above the symphysis pubis to a depth of 1–2 cm.
- Withdraw urine and remove the syringe.
- Spray the puncture site with collodion.

Caution: The procedure is done only if the bladder is full.

Urine examination

A number of simple laboratory tests can be done on freshly voided urine (Table 17.1). The selection depends on the indication for examination.

Paper strips, like Dipstix™ and Phenistix™, are dipped into urine and then read.

Microscopic examination is done on the sediment, which is obtained after centri-fuging urine at 3 000 rpm for one minute.

The specific gravity is usually low (1 002–1 006) in the early weeks of life.

A trace of protein may be detected for several days after birth. This transient feature occurs in 20% of babies, mostly preterm ones. Transient glycosuria may also be noted in 25% of normal babies.

A pink stain may appear in the nappy. This is caused by urates, which are present for several days. A mother needs reassur-ance that this is not blood.

Important causes of abnormal contents are listed in Table 17.1.

CONGENITAL RENAL MALFORMATIONS

Important malformations of the renal system are listed in Table 17.2.

Presentation

Suspect a renal malformation if the following disorders are present:

- Oligohydramnios, e.g. renal agenesis.
- Ear deformities.
- Potter facies (p. 238), e.g. renal agenesis.
- Anorectal malformations.
- Abdominal muscles defects.
- Spina bifida (p. 136).
- Cardiac defects.

Signs and symptoms

Any of the following may be present:

Visible abnormality – e.g. exstrophy of bladder.

Disorders of micturition:

Failure to pass urine – e.g. kidney agenesis, urethral obstruction.

Inadequate output – e.g. hypoplastic kidneys.

Constant dribbling – e.g. urethral valves.

Palpable renal masses – e.g. polycystic kidney, hydronephrosis.

Ascites.

General features

- Failure to thrive. ▪ Persistent vomiting.
- Lethargy. ▪ Dehydration.

Laboratory features

- Urine – pyuria, proteinuria, glycosuria; bacteruria.
- Blood – raised levels of urea and creatinine, high or low potassium and sodium levels.

Ultrasonography

The kidney and renal tract can be clearly visualised with ultrasound imaging. This method enables a rapid and accurate diagnosis to be made of many congenital abnormalities.

TABLE 17.1

Simple laboratory tests on urine			
Test	*Objective*	*Outcome*	*Important reasons*
Dipstix	Protein	More than trace	Asphyxia, infection
	Glucose	More than trace	IV dextrose, diabetes, Fanconi syndrome
	Haemoglobin	Present	Asphyxia, haemolytic disease
	Bilirubin	Present	Obstructive hyperbilirubi-naemia
	Urobilin	Present	Haemolytic disease, liver disease
	Specific gravity	More than 1 012	Underhydration, solute load
		Less than 1 008	Overhydration, renal disease
Refraction	Osmolality	More than 400 mOsm	Underhydration
		Less than 100 mOsm	Overhydration
Clinitest	Reducing substances	Present	Galactosaemia, fructosaemia in absence of glycosuria
Phenistix	Phenylpyruvic acid	Present	Phenylketonuria
Litmus	pH	Persistently over 7	Infection, tubular acidosis
		Persistently under 6	Metabolic acidaemia
Microscopy	Pus cells	Present	Infection
	Casts	Red or white cell types	Glomerular disease, dehydration, infection
	Crystals	Orotic acid	Hyperammonaemia
	Red cells	Present	Asphyxia, renal vein thrombosis, haemorrhagic disease, DIC
	Epithelial cells	Inclusion bodies	Cytomegalovirus
Culture	Bacteria	More than 10^5 colonies	Infection
Latex agglutination	Group B streptococcal antigen	Present	Group B streptococcal disease

TABLE 17.2

Congenital malformations of the renal system			
Kidney	*Ureter*	*Bladder*	*Urethra*
Agenesis	Megaloureter	Exstrophy	Valves
Single cysts	Duplication		
Hypoplasia			
Multicystic kidney			
Horseshoe kidney			
Polycystic kidney			
Ectopic kidney			
Hydronephrosis			

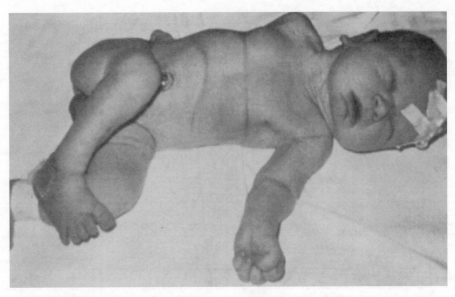

Fig. 17.2 *Renal agenesis. Note the prominent skin folds under the eyes, the low-set ears and the characteristically large hands*

Specific malformations

Renal agenesis (Fig. 17.2)

The kidneys are absent in 1 in 4 000 babies, mostly male. Many are stillborn (40%) and the others die soon after birth as a result of pulmonary hypoplasia.

The following features are characteristic of renal agenesis:

- *Pregnancy:* Oligohydramnios.
- *Placenta:* Amnion nodosum.
- *Infant:*
  - 'Potter facies' (wide-set eyes, prominent epicanthic folds, flat bridge of nose, low-set ears).
  - Hypoplastic lungs.
  - Skeletal abnormalities.
  - Large spade-like hands, bow legs and club feet.

Hypoplastic kidney

Underdeveloped kidneys are usually associated with other abnormalities of the urinary tract, such as kidney cysts. One or both kidneys may be affected and the outcome depends on the total functioning mass of kidney tissue.

Horseshoe kidney

The ureteric buds may fuse in the embryo to produce a midline kidney, which is shaped like a horseshoe when the lower poles are united.

The flow of urine can be obstructed where the ureters cross the isthmus. This may lead to pyelonephritis.

Diagnosis
Ultrasonography.

Treatment
- Control of urinary infection.
- Correction by surgery in selected cases.

Ectopic kidney

The kidney ascends from the fetal position in the pelvis to its permanent site in the abdomen. This process can be arrested at any stage. Obstruction to the flow of urine may occur and result in infection.

Treatment is usually conservative, but nephrectomy is occasionally required.

Kidney cysts

Single cysts

These occur in 3–5% of infants and are rarely detected on clinical examination. They are usually of no significance, but large ones require excision.

Multicystic kidney

A kidney may be composed of multiple cysts and have limited amounts of functional tissue. The organ loses its characteristic shape and may be palpated as a mass in the abdomen.

Diagnosis can be confirmed by ultrasonography and intravenous pyelography.

A nephrectomy is performed if one kidney is affected and the outlook is excellent.

Polycystic kidney

This is usually inherited as an autosomal recessive malformation.

Cysts are uniformly distributed throughout both kidneys, giving them a sponge-like appearance. They may also occur in the liver, lungs and pancreas.

Labour can be obstructed owing to massive distension of the abdomen.

Many affected infants are stillborn or die shortly after birth. Survivors have varying degrees of renal failure in infancy and childhood.

Hydronephrosis

This denotes a dilation of the renal pelvis which usually results from an obstruction at the ureteropelvic junction. It may be uni- or bilateral and can be associated with other renal tract abnormalities, for example urethral valves.

Pyelonephritis commonly occurs as a result of infection.

The presenting features vary from palpable masses in the abdomen to a urinary tract infection. Diagnosis is confirmed by ultrasonography. The treatment and outlook depend on factors such as the nature of the obstruction, e.g. stricture or aberrant blood vessel; the extent of the lesion, e.g. uni- or bilateral; the presence of infection and the functional state of the kidneys.

Megaloureter

The ureters and bladder can be grossly dilated without obvious signs of obstruction. This is sometimes associated with spinal lesions such as meningomyelocele.

Pyelonephritis commonly occurs and can be difficult to control.

Duplication of ureters

The ureters may be doubled on one or both sides. Urinary tract infection is common. Treatment is usually conservative and surgery is indicated on occasion.

Exstrophy of the bladder (Colour plate X)

This rare abnormality usually occurs in males. The mucosal surface of the bladder is exposed through a defect in the lower abdominal wall. The pelvic bones are widely separated and an epispadias is present.

Urinary incontinence frequently persists despite reconstructive surgery.

Urethral valves

Structures resembling valves can form in the posterior urethra and obstruct the flow of urine at the bladder neck. The resultant back pressure causes hypertrophy of the bladder, dilation of the ureters and hydronephrosis. These features can be present at birth. Pyelonephritis is a common complication and the renal tract may rupture and produce ascites.

Urine may dribble continually from the meatus and the distended bladder is palpable above the symphysis. The condition is virtually restricted to males and can be detected by ultrasonography and a voiding cystourethrogram (Fig. 17.3).

Treatment

Prolonged back pressure can cause irreparable damage to the kidneys and the valves should be resected as soon as possible.

URINARY TRACT INFECTION

Renal tract infections are usually blood-borne and caused by *E. coli*, enterococci or *Klebsiella* organisms.

Specific predisposing factors in the postnatal period include:

- renal tract abnormality, for example double ureter
- neurogenic bladder, such as in association with meningomyelocele.

Clinical features
The infant is often asymptomatic in the early stages or may show non-specific signs of infection (p. 91). The urine may smell offensive. Enlarged kidneys may be palpated.

Diagnosis
A pure growth of bacteria with a colony count of 10^5/ml is very significant, particularly if obtained from repeated

samples of a 'clean catch' specimen of urine. In a doubtful case or in the case of an extremely ill infant the urine specimen can be collected by bladder puncture (p. 236).

Treatment
Ceftriaxone is used until culture results are known.

Appropriate therapy is given for two weeks.

Follow-up
Repeat checks on urine should be made over the subsequent six months.

Ultrasound examination is advisable in the event of a relapse, as there may be an underlying congenital abnormality.

Note
Examine the urine for pus cells and organisms in all infants who do not thrive, who have prolonged jaundice or who appear to be ill.

RENAL VEIN THROMBOSIS

The risk of vascular thrombosis is increased by the following factors:

- Dehydration.
- Polycythaemia.
- Birth asphyxia and shock.
- Bacteraemia.
- Infant of a diabetic mother.

Diagnosis
Renal vein thrombosis is characterised by sudden enlargement of a kidney that is palpable. Associated signs include oligaemia, anuria, haematuria, abdominal distension and vomiting.

Confirmation can be obtained from ultrasonography, intravenous pyelography and photoscanning.

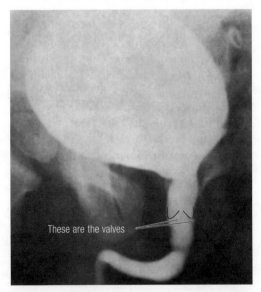
These are the valves

Fig. 17.3 *Urethral valves. Dye has been instilled into the urethra and bladder to demonstrate urethral valves and dilated prostatic urethra*

Treatment
The primary disorder, like dehydration, needs to be corrected and a careful check

kept of urinary output, weight, urea, electrolytes and acid-base balance. Renal failure usually responds to conservative management.

Long-term complications such as hypertension may necessitate nephrectomy.

ACUTE RENAL FAILURE

Various prerenal, renal or post-renal factors can cause acute failure of glomerular and tubular function.

Prerenal factors
Perinatal insults that result in ischaemia of the kidneys and hypoperfusion account for most cases of acute renal failure.

Important conditions are:
- dehydration
- acute haemorrhage
- perinatal hypoxaemia
- septicaemia
- drugs, for example indomethacin.

Renal factors
Intrinsic lesions of the kidney can be caused by congenital or acquired factors.
Examples:
- *Congenital:* Hypoplastic renal tissue, cysts.
- *Acquired:* Nephrotoxic drugs, like aminoglycosides and indomethacin

Postrenal factors
Obstructive lesions of the renal tract can impair function by causing back pressure on the kidneys.

Important conditions are:
- posterior urethral valves
- megaloureter.

Diagnosis
Characteristic features are:
- oliguria (urine output less than 0,5 ml/kg/hour)
- anuria
- raised blood urea.

Other findings include:
- haematuria
- proteinuria
- oedema
- raised serum creatinine
- raised serum potassium (> 7 mmol/l)
- low serum sodium (< 120 mmol/l)
- metabolic acidaemia ($HCO_3 < 20$ mmol/l).

These abnormalities, if not corrected, can result in cardiac arrhythmias, seizures, coma and death.

Treatment
The primary cause of renal failure requires urgent treatment.

Prerenal: Hypovolaemia is the major cause of poor renal perfusion and can be corrected by:
- plasma volume expanders, such as normal saline or stabilised human serum (10–20 ml per kg)
- blood transfusion, if severe blood loss has occurred.

Use a diuretic, furosemide (2 mg/kg), to increase urine flow once hypovolaemia has been corrected.

If this is unsuccessful then institute a strict intake and output regimen. The urine output is estimated by weighing nappies before and after micturition.

Fluid restriction: A total amount of 25 ml/kg/day will cover insensible fluid losses.

Energy: Requirements are provided by dextrose water 10% to minimise fat and protein catabolism.

Protein restriction: Essential amino acids may be added to the fluid to maintain positive nitrogen balance, for example Vamin 5–10 ml.

Weight: The infant is weighed at least three times a day and a loss of 1% bodyweight is permitted. A gain in weight usually indicates overhydration.

Many renal and postrenal abnormalities

are correctable and an accurate diagnosis, such as urethral valves, should be established. Ultrasonography plays an important role in this respect.

Correction of electrolyte imbalance
Hyperkalaemia: Potassium accumulates in the baby's serum and may cause cardiac arrhythmia and death, especially when associated with ECG abnormalities (high T waves, prolonged QRS, depressed ST segments).

The ion-exchange resin Kayexalate® can be used to reduce the level of serum potassium when it exceeds 7 mmol/l. It is given orally or rectally (1 g/kg) and is retained for 30 minutes.

If it is not effective, or in an emergency, a rapid reduction of serum potassium may be achieved by administering:

- sodium bicarbonate 4% 2,5 mmol/kg IV, or
- calcium gluconate 10% 0,5 ml/kg IV.

Give the latter slowly, together with ECG monitoring.

Use peritoneal dialysis if these measures are unsuccessful. It is also indicated for:

- intractable fluid overload
- coma.

Hyponatraemia: The level of serum sodium is usually low as a result of fluid retention and may be corrected by restricting the intake of water.

Correction of acid-base imbalance
Metabolic acidaemia is corrected with sodium bicarbonate (p. 175).

Outcome
The prognosis depends on the primary cause and the overall mortality is 50%.

Recovery from acute renal failure occurs within two weeks, but many survivors have impaired renal function.

GENITALIA – MALE
Penis

The normal penis when stretched has a length of 3,5 cm (± 0,4) from base to tip of glans in the full-term baby. The foreskin adheres to the glans and cannot be fully retracted. It tapers beyond the glans to a narrow opening that permits a good stream of urine. This is not an indication for circumcision, which is done mostly for religious or parental reasons.

Hypospadias (Fig. 17.4)
Suspect hypospadias if the newborn appears to have been circumcised or if the penis has a 'hooded' appearance. In severe cases the shaft of the penis is bent (chordee).

Incidence
This defect occurs in 2 to 3 per 1 000 births.

Types
Mild: The urethra opens on the glans, but ventral to its normal position.

Moderate: The urethral opening is situated on the shaft of the penis. There is usually some degree of chordee.

Severe: The urethra opens at the base of the penis. Chordee is marked and penis is small. The testes may be undescended.

Treatment
The majority of cases are mild and require no treatment.

Moderate and severe lesions are repaired when the child is three to four years of age.

Circumcision is never done as the foreskin may be required for the plastic repair operation. Meatotomy may be necessary.

Infants with severe hypospadias should be investigated for intersex, especially if the testes are undescended (p. 245).

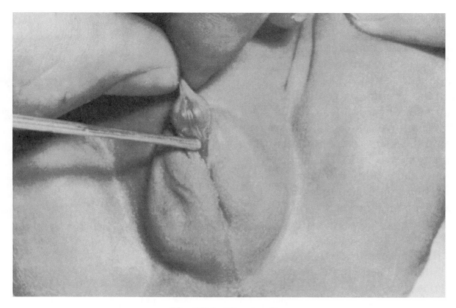

Fig. 17.4. *Hypospadias.*

Epispadias

The urethra opens on the upper surface of the penis. This rare defect is usually associated with other abnormalities, like exstrophy of the bladder.

Treatment
Surgical repair.

Micropenis

An apparently small penis is usually owing to an excessive amount of suprapubic fat. When this is retracted the penis is noted to be of normal size. Micropenis is rare and often found in association with other defects.

Testes

Undescended testis

The testes develop from the medial aspects of the urogenital ridge in the abdomen. From this position they descend to reach the deep inguinal ring at 12 weeks and the inguinal canal by about 28 weeks. They are present in the scrotum after 32–36 weeks.

Scrotal temperature is 4° C less than body temperature. This is essential for the normal function of the testes.

In the condition of undescended testis, one or both testes may be arrested in the abdomen or in the inguinal canal.

Associated deformities
- Small, underdeveloped scrotal sac.
- Indirect inguinal hernia in 90% of cases.

Prognosis
The testes may descend spontaneously, especially if the infant is preterm. If a testis fails to reach the bottom of the scrotum by six weeks of age, it is likely to remain permanently higher.

Undescended testes can atrophy, and in rare cases malignant changes may occur.

Treatment
An associated inguinal hernia will require repair and the testes can be anchored in the scrotum at the same time.

In uncomplicated cases the testes may be relocated after the age of two years.

Retractile testis

Testes may normally be drawn out of the scrotum by the cremaster muscles. This often happens if the infant is cold or when the thigh is touched. A testis can be relocated in the scrotum by gently pushing it with a finger towards the scrotum, starting at the inguinal canal. Obtain a surgical opinion if the testes are not located in the scrotum by six weeks. At this stage retractile testes may require hormone therapy, human chorionic gonadotrophin or surgery to maintain them in the sac.

Ectopic testis (Fig. 17.5)

Testes have passed through the inguinal canal but have settled in an abnormal position, such as in the perineum, inner surface of thigh or even in the abdominal wall.

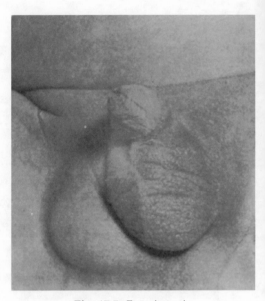

Fig. 17.5 *Ectopic testis*

Congenital hydrocele (Fig. 17.6)

In the fetus, the peritoneum continues as the 'processus vaginalis', which precedes the testes into the scrotum. Normally the testes are surrounded by the lower extremity of this structure, termed the 'tunica vaginalis'. The upper portion is obliterated. Hydrocele of the tunica vaginalis is the result of the persistence of the processus vaginalis, enabling peritoneal fluid to accumulate around the testes.

The right side is affected more often than the left, but the hydroceles may be bilateral.

An indirect inguinal hernia can occur if the whole canal remains patent.

Clinical picture

The hydrocele presents as a soft cystic swelling that is translucent.

Prognosis and treatment

The majority of hydroceles disappear spontaneously as the processus vaginalis undergoes obliteration. Surgery is indicated if the swelling persists.

Inguinal hernia

In babies these herniae are usually indirect and result from the partial or complete persistence of the processus vaginalis. The right side is more frequently affected and the incidence among boys is nine times greater than among girls.

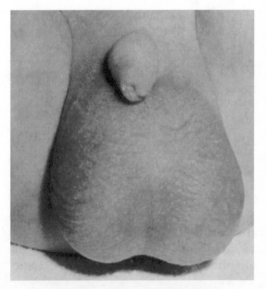

Fig. 17.6 *Congenital hydrocele*

Signs

A soft mass develops in the groin or in the scrotum, or an existing mass enlarges as soon as the baby cries.

Treatment

Surgical repair is done at the age of two or three months. Irreducible or strangulated herniae must be repaired immediately.

Torsion of testis

Torsion may occur *in utero* and presents as a painless firm swelling of the scrotum at birth.

The testis is not removed, but may be untwisted at operation to preserve functional tissue.

GENITALIA – FEMALE
Labia

A full-term baby has well-developed labia majora, which cover the labia minora. The latter are exposed in a preterm infant and the clitoris is prominent owing to under-developed labia majora.

Fused labia

Connective tissue adhesions between the labia majora may obscure the vaginal orifice. These connections are fragile at birth and can be broken by a probe without discomfort to the infant.

This must be distinguished from true fusion in which the labia resemble a scrotum. This occurs in intersex states (p. 246).

Vagina

A white discharge is noted on the second day. It contains cells and secretions from the vagina and uterus and persists for several days (Colour plate XI).

Bleeding can occur at the end of the first week as a result of endometrial shedding. This is present in approximately 10% of normal babies.

Hymenal tag (Colour plate X)

Baby girls can have a pink fleshy append-age at the vaginal opening. It gradually shrinks and disappears.

Hydrocolpos

In cases of a vaginal membrane, vaginal atresia or imperforate hymen, the uterus can distend due to excessive accumulation of mucus from cervical glands. This presents with:

- acute retention of urine due to pressure on the urethra
- rectal obstruction due to pressure on the bowel
- a suprapubic mass.

Treatment

In most cases perforation of the hymen or vaginal membrane is all that is required.

SEX DIFFERENTIATION

Embryology

The primitive gonads are indistinguish-able in male and female embryos before seven weeks. Their subsequent differentiation and development depend on the sex chromosomes (XY and XX) acquired at fertilisation. The Y chromosome is essential for testicular formation and in its absence the indifferent gonads will develop into ovaries. Normal ovarian development is dependent on two X chromosomes (XX), and ovarian dysgenesis (Turner syndrome) results when one X chromosome is absent (XO).

The external genitalia also pass through an indifferent stage and acquire their sexual characteristics between 6 and 12 weeks. Masculinisation is caused by androgens, which are produced by the testes. Feminisation occurs in the absence of androgens.

Development disorders:
(see p. 118). (Colour plate X)

Infants with ambiguous genitalia are classified into three groups:

1   Virilised females.
2   Undervirilised males.
3   True hermaphrodites.

Two factors are of prime importance in the diagnosis and treatment:
1   The presence or absence of gonads.
2   The size of the phallus.

Infants who lack gonads are considered to be virilised females. Those with gonads may be undervirilised males or true hermaphrodites with testicular and ovarian tissue.

Virilised females

Excessive amounts of androgen can cause masculinisation of the external genitalia. The features range from fusion of the labia and enlargement of the clitoris, if the genitalia were stimulated before 14 weeks, to clitoral enlargement only if the insult occurred later.

Androgens may have been ingested by the mother during pregnancy or over-produced by the fetal adrenal gland as a result of congenital adrenal hyperplasia. The latter accounts for most cases and an infant without gonads is considered to have this syndrome until disproved. Characteristic findings of masculinisation are listed in Table 17.3.

Undervirilised males

Genital development in males depends on an adequate production of androgen by the fetal testes and adrenal gland. Defects in virilisation can occur as a result of inadequate formation of androgen due to enzymatic defects in the testes or adrenals. In some, the testes may fail to respond to adequate amounts of androgen.

Characteristic features of the undervirilised male are indicated in Table 17.3. Inform parents of the uncertainty and indicate that expert evaluation is essential before gender can be assigned.

True hermaphrodite

These infants have ovarian and testicular tissue in one or both gonads.

The external genitalia usually consist of an enlarged phallus with hypospadias and fused labia. Diagnosis requires laparotomy and a biopsy of the gonads. Features are listed in Table 17.3.

Investigations

Establish whether androgenic drugs were ingested during pregnancy or if similar problems had occurred in the family.

Clinical

Examine the baby's external genitalia to determine:

TABLE 17.3

Factors that may be associated with intersex			
Features	Virilised female	Undervirilised male	Hermaphrodite
Sex chromatin	Positive	Negative	Variable
Sex chromosomes	XX	XY	Variable
Gonads	Absent	Present	Present
Phallus	Enlarged clitoris	Hypospadias	Hypospadias
Uterus	Present	Absent	Usually present
Medication	Androgens or progestins	Nil	Nil
Urine	Raised 17-ketosteroids	Raised 11-ketopregnanetriol	–
Plasma	Raised pregnanetriol, low sodium, high sodium	Raised 17-hydroxy pregnenolone	–

- presence and site of gonads
- size and shape of the phallus
- site of the urethral meatus
- presence of a vaginal opening
- appearance of the scrotum or labia.

General examination includes a measurement of blood pressure.

The infant without gonads is viewed with urgency. A salt-losing form of adrenal hyperplasia must be excluded.

Serum electrolytes. Sodium and potassium levels are determined immediately.

Less urgent investigations include:

Urine: 24-hour collection for 17-keto-steroids (normal less than 1,0 mg).

Buccal smear: Sex chromatin.

Leukocyte culture: Sex chromosomes x and y specific probe detection.

Ultrasonography: Presence of uterus and ovaries.

Radiography: Radiopaque dye can outline the vagina and uterus.

A laparotomy and gonad biopsy may be needed when the above investigations are inconclusive.

Additional investigations may include 17-Hydroxyprogesterone, gonadotropins, testosterone and anti-mullerian hormone levels.

Treatment

Virilised females will almost always be reared as girls and those with congenital adrenal hyperplasia require lifelong therapy with steroids (p. 275).

The management of other cases should be conducted only by experts in the fields of paediatric endocrinology, psychology and surgery.

CHAPTER 18

Skin and Tissue Disorders

EPIDERMIS AND DERMIS

Embryology

The skin is formed from two embryonic layers during the third week of gestation. The epidermis is derived from ectoderm and the dermis from mesenchyme. Neural crest elements provide pigmented cells.

The surface cells proliferate to form a periderm, which contains microvilli. These can transfer fluid and substances between the fetus and the amniotic fluid. The periderm is shed before birth.

Cells at the base of the epidermis extend into the dermis to form ridges. These produce characteristic grooves on the surface of the skin (fingerprints). The pattern is specific for each baby and can be used for identification at birth. It is altered in a characteristic way in various chromosomal abnormalities.

A multilayered epidermis has formed by the time the fetus is mature.

Sebum is secreted by sebaceous glands during the second trimester and covers the skin to form vernix caseosa (Fig. 18.1). This greasy-white substance protects the fragile skin and acts as a lubricant during birth. It also contains fetal hair and squamous cells from the epidermis and the amnion.

Sweat glands are active after birth in the full-term baby, but do not function in the preterm infant. This has important implications for thermoregulation (p. 267).

Miscellaneous features

Milia (Fig. 18.2)

White papules, the size of pinheads, are frequently seen on the nose, cheeks or chin. They are caused by keratin cysts in sebaceous glands and disappear within three weeks.

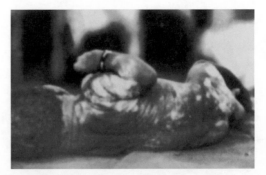

Fig. 18.1. *Normal newborn infant with vernix caseosa*

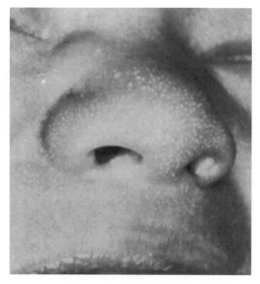

Fig. 18.2 *Milia of the nose*

Erythema toxicum (Colour plate XI)

This rash may appear on the trunk, face or limbs within hours or days of birth. It consists of multiple erythematous areas that have a central yellowish papule. The eruption fades rapidly and may reappear at different sites. The papules are packed with eosinophils, but the aetiology is unknown. This common rash can be alarming for parents, who should be reassured of its benign nature.

Peeling

The skin of the hands and feet may peel within days of birth, particularly in growth-retarded, meconium-stained and post-term babies. Excessive peeling is also a feature of infections such as syphilis.

Miliaria (heat rash)

Fine red papules may occur over the chest and neck from overheating. This reflects immaturity of the sweat glands. The rash resolves when appropriate steps are taken to prevent hyperthermia.

Harlequin colour change (Colour plate XI)

This is characterised by reddening of one half of the body and blanching of the other half. A distinct demarcation of colour is noted along the midline. The condition is likely to occur in a preterm baby and is not significant. The reason for flushing and blanching is unknown.

Jaundice

Yellow staining is commonly seen after the third day of life (p. 99).

Peripheral cyanosis

The hands and feet may remain blue for one to two days after birth. This is unrelated to hypothermia and is probably due to a sluggish peripheral circulation.

Oedema

The newborn infant has a high extracellular water content that can be exaggerated to result in oedema. During pregnancy various diseases can cause fetal oedema (hydrops fetalis). They are listed in Table 18.1.

Oedema confined to the hands and feet is a feature of Turner syndrome (p. 120). Oedema of the scalp (caput) can result from pressure on the presenting part during birth (p. 257).

Oedema frequently occurs after birth, especially in preterm babies.

Important causes are listed in Table 18.2.

Sclerema

This is characterised by non-pitting swelling of the skin and subcutaneous

TABLE 18.1

Important causes of hydrops fetalis	
Isoimmunisation	Rhesus disease, ABO, G6PD deficiency
Cardiac failure	Congenital heart defects, atrial tachycardia
Nephrotic syndrome	
Intrauterine infection	Toxoplasmosis, parvovirus, syphilis

TABLE 18.2

Generalised oedema after birth: important causes
Prematurity
Hyaline membrane disease
Hypomagnesaemia
Sepsis
Circulation overload
Cardiac failure

tissue. It may occur during severe illness, like septicaemia, or with shock or hypothermia.

The induration usually starts on the thighs and buttocks, but can encase the whole infant. No specific histological abnormality can be demonstrated in the skin or subcutaneous fat.

The efficacy of steroids in treatment is doubtful. The prognosis is poor as it depends on the underlying disease.

Subcutaneous fat necrosis

Sharply defined red or purple nodules may be palpated under the skin of the cheeks, shoulders or buttocks several days or weeks after birth. Trauma and hypothermia may play a role in the aetiology of fat necrosis. Do not mistake the swellings for abscesses. They are painless and may fluctuate, but are not associated with systemic illness. Resolution occurs within months.

Caution: Occasionally, particularly if widespread, the condition may be associated with hypercalcaemia. Check serum calcium level at intervals. Diuretics and steroid treatment may be needed for hypercalcaemia.

The distinguishing signs of oedema, sclerema and fat necrosis are tabulated in Table 18.3.

Buttock rashes

Contact dermatitis and physical irritation
Washing-powder, bleach or soap residues in the nappy can all result in an erythematous rash on the convex surface of the buttocks.

A similar rash can occur in skin folds as a result of irritation from dried vernix, faeces or powder that has been applied to wet skin. This is termed intertrigo. The area can become excoriated and may be infected with bacteria or *Candida albicans.*

Treatment: Remove the offending agent. Wash the buttocks with soap and water and dry after each nappy change. Apply a barrier cream, for example pure lanoline, to the red or excoriated regions.

Perianal dermatitis

The skin around the anus may become red and excoriated within the first few weeks of birth. This is more likely to occur in the bottle-fed than in the breast-fed infant. The cause usually is irritation by dry faeces.

Treatment: Do not allow stools to be in contact with the skin for long. Change the

TABLE 18.3

Distinguishing features of oedema, sclerema and fat necrosis						
	Sites	Skin	Skin temperature	Pitting	illness	Outlook
Sclerema	Buttocks thighs, general	Hard white	Cold	No	Yes	Poor
Oedema	Usually lower limbs	Normal, shiny	Normal	Yes	Usually not	Variable
Subcutaneous fat necrosis	Face, shoulders, buttocks	Red raised areas	Normal	No	No	Excellent

nappy as soon as it is soiled. Wash the buttocks with soap and water, rinse and dry and protect with Vaseline.

If excoriations are present either of the following ointments can be applied:

- glycerine acid tannic 1 part
- acriflavine emulsion 4 parts.

Should these measures fail to heal the ulcers, lie the infant prone with buttocks exposed to the air.

Moniliasis

Thrush infection of the skin is usually confined to the nappy region and is often secondary to *Candida* infection in the mouth or gut.

Erythematous streaks appear on the convex surface of the buttocks away from the anus. These become vesicular and confluent and may spread to involve the whole perineum. Lesions on the buttocks usually remain dry, whereas the lesions in skin folds become moist and covered with a pseudomembrane. Satellite papules often surround the lesions. The regional lymph glands are not enlarged.

Diagnosis: Fungal spores and hyphae may be seen under the microscope from scrapings of a lesion, and the organism *Candida albicans* can be cultured on selective media.

Treatment: Apply Nystatin ointment to the lesions for five to seven days. Give Nystatin suspension (1 ml, four times a day) to infants with oral or intestinal thrush.

Note: Any perineal rash may be infected with *Candida* and the fungus should be sought in every case.

Seborrhoeic dermatitis

This occurs during the early weeks as 'cradle cap'and later as generalised seborrhoea of the scalp, ears, forehead, neck, axillae and perineum. The aetiology is unknown and may be associated with a deficiency of zinc.

Cradle cap

Seborrhoea of the scalp usually starts over the anterior fontanelle and consists of greasy yellow scales.

Treatment: Mild cases can be controlled by washing the scalp daily with a bland shampoo. This is done following the application of a 2% solution of sodium bicarbonate to soften the scales.

Treat severe cases with a preparation that promotes desquamation. This contains liq. picis carb. 2% and salicylic acid 2% in Vaseline. Rub it into the scalp each morning. The hair is then shampooed and the ointment reapplied.

Generalised seborrhoea (Colour plate VIII)

The lesions in skin folds can become excoriated and infected. Widespread seborrhoea occasionally develops into atopic eczema.

Treatment: Resolution can be hastened by the application of 1% hydrocortisone cream four times a day for a week. The course may need to be repeated, but steroids should not be applied continuously for prolonged periods.

Use a bland soap, such as Neutrogena™, to wash the infant.

Any secondary infection will need appropriate treatment.

Excoriated skin can become infected with *Candida albicans* and this fungus should be sought in scrapings from the lesions.

Congenital abnormalities

Aplasia cutis

Congenital absence of the skin usually presents as a midline defect of the scalp (Fig. 18.3). The sharply defined lesion is round or oval and varies in depth depending on the degree of aplasia. All layers of the skin can be absent.

Defects also occur on the trunk or extremities and multiple ones often have a symmetrical distribution.

The cause is unknown. Sporadic as

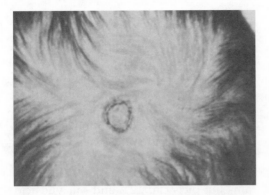

Fig. 18.3 *A midline ectodermal defect of the scalp*

well as autosomal dominant occurrence has been reported. Spontaneous healing occurs within months and results in a hairless atrophic scar. It may be associated with a defective gene for keratinocyte transglutaminase.

Ichthyosis

This autosomal recessive disorder is characterised by excessive scaliness of the skin and occurs in various forms.

Collodion skin (Fig. 18.4)

A parchment-like membrane, the fetal periderm, encases the baby and impairs sucking, breathing and movement. The eyes are occluded, the mouth is rigid and open, the nose and ears are compressed, and the fingers and toes are immobilised. The membrane cracks within days and peels to reveal normal skin. In later life the skin may be hyperkeratotic.

Harlequin fetus

This severe form results in death, as the constricting membrane does not separate. The infant is unable to breathe adequately and cannot regulate body temperature.

Albinism

This occurs in a partial or complete form.

The complete variety shows hypopigmentation of the skin, hair and eyes.

The following features occur:
- Photophobia.
- Nystagmus.
- Impaired visual acuity.

A white forelock is commonly seen in the partial form.

Cutis laxa

This is an autosomal dominant, recessive or x-linked abnormality of elastic tissue. The fibrillin 5 gene may be involved. The skin has poor elasticity and hangs in folds. Systemic manifestations include hernias,

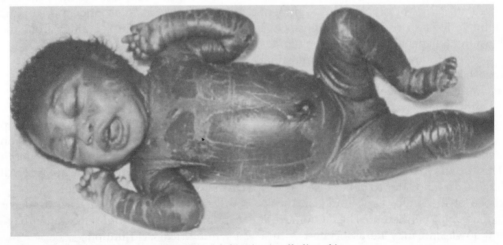

Fig. 18.4 *Ichthyosis: A collodion skin*

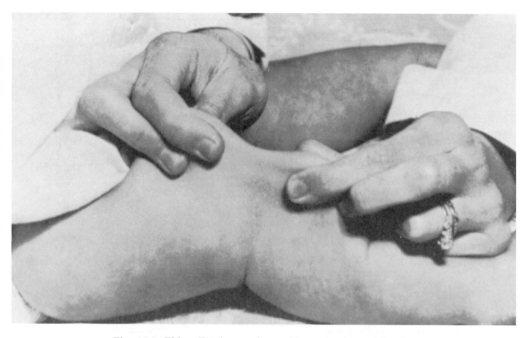

Fig. 18.5 *Ehlers-Danlos syndrome: Hyperelasticity of the skin*

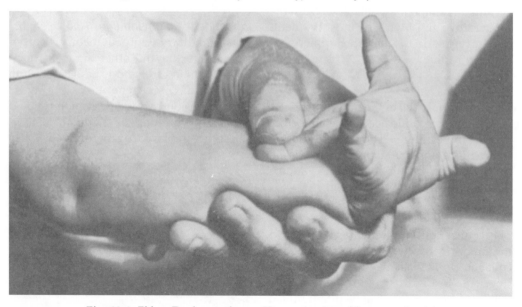

Fig. 18.6 *Ehlers-Danlos syndrome: Hyperextension of fingers and wrist*

cardiovascular disease and emphysema. The prognosis depends on the extent of the disorder.

Ehlers-Danlos

An abnormal gene in fibrous collagen causes the skin to be easily stretched (Fig. 18.5). It looks normal, but heals poorly when traumatised. The joints are excessively mobile (Fig. 18.6). Vitamin C, a co-factor for collagen fibre synthesis may offer some relief.

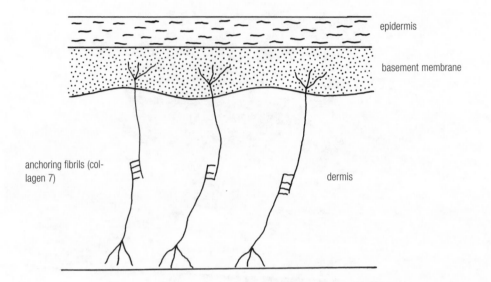

Fig. 18.7 *The connection between the dermis and epidermis is weakened by defective collagen (type 7)*

Epidermolysis bullosa (Colour plate IX)

The skin can blister after birth if genes for keratin or collagen are defective. Mutants for keratin 5 and 14 are the most frequent. Three types occur: simplex, junctional and dystrophic

Epidermolysis bullosa simplex

The epidermal cells in the outermost layer of the skin are fragile because of abnormal keratin (types 5, 14). They break apart if traumatised and the gaps fill with tissue fluid to form blisters. These are superficial and heal without scarring.

Dystrophic epidermolysis bullosa

The connection between the dermis and the epidermis is weakened by defective collagen (type 7) in the anchoring fibrils (Fig. 18.7). Light stroking causes the epidermis to peel off. The resultant bullae may fill with blood and can scar.

A generalised form that also involves the mucous membranes has a poor prognosis. Structures like hair and teeth are defective and many babies die of infection in the early months.

Treatment of the severe forms is unsatisfactory and genetic counselling is important because the disease may be inherited.

Incontinentia pigmenti (Fig. 18.8)

This hereditary neurocutaneous disorder affects the skin and other organs. It usually occurs in girls and is associated with a defective NEMO gene.

Skin lesions are present at birth and consist of bullous or papular lesions. These are replaced by pigmented warty

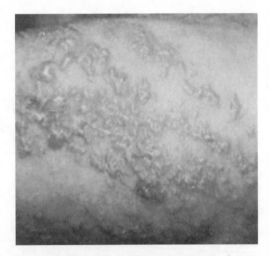

Fig. 18.8 *The early papular lesions of incontinentia pigmenti*

lesions which gradually resolve to form flat, hyperpigmented areas, usually arranged linearly. The disorder is a sex-linked dominant one.

Differential diagnosis: Erythema toxicum in early stages.

Treatment: Nil.

Prognosis: Some cases of this disorder are associated with microcephaly and mental retardation.

Congenital ectodermal dysplasia

This is characterised by the incomplete development of the epidermis and its appendages.

- The hair is fine and thin or absent.
- The teeth are absent or may be only a few misshapen stumps.
- The nails are atrophic or absent.
- The sweat glands may be absent, causing hyperpyrexia in hot weather.
- The sebaceous glands and lachrymal glands may be absent.
- The skin is dry, smooth, white and shiny.
- The face is typical: The bridge of the nose is flattened, the supraorbital ridges prominent, the external angles of the eyes lifted and the lower jaw underdeveloped.

Aetiology: The condition is apparently hereditary. Boys are affected more often than girls, especially in cases without sweat glands. In these, there is a sex-linked inheritance, as in haemophilia.

NAEVI (BIRTHMARKS)

Haemangiomas, vascular malformations and pigmented lesions are the most common form of birthmarks.

Haemangiomas

These include capillary and cavernous naevi and are characterised by proliferation and involution.

Capillary naevi (Colour plate XI)

Vascular pink blemishes are seen on the skin at birth in approximately 50% of babies. They usually occur on the upper eyelids, where they are known as 'stork bites', the midline of the forehead, and the nape of the neck, where they are described as 'salmon patches'. These flat birthmarks are more noticeable during crying.

The facial blemishes disappear within two years. Those on the neck persist into adulthood, but are concealed by hair.

Cavernous naevi
Strawberry mark (Colour Plate XII)

This superficial angioma is not present at birth. It arises from a blanched area of skin and develops into a bright red swelling. Multiple lesions may occur anywhere on the body and they vary in size.

Vascular growth ceases after several months and depigmented areas appear in the swelling. This heralds the stage of resolution and an uncomplicated naevus heals without scarring. Most resolve within seven years.

Complications: Ulceration, bleeding, infection or scarring may occur if a large haemangioma is in an area that is easily traumatised, such as the buttock. Antibiotic therapy may be needed to treat infection.

Cavernous naevi can extend into deeper tissues to cause extensive swelling. The superficial portion may be purple or blue. Swelling can impair the function of a vital organ, e.g. vision may be impaired by a naevus of the eyelid. Cardiac failure or thrombocytopenia may occur when the lesion involves a large area like a limb.

Treatment: Large haemangiomas and those with complications can be reduced in size by steroid therapy. Prednisone may be given systemically or injected into the lesion. It probably acts by blocking the enzyme glutamine transferase, which is present in all haemangiomas. Interferon alpha is an alternative treatment.

Vascular malformations

These developmental errors are present at birth and involve veins, arteries, capillaries, lymphatics or a combination thereof. The 'fast flow variety are arterio-venous connections, while the 'slow flow' group comprise capillaries, veins or lymphatics.

Capillary malformation

Port-wine stain

This capillary malformation, also known as 'naevus flammeus', is obvious at birth. The superficial dermal capillaries that extend to a depth of half a centimetre are hyperplastic. This mark differs from the innocuous 'stork bite' in the following ways:

- The stain occurs on the face, limbs or body. On the face it does not cross the midline.
- Its size varies and so does the colour, from pink to purple.
- It is flat at birth, but later can become raised.
- It does not regress and can darken and become nodular.

An angioma in the trigeminal area of the face may also involve the meninges of the brain. The resultant Sturge-Weber syndrome is associated with seizures, hemiparesis and intracranial calcification.

Treatment: The capillary angioma can be removed by flashlamp pulsed tunable dye laser. The laser energy is absorbed by the red blood cells in the dermal capillaries and transferred to the endothelium, which is destroyed. The perivascular tissues are unaffected. Six to ten treatments are needed for a satisfactory cosmetic result. The optimum time to treat is soon after birth.

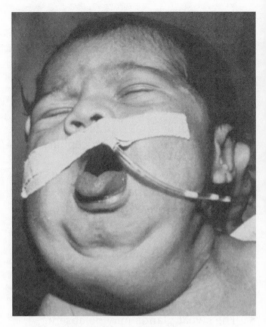

Fig. 18.9. *A cystic hygroma.*

Lymphatic malformation

This consists of dilated lymph channels that coalesce into a cystic mass.

Cystic hygroma (Fig. 18.9)

This multiloculated lesion involves the face, neck or shoulder. It can compress underlying structures.

Treatment: Localised lesions are excised or treated with carbon dioxide laser. Large ones may only be partially resectable.

Pigmented naevi

These vary considerably in size, site and colour.

Mongolian spot (Colour plate XI)

Dark-skinned babies frequently have blue-grey areas over the buttocks, back or shoulders, which are produced by melanocytes in the dermis. They should not be mistaken for bruises.

Naevi (moles) are rarely present at birth and usually appear after two years of age.

Café-au-lait spots

Light-brown patches may be seen anywhere on the skin at birth. They are caused by melanocytes in the epidermis and usually persist into adulthood.

An excessively large area or more than six small patches may indicate neurofibromatosis – these ultimately form tumours that contain perineural elements and may involve many organs. This is an autosomal dominant condition.

Giant hairy mole (Fig. 18.10)

Dark-brown or black patches of skin may be noted at birth. The areas are usually thickened and rough and may be hairy. Common sites include the buttocks, back and scalp. Lesions are excised when possible as there is a chance of malignancy in later life.

Sebaceous naevus

A cluster of yellow papules may be noted on the scalp or forehead. This wart-like lesion rarely exceeds 1 cm in diameter and may be excised if it persists into adulthood.

TRAUMA

Tissue injuries of scalp

Caput succedaneum (Fig. 18.11)

The forces applied to a fetus prior to rupture of the membranes are equal in

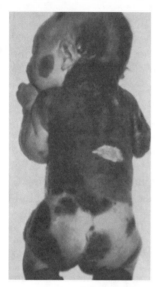

Fig. 18.10 *A widespread non-vascular naevus. This hairy mole is probably too diffuse for surgical removal to be contemplated*

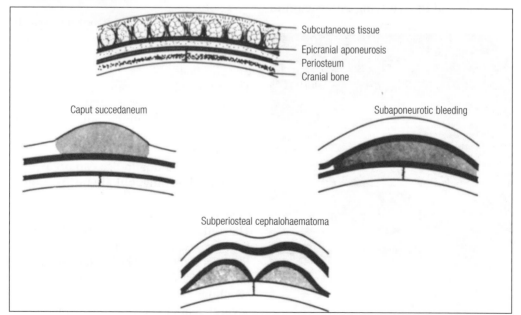

Fig. 18.11 *Sites of head injuries*

all directions. Once the membranes have ruptured, the presenting part of the fetus fills the cervical opening and is exposed to atmosphere pressure. The rest of the fetus is subjected to greater pressure during labour from uterine contractions and this may result in venous congestion and extravasation of fluid and blood into the tissues of the presenting part. In vertex presentations an oedematous swelling usually appears over the parietal region of the head and is termed the caputsuccedaneum. In breech presentations the perineal region and genitalia may be swollen and bruised (Colour plate XII), whereas in a face presentation the eyes and facial tissues are affected.

Treatment
Nil.

Prognosis
Excellent. The swelling subsides within a few days.

Cephalhaematoma (Fig. 18.12)
Blood may accumulate between a cranial bone and its overlying periosteum to

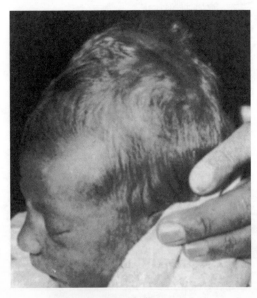

Fig. 18.12 *Cephalhaematoma*

cause a subperiosteal cephalhaematoma. The bleeding occurs slowly from damaged capillaries so that a swelling is not obvious at birth.

This type of injury may occur in normal vertex deliveries, particularly in primiparae and in cases of cephalopelvic disproportion. It is more common in infants who are delivered by forceps or vacuum extraction.

A cephalhaematoma usually develops over a parietal bone and may be unilateral or bilateral. It never crosses a suture line as the periosteum is firmly adherent to the edges of bone. An underlying linear fracture of the bone may be present.

Occasionally the occipital region is involved, in which case the cephalhaematoma must be distinguished from other midline swellings in that area, for example encephalocele.

Certain features distinguish a cephalhaematoma from a caput succedaneum:
- *Onset:* The swelling is not present at birth and may be obvious only after six to 12 hours.
- *Site:* The swelling does not cross over a suture.
- *Skin:* Overlying skin is not necessarily bruised or oedematous.

Complications
These are extremely rare.
Infection: Bacteria may enter the haematoma through an overlying skin abrasion or as a result of needle aspiration.

Anaemia and jaundice can occur from excessive bleeding, but are uncommon.

Course
The outer base often calcifies to form a firm rim, while the centre of the swelling remains fluctuant. The cephalhaematoma may persist for six to eight weeks. A few swellings actually ossify and may take several years to become inconspicuous.

Treatment
Nil, in the majority of cases. Phototherapy may be needed if severe jaundice is present.

Note
Do not aspirate a cephalhaematoma. It is unnecessary and can introduce infection.

Skin and soft tissue injuries
Damage to the skin and soft tissue can range from mild abrasions to deep and more serious wounds.

Such injuries may be the result of:
- the application of forceps
- vacuum suction apparatus
- scalp electrode clips
- scalp blood sampling
- rupture of membranes with toothed forceps
- scalpel cut at Caesarean section.

Vacuum haematoma
Vacuum suction can produce a characteristic 'suction haematoma' consisting of a purple swelling over the site of application of the cup. The edge of the swelling may be excoriated or blistered (Fig. 18.13). Jaundice may develop owing to absorption of blood.

Treatment
An open skin lesion is a site for infection. Clean abrasions on the scalp by shaving off the surrounding hair and applying an antiseptic agent, such as mercurochrome. Deep cuts may need to be sutured. Most lesions heal within days.

Subaponeurotic bleeding
Extensive bleeding can occur beneath the epicranial aponeurosis from trauma to the head. This is likely to occur after failed vacuum extraction, poorly applied forceps to the head, or in association with bleeding disorders, such as haemorrhagic disease.

Signs
The head may be swollen, fluctuant and oedematous and head circumference can be increased (Fig. 18.14). Blue discoloration of upper eyelids and of the skin behind the ears may appear after a few days (Fig. 18.15).

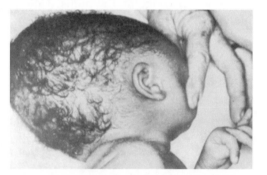

Fig. 18.14 *Subaponeurotic bleeding can cause marked swelling of the scalp*

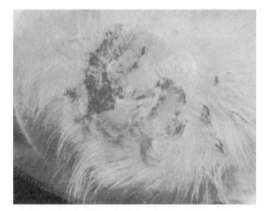

Fig. 18.13 *Vacuum haematoma*

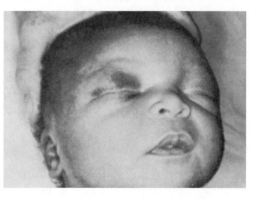

Fig. 18.15 *Bruising of eyelids owing to subaponeurotic bleeding*

Treatment
Bleeding subsides without specific treatment in the majority of cases. Anaemia and jaundice can result from large bleeds and may require correction.

Prognosis
Good, if complications such as anaemia are promptly corrected.

INFECTIONS
Intrauterine infection
Skin eruptions may be a manifestation of various fetal infections. Dermal erythropoiesis occurs in rubella and cytomegalovirus infections and produces purple lesions known as blueberry muffin spots.

Copper-coloured macules or bullae may appear on the baby's buttocks, palms and soles in congenital syphilis (Colour plate II).

Vesicles are seen in chickenpox and herpes simplex.

Postnatal infection
Sepsis
Clinical presentation
■ Bullous impetigo.
■ Abscess.
■ Paronychia.
■ Scalded skin syndrome.

Bullous impetigo: Single or multiple blisters may appear around the umbilicus or on the buttocks from staphylococcal infection. The vesicles, which are filled with clear or turbid fluid, rupture to reveal a moist base. Gram-positive cocci can be demonstrated in the blister fluid. The infection is highly contagious and strict asepsis must be practised. The bullae heal without scarring in response to antibiotic therapy.

Paronychia: A nail fold infection forms swelling and redness. Later a bead of pus forms under the nail at the lateral margin.

Scalded skin syndrome: A staphylococcal infection at any site may be associated with generalised erythema. The organisms release an erythrotoxin that causes the skin to blister and exfoliate. Complications such as fluid loss and septicaemia can be prevented by prompt antibiotic therapy.

Treatment
All traumatised areas of skin should be cleaned immediately to prevent sepsis. Hair which surrounds a scalp wound is shaved off and aqueous mercurochrome 1% is applied to the lesion.

Systemic antibiotic therapy is used for most skin infections, particularly in the preterm baby. A penicillinase-resistant drug, cloxacillin, is given for a week.

Thrush
Cutaneous thrush is usually confined to the perineum (p. 251), but can occur in moist skin folds of the neck and axilla. Lesions are papular or erythematous and may ulcerate.

Spores and hyphae can be identified in scrapings from the lesions.

Mastitis (Colour plate II)
Engorged breasts may become infected if they are squeezed or massaged. This complication usually occurs after the second week of life and is likely to be caused by *Staphylococcus aureus*. The affected breast is red, swollen and tender, and an abscess may form.

Treatment
Antistaphylococcal penicillin, e.g. cloxacillin. Incision and drainage of abscess.

Note
Breasts that show physiological engorgement with milk are not red and tender and should never be expressed.

CHAPTER 19

Metabolic and Endocrine System Disorders

GLUCOSE

This is the main source of energy for the fetus and newborn baby and is of prime importance in brain metabolism.

During pregnancy, sugar is constantly transported across the placenta and the fetus maintains the plasma glucose at 75% of the maternal level.

In the last month glucose is stored as glycogen in the liver and heart. This reserve is usually inadequate in preterm babies and can become depleted in those who are growth-retarded or hypoxaemic.

After birth the rate of production and utilisation of glucose determines the level of glucose in plasma. The initial energy requirements are high and the blood level of glucose in plasma falls to approximately 3,3 mmol/l. Most of the glycogen in the liver is converted to glucose (glycogenolysis) and this sugar is also derived from amino acids and glycerol (gluconeogenesis).

Glycogenolysis and gluconeogenesis are regulated by hormones such as glucocorticoids, insulin and glucagon.

Glycogen is steadily replenished by sugar from food and the plasma level of glucose reaches the adult range within a week.

Hypoglycaemia

An adequate supply of glucose is essential for normal brain function since hypoglycaemia can cause extensive neuronal damage. Signs of hypoglycaemia rarely develop when the glucose level is above 2,5 mmol/l and this is considered to be the lower limit of normal. Hypoglycaemia is often asymptomatic, but should be viewed with concern because of the possible consequences.

Clinical features

The signs of hypoglycaemia are non-specific and include:

- seizures
- apnoea and cyanosis

TABLE 19.1

Hypoglycaemia	
Causes	*Mechanism*
Common:	
Intrauterine growth retardation	Inadequate glycogen
Prematurity	Inadequate glycogen
Stress, e.g. respiratory distress, asphyxia, hypothermia	Depletion of glycogen
Infant of diabetic mother	Hyperinsulinism
Less common:	
Post-exchange transfusion	Hyperinsulinism
Rhesus disease	Hyperinsulinism
Beckwith syndrome	Hyperinsulinism
Nesidiodysplasia	Hyperinsulinism
Leucine sensitivity	Hyperinsulinism
Galactosaemia	Defective release of glucose from the liver

- lethargy, hypotonia, poor sucking
- lachycardia

Causes

Hypoglycaemia results from inadequate or depleted stores of glycogen, hyperinsulinism, defective gluconeogenesis, or impaired formation of glucose. Important causes are listed in Table 19.1.

Measurement of blood glucose

Test strips provide a semiquantitative estimation of blood sugar and are ideal for screening babies who are at risk for hypoglycaemia. These include infants of diabetic mothers and those who are preterm, growth-retarded or stressed (Table 19.1).

This group is likely to develop transient hypoglycaemia within 24–48 hours of birth, the most critical period being the first six hours.

Frequency: Determine the level of blood sugar hourly for the first six hours and then test it three-hourly for the next 24–48 hours.

Subsequent frequency and duration of monitoring depends on the stability of blood glucose.

The test can be discontinued when the infant is receiving adequate milk feeds

and shows no significant fall in blood glucose between feeds.

Cover the test zones of a Haemo-Glukotest strip with a drop of blood for a minute. Wipe off the blood with clean cotton wool and insert the strip into a Refrolux meter. The level of blood glucose will be displayed by the meter after two minutes.

A low reading (less than 2,5 mmol/l) should be confirmed by a quantitative test for plasma glucose in the laboratory. If this is associated with clinical signs, sufficient venous blood should be taken for the investigation of hypoglycaemia before treatment is given.

Prevention

Transient hypoglycaemia is preventable and the following steps are taken to avoid it in those at risk, that is infants suffering from the common conditions in Table 19.1.

Intravenous feeding: Use dextrose water 10% intravenously as soon after birth as possible. Control the rate of flow with an infusion pump and give 60–90 ml/kg for the first day.

Oral feeding: The introduction of milk feeds depends on the size and state of the infant. Commence feeding within 24 hours whenever possible.

The weaning from intravenous to oral nutrition is gradual and may last from 24 to 48 hours. Discontinue the dextrose drip when milk feeding is fully established and the level of blood sugar is stable.

Treatment
Hypoglycaemia with or without symptoms is a neonatal emergency.

Glucose bolus injection: Transient hypoglycaemia usually responds rapidly to an intravenous injection of concentrated glucose. Dextrose water 10% is suitable and contains 0,1 g of glucose per millilitre. Slowly inject 5 ml/kg of this water into a peripheral vein.

Continuous IV infusion: Follow the bolus injection with a continuous infusion of dextrose water 10% at a volume of 90–120 ml/kg/day. The rate of flow, which is controlled by an infusion pump, depends on subsequent plasma levels of glucose.

Monitor blood glucose levels every half an hour until stable. Avoid reactive hypoglycaemia by ensuring that the intravenous infusion is not discontinued before adequate milk feeds have been established.

Hormone therapy: This is seldom necessary but can be used to stimulate sugar production if the glucose infusion is inadequate or not successful.

Hydrocortisone: This drug stimulates gluconeogenesis and is usually effective in all forms of transient hypoglycaemia. Dose 1–3 mg/kg/dose IV or IM.

Glucagon: This is helpful if hepatic glycogen is present and consequently works best in infants of diabetic mothers.

Dose 50–100 μg/kg IV or IM. This can be repeated after 6 to 12 hours.

Intractable hypoglycaemia
Some uncommon forms of hypoglycaemia, like hyperinsulinism, may not respond to the usual therapeutic measures.

The initial blood sample obtained during investigation for hypoglycaemia should be sent to a laboratory for the cause to be found. A hormone profile may be required and includes levels of insulin, ACTH, TSH. An amino acid profile may also be necessary. Urine is examined for amino acids and reducing sugars.

A condition such as nesidiodysplasia (involving excessive numbers of misplaced endocrine cells in the pancreas) may necessitate partial pancreatectomy if hypoglycaemia is resistant to drugs such as ACTH, somatostatin and diasoxide.

Outcome
Asymptomatic hypoglycaemia has a good prognosis, but the symptomatic variety is associated with neurological deficits in 30% of cases.

CALCIUM

This mineral accumulates in the fetus during the last 10 weeks of pregnancy and is stored in bone, which coincides with ossification.

After birth the serum level of calcium declines owing to a reduced intake. This is soon rectified by the activity of the parathyroid glands. They release parathormone (PTH), which mobilises calcium from bone, increases its reabsorption by the kidneys and improves absorption from the gut. Vitamin D has a similar action, whereas calcitonin has an opposing effect on calcium homeostasis.

Hypocalcaemia
Two fractions of calcium are present in serum: one is bound to albumin, the other is free or ionised. A decrease in the latter can result in excitability of nerves. The level of ionised calcium is rarely measured in laboratories and hypocalcaemia is defined as a serum level of less than 1,8 mmol/l of total calcium.

Causes

Hypocalcaemia can occur early or late and the factors that have been implicated include:

- inadequate amounts of parathormone or vitamin D
- excessive amounts of phosphate
- lack of magnesium.

Early hypocalcaemia

Parathormone levels remain low after birth in certain babies. Those at risk include:

- preterm babies
- infants of diabetic mothers.

Late hypocalcaemia

Some milk formulas contain high levels of phosphate, which can lower serum calcium within a week.

Hypocalcaemia can also occur in infants who are depleted of magnesium and in those who have undergone exchange transfusions with citrated blood. Rare causes include the Di George syndrome (absent parathyroid glands) and maternal hyperparathyroidism.

Treatment

Asymptomatic hypocalcaemia can be corrected with oral supplementation of calcium gluconate (p. 308).

Signs of hypocalcaemia, such as convulsions, tetany or carpopedal spasms, need urgent correction.

Immediate: Give calcium gluconate 10% solution 1 ml/kg into a peripheral vein. The rate of injection should not exceed 1 ml per minute and continuous ECG monitoring must be done. The hazards of intravenous injection include:

- bradycardia or cardiac arrest
- tissue necrosis and calcification.

Subsequent treatment: A continuous IV infusion is used for 24–48 hours. Add calcium gluconate 10% to the maintenance solution (2 ml calcium gluconate 10% per

100 ml) and control the calcium rate with an infusion pump.

Use a peripheral vein rather than the umbilical artery or vein because of the potential hazards of calcium. Do not add sodium bicarbonate to the IV solution as it can cause calcium to precipitate.

Hypercalcaemia (p. 250)

MAGNESIUM

This important intracellular ion is transferred across the placenta in the last trimester and the level in the fetus depends on that in the mother.

Hypomagnesaemia

Maternal diseases such as toxaemia, hyperparathyroidism and diabetes mellitus can cause hypomagnesaemia in an infant.

After birth, the causes include:

- high phosphate load from milk
- prolonged parenteral nutrition
- exchange transfusion.

Hypomagnesaemia can inhibit parathormone secretion and is associated with hypocalcaemia. Hypocalcaemic infants who fail to respond to calcium therapy may need magnesium supplementation.

The signs of hypomagnesaemia are similar to those of hypocalcaemia and are likely to occur when the blood magnesium level is below 0,6 mmol/l. Generalised oedema often occurs when the imbalance has been caused by a high phosphate load from cow milk.

Treatment

Give magnesium sulphate 50% by intramuscular injection. Dose 0,1 ml/kg. Repeat this after 24 hours if necessary.

TABLE 19.2

Important causes of dehydration				
Inadequate intake	*Diarrhoea*	*Vomiting*	*Insensible loss*	*Urine loss*
Poor sucking	Gastroenteritis	Necrotising entero-colitis	Phototherapy	Diuretics
Blocked IV drip	Lactose intolerance	Bowel obstruction Septicaemia	Radiant heating Epidermolysis bullosa Poor humidification during IPPV Extreme prematurity	Diabetes mellitus Tubular dysfunction

FLUID AND ELECTROLYTE IMBALANCE

Dehydration

This results from an inadequate intake or an excessive loss of fluid and occurs rapidly in a baby because the fluid requirements, extracellular fluid volume and surface areas are relatively large.

Gastroenteritis is the most significant and hazardous cause of dehydration.

Other factors are listed in Table 19.2.

Clinical signs
- A loss of more than 5% body weight.
- Dry tongue.
- Sunken fontanelle.
- Depressed eyeballs.
- Loss of tissue turgor – skin loses its elasticity and does not spring back when lifted between a thumb and forefinger.
- Hypotonia.
- Oliguria – urine output is less than 1 ml/kg/hour.
- Shock – this may occur if more than 10% of body weight is lost.

Features of shock include:
- hypotension
- weak peripheral pulses
- hypothermia
- tachycardia
- poor skin perfusion – blanching is prolonged when the skin is pressed with a finger
- anuria
- coma.

Laboratory findings
- Urine osmolality is more than 400 mmol/l; specific gravity is more than 1 012.
- Haemoglobin is raised.
- Haematocrit is raised.
- Electrolyte disturbance – electrolytes are frequently lost.

Three types of dehydration are described, depending on serum osmolality and sodium level:

Isotonic dehydration: The amounts of fluid and electrolytes that are lost are balanced and the serum sodium remains normal (± 140 mmol/l). This is the most common form.

Hypertonic dehydration: Loss of fluid exceeds that of electrolytes and as a result serum sodium is raised (more than 150 mmol/l). This can cause sludging of the red cells and cerebral venous thrombosis.

Hypotonic dehydration: Loss of electrolyte exceeds that of fluid and serum sodium is lowered (less than 130 mmol/l). This may cause cerebral oedema and shock.

Potassium: Large amounts of potassium may be lost in stools to produce hypotonia and ECG abnormalities.

Chloride: This can be lost from the stomach through persistent vomiting, e.g. pyloric stenosis. It may result in a metabolic alkalaemia.

Bicarbonate: A metabolic acidaemia may result from the loss of bicarbonate in stools or urine.

Rehydration treatment
Fluids suitable for the correction of dehydration from diarrhoea are listed in Table 19.3.

Dehydration due solely to vomiting should be treated with 0,45% saline dextrose solution containing no lactate.

Severe dehydration: An infant who has lost more than 10% of weight needs approximately 200 ml/kg of fluid in 24 hours. Give half of this (100 ml/kg) to correct shock and dehydration and half for maintenance.

Run the fluid through a scalp, peripheral or umbilical vein. The latter remains patent until about 10 days of age and can be catheterised if attempts at other sites have failed.

A scheme for rehydration is presented in Table 19.4.

Mild dehydration: An infant who has lost less than 5% of body weight requires 150 ml/kg of fluid in 24 hours. Use a third (50 ml/kg) over eight hours, to correct hydration and the remainder (100 ml/kg) provides maintenance for the day. Half-strength Darrow/dextrose is suitable.

The intravenous route is preferable, but occasionally a nasogastric drip can be used provided there is no vomiting and attempts to set up a venous drip have been unsuccessful. Control the rate of flow with a constant infusion pump.

Complications during treatment
- Overhydration.
- Convulsions.

Overhydration
This is a greater hazard at this stage than underhydration.

Signs:
- Liver enlargement.
- Tachycardia.
- Oedema.

Prevention of overhydration: Examine the infant frequently and constantly assess fluid requirements. The initial estimates are approximations only and may need adjustment. Keep an intake and output chart for each infant. Use only bottles or packs of 200 ml capacity to reduce the chances of overload.

Regulate the rate of flow through a constant infusion pump. If such an appa-

TABLE 19.3

Fluids suitable for correction of dehydration due to diarrhoea					
			mmol/l		
	Na	*K*	*Cl*	*HCO₃*	*Lactate*
Stabilised human serum	146	5	75	60	–
Half-strength Darrow/5% dextrose	61	17	52	–	26

TABLE 19.4

Treatment of severe dehydration and shock			
Purpose	*Fluid*	*Amount*	*Time*
Correction of shock and acidaemia	Stabilised human serum or Normal saline Half-strength Darrow/dextrose Sodium bicarbonate 4%	10 ml/kg 10 ml/kg 4 ml/kg	within 15 minutes 15–30th minute 30th minute–8th hour
Rehydration	Half-strength Darrow/dextrose	80 ml/kg	30th minute–8th hour
Maintenance	Half-strength Darrow/dextrose	100 ml/kg	8th–24th hour

ratus is not available, check and record the drip rate every 15 minutes.

Convulsions

Seizures may occur during the period of rehydration, particularly with metabolic acidaemia. They are most likely caused by hypocalcaemia and hypomagnesaemia.

Treatment:
- Magnesium sulphate 50% (p. 308).
- Calcium gluconate 10% (p. 308).

Convulsions may occasionally occur in hypernatraemic states, despite a slow correction of electrolyte imbalance. Anticonvulsant treatment will be required, e.g. Phenobarbitone (p. 306) or Diazepam (p. 306).

Further treatment

Rehydration should be completed within 24 hours and oral fluids can then be introduced. Give half-strength Darrow/dextrose by bottle or nasogastric tube and introduce milk after a further 12 hours.

Give half the maintenance requirements by mouth, that is, 50 ml/kg, and the rest intravenously.

By the third day, the infant should be able to take all requirements by mouth.

Intravenous drip

Blood, plasma, electrolytes and dextrose water are given into a scalp or peripheral vein. The umbilical vein, which remains patent for about 10 days, may be catheterised in an emergency, but this route should not be used for longer than 24 hours as venous thrombosis can occur.

Peripheral vein drip

Suitable veins are found on the dorsum of the hand, in the elbow flexure and on the medial malleolus of the foot.

A needle set or plastic cannula (size 24- or 26-gauge) may be used. A cannula is easily immobilised and is less likely to cause phlebitis.

Tie an elastic band around the limb to promote venous distension and insert the cannula into the vessel. When the stylette is removed, blood should flow into the hub. The drip set is attached, the elastic band is removed and the electrolyte or water solution is run into the vein. Advance the cannula into the vessel until only the hub remains visible. Fix it to the skin with strips of plaster and immobilise the limb onto a plastic drip pack with plaster strips.

THERMOREGULATION

Heat is produced constantly in the body from metabolic reactions and then lost from the skin to the environment. A baby, being homeothermic, can usually maintain a normal deep body (core) temperature by balancing the amount of heat produced with that lost.

Thermoneutral state

A desirable situation is attained when heat production is minimal and oxygen consumption is low. This enables optimum use to be made of energy for growth. In this state, the body's temperature is controlled by vasomotor adjustments alone. Peripheral vessels, regulated by the hypothalamus, are either constricted to conserve heat or dilated to promote the loss of heat.

The rate of metabolism is more accurately reflected by changes in temperature at the periphery, for example on the skin of the abdomen, than by changes in the depth of the body, such as in the rectum. A baby can be severely stressed by cold and yet maintain a normal rectal temperature. This is achieved by an increase in oxygen consumption.

A baby is considered to have attained a thermoneutral state when the temperature of the exposed skin over the abdomen is 36,2 °C to 36,8 °C. Oxygen consumption is minimal and deep body temperature is kept normal by variations in the flow of peripheral blood. The environmental temperature needed to maintain this state depends on the weight and age of a baby as well as on the degree of humidity, air currents and clothing.

Response to excessive heat
When the body is overheated, vasodilation alone cannot cope with heat loss and sweating provides rapid evaporative cooling. In the full-term infant this occurs when the abdominal skin temperature exceeds 37–37,5 °C. The preterm infant cannot sweat effectively, if at all, and may easily overheat.

Response to excessive cold
Peripheral vasoconstriction increases the total insulation of the body, thereby preventing a fall in deep body temperature. This mechanism is inadequate when the abdominal skin temperature falls below 35,5 °C . The infant cannot shiver to provide extra heat and at this 'critical' tem-perature oxygen consumption increases from non-shivering thermogenesis.

Heat production
Non-shivering thermogenesis takes place in brown adipose tissue. Deposits of brown fat are laid down in the fetus after 28 weeks' gestation. They are found mainly in the cervical region between the scapulae, in the axillae and mediastinum and around the kidneys and adrenal glands (Fig. 19.1). The cells of brown fat are smaller than those of white fat and have an abundant blood and sympathetic nerve supply. The metabolism of the brown fat is stimulated by noradrenaline with the release of fatty acids and glycerol, and the heat produced is conveyed throughout the body by the bloodstream. Brown fat gradually disappears during the first year of life.

Heat loss after birth
The fetus *in utero* has a body temperature about 0,5 °C higher than that of the

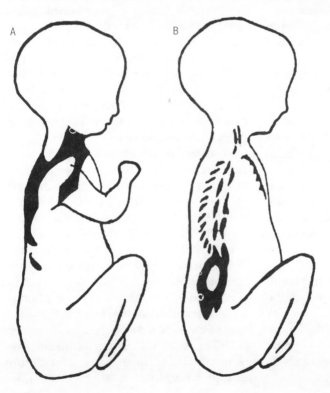

Fig. 19.1 *The distribution of brown adipose tissue:*
A. Superficial sites; B. Deep sites. (From Aherne, W and Hull, D. 1964. Proceedings of the Royal Society of Medicine **57**: *1172)*

mother. After birth there is a sharp drop in body temperature, caused by radiation, conduction, convection and evaporation. The temperature fall may average 0,3 °C a minute and is more marked in preterm than in term babies.

Cold injury
This is the consequence of severe hypothermia and is likely to occur in a low-birthweight baby who is born at home in winter.

Clinical features
Thermoregulation ceases when the core temperature has fallen below 32 °C and the following signs may be noted:

- Hypothermia: The infant feels cold and usually has a skin temperature below 32 °C. It may be as low as 27 °C.
- Lethargy.
- Inability to suck
- Depressed or absent reflexes.
- Bradycardia – heart rate is usually below 100 per minute.
- Oliguria.
- Pink skin: The cheeks are often ruddy and look deceptively healthy. This is due to oxygenated red cells being trapped in the skin capillaries.
- Oedema: Swelling may be noted over the lower limbs and later spreads to involve the whole body. In severe cases, it is non-pitting and encases the infant to produce sclerema.
- Purulent nasal discharge: Respiratory infection is common.

Complications
Hypoglycaemia: This is likely to occur during the stage of rewarming and may present with convulsions.

Hypoxaemia: Bronchopneumonia is common and may present with cyanosis.

Acidaemia: A metabolic acidaemia may occur from hypoxaemia.

Gangrene: Extremities, i.e. fingers and toes, may be affected.

Kernicterus: Fatty acids are released and these may bind to albumin to release bilirubin. Brain damage has been noted in hypothermic infants, particularly those below 1 000 g in weight.

Pulmonary haemorrhage: Intrapulmo-nary bleeding is often fatal.

Treatment
Prophylactic: Dry the low-birthweight baby who is born at home with a clean towel and then place the infant between mother's breasts. Ensure skin to skin contact to maintain normal body temperature. Transport both to hospital this way. If this is not possible, wrap the infant in a dry towel, cover the head with a woollen cap and transfer the baby to hospital in a heated portable incubator. If this is not available, wrap the baby in an aluminium plastic pack, the 'Silver Swaddler'. This sterile wrap effectively reduces radiant heat loss and is soft and disposable. It is best used for transportation and not for routine nursing as it can cause overheating.

Specific: The infant who shows signs of cold injury must be rewarmed rapidly. This can be achieved by a servo-controlled radiant heater.

If this device is not available wrap the baby in a clean dry towel, cover with cotton wool and place in an incubator. Check the abdominal skin temperature every 15 minutes and undress the infant when the temperature reaches 35 °C , to prevent overheating.

Hypoglycaemia
The level of blood sugar can fall during rewarming and must be kept normal by a 10% dextrose drip. This is preferably given into a peripheral vein.

Infection
Antibiotics are recommended in view of the high risk of infection.

Hypoxaemia

Many infants are hypoxaemic, which can be exaggerated during the process of rewarming as oxygen consumption increases. Give sufficient oxygen to maintain SaO_2 between 89–92%.

Steroids are of doubtful value and are recommended only if sclerema is present.

Prognosis

Cold injury has a mortality of 25% and survivors have a 10% chance of brain damage from hypoxaemia, hypoglycaemia or hyperbilirubinaemia.

INHERITED METABOLIC DISORDERS

These are caused by the malfunction or absence of single-gene products such as enzymes. They occur in approximately 1% of live births and most are transmitted in a recessive manner.

The body contains thousands of enzymes and proteins, but individual disorders are rare. Several that are important in the neonatal period are listed in Table 19.5.

Enzymes act as catalysts in chemical reactions, that is, they promote the rapid conversion of precursors to end-products without partaking in the reaction.

Enzyme (X)

Precursor (A) ——→ End-product (B)

TABLE 19.5

Inherited metabolic disorders	
Carbohydrate	Galactosaemia (p. 273)
	Glycogen storage disease (p. 273)
	Lactose intolerance (p. 274)
Amino acids	Phenylketonuria (p. 272), albinism
	Urea cycle defects
	Organic acid defects
Steroids	Congenital adrenal hyperplasia (p. 275)
Red cells	Methaemoglobinaemia (p. 227)

The absence of a specific enzyme (X) may result in:

- accumulation of the precursor (A), which may or may not be toxic
- conversion of precursor (A) through other pathways to products that may be toxic or metabolically active
- deficiency of end-product (B).

Explanation of phenylketonuria, albinism and alcaptonuria

Phenylketonuria

Phenylalanine is an essential amino acid present in various foodstuffs. Normally it is changed by an enzyme (phenylalanine hydroxylase) to tyrosine (reaction 1 in Fig. 19.2). When this enzyme is absent, phenylalanine and its metabolites accumulate in the body. These substances can 'poison' the brain to cause feeble-mindedness. The breakdown products, phenylketones, are excreted in the urine, hence the name phenylketonuria.

Albinism

Tyrosine is normally converted to melanin (reaction 2 in Fig. 19.2), a pigment responsible for the colour of the skin, hair and iris. When the specific enzyme tyrosinase is absent, melanin is not formed and there is a lack of colouring, a condition known as albinism.

Alcaptonuria

Tyrosine is also changed to homogentisic acid and then to aceto-acetic acid (reactions 3(a) and 3(b) in Fig. 19.2).

When the enzyme for reaction 3(b) is absent, homogentisic acid accumulates and is excreted in the urine, which darkens on standing.

This disorder, known as alcaptonuria, is not serious in the newborn period, but it is associated with arthritis in later years.

Diagnosis

This can be difficult owing to the varied

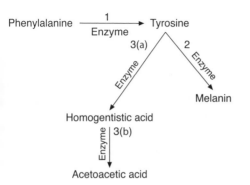

Fig. 19.2 *Metabolism of phenylalanine*

metabolic pathways that may be involved in the numerous diseases.

A family history of a metabolic disorder or clinical features as listed in Table 19.6 should arouse suspicion and prompt further investigation.

Table 19.6

Clinical features of metabolic disorders
Unusual appearance of skin, hair, eyes or genitalia
Unusual odour of body or urine
Persistent vomiting or diarrhoea
Lethargy, hypotonia, seizures or coma
Persistent jaundice

When these features are present, biochemical manifestations should be sought. The time of onset is critical. Many signs appear after the onset of breast-feeding and not at birth. The disorders of protein and carbohydrate metabolism usually manifest at this stage and may progress relentlessly to critical illness. Many are labelled as sepsis but in each

Table 19.7

Tests for metabolic disorders	
Urine	Colour and odour
	Reducing substances, Phenistix
	Microscopy for crystals
Blood	Acid-base status
	Sodium, potassium, calcium
	Urates, urea, ammonia
	Glucose
	Bilirubin

case of presumed infection where no pre-existing risk factors are applicable, exclude a metabolic disorder. Important screening tests are listed in Table 19.7.

A specific diagnosis can usually be concluded on further biochemical analyses of blood, urine or cultured skin fibro-blasts.

Treatment
This is exacting and should be conducted by experts in metabolic diseases. In a critical case of unknown cause the following must be addressed:
* Metabolic acidosis – if the pH is less than 7.25 use sodium bicarbonate for correction (p. 175).
* *Hypoglycaemia* – initially use a bolus injection of 10% Dextrose water followed by a constant infusion.
* *Hyperammonemia* – sodium benzoate promotes the elimination of nitrogen. If the serum ammonia exceeds 500 mmol/l consider peritoneal dialysis.

Many conditions listed in Table 19.8 are amenable to therapy.

The timing of intervention is critical because the consequences of a disease such as phenylketonuria, when left untreated, can be disastrous.

Prenatal treatment has become feasible for diseases such as methylmalonic acidaemia, an organic acid defect.

Mass screening for metabolic disorders
This was made possible by the development of a simple test for phenylketonuria. Early detection enabled therapy to be started promptly, thereby preventing neurological damage.

It proved to be cost-effective in industrialised countries and was extended to include disorders such as galactosaemia and congenital hypothyroidism.

There is no consensus regarding the feasibility of screening programmes in

TABLE 19.8

Treatment of inherited metabolic disorders	
Reduction of toxic metabolites by dietary means	
Phenylalanine-free	Phenylketonuria (p. 272)
Lactose-free	Lactose intolerance (p. 274)
Galactose-free	Galactosaemia (p. 277)
Reduction of toxic metabolites by substrate depletion	
Sodium benzoate	Urea cycle defect (ornithine decarboxylase)
Co-factor stimulation of defective enzyme	
Vitamin B_{12}	Methylmalonic acidaemia
Supplementation of end-product	
Thyroxine	Hypothyroidism (p. 276)
Steroids	Adrenal hyperplasia (p. 275)

southern Africa. They are probably not cost-effective owing to the rarity of phenylketonuria and the demands made by other treatable conditions in infancy.

Specific metabolic diseases

Phenylketonuria

Incidence
The disorder, due to mutations in the PAH gene, occurs in every 10 000 to 20 000 births.

Clinical presentation
The baby appears normal at birth, but is liable to develop irreversible brain damage within a few weeks if the blood level of phenylalanine exceeds 1,5 mmol/l.

Early features include vomiting and eczema and the urine has a characteristic 'mousy' odour. The infant may develop convulsions, hyperactivity, microcephaly and growth retardation. The majority of children are blue-eyed and blond, owing to a lack of melanin, and show varying degrees of mental retardation.

Diagnosis
Screening tests: The widely used Guthrie test is recommended for newborn infants. It is based on a bacterial inhibition test of serum phenylalanine levels. The test should be performed only when a baby is established on a milk diet, that is between the fifth and seventh day. Drops of heel blood are collected on filter paper, which is dried and dispatched to a special regional laboratory.

Simple bedside tests can be used for individual babies.

Ferric chloride test: One drop of a 10% solution is added to a freshly wet nappy. An intense green-blue colour develops if phenylketones are present in the urine.

Phenistix: A paper strip impregnated with ferric ammonium sulphate is dipped into urine or pressed on a wet nappy. A green colour signifies the presence of phenylketones.

These investigations are essential for small babies with eczema.

Screening tests are not specific and the blood level of phenylalanine must be determined in every positive case.

Treatment
A phenylalanine-free diet. This should be designed by a dietician as hidden sources of the amino acid like aspartame, a common sweetener, must be avoided. In the early months breast-feeding can usually be continued.

Frequent checks are made of the

blood phenylalanine level which should be maintained between 0,24 and 0,48 mmol/l. Continuation of the diet becomes exceedingly difficult when the infant gets older, as staple products such as eggs, milk, meat, fish and certain vegetables are either forbidden or allowed in small quantities. Dietary control should be maintained into adulthood as it remains uncertain at what stage treatment can safely be stopped.

Prognosis
Mental retardation can be avoided if treatment is commenced within the first few weeks of life. Once mental deficiency is present, it is unlikely to be cured, but further retardation can be prevented.

Phenylketonuria is transmitted by a recessive gene and the chances of a recurrence in future children of the same parents are one in four.

Galactosaemia
Lactose, the sugar present in milk, is changed to glucose and galactose in the digestive tract. The galactose is absorbed and normally converted to glucose in the liver. In the absence of the specific enzyme necessary for this conversion, galactose-1-phosphate accumulates in the body fluids.

Clinical features
The infant appears normal until milk feeds are commenced. Within a few weeks there may be jaundice, listlessness, vomiting, hypoglycaemia and failure to gain weight. The liver and spleen enlarge, cataracts develop and signs of mental retardation may be noted. These features can be delayed for several months in mild cases.

Diagnosis
Screening test: A test reveals reducing sugars present in the urine, which may also contain albumin.

Test for reducing substances: Clinitest tablets or Benedict reagent. Confirmation is obtained by the measurement of galactose-1-phosphate uridylyltransferase activity in red cells.

The activity of this enzyme can also be determined in amniotic cells obtained by amniocentesis so that a diagnosis can be made in the antenatal period.

Treatment
The infant is maintained for life on a galactose-free diet. The outlook is good and mental deficiency can be prevented provided treatment is started early.

Glycogen storage disease
The glycogen molecule consists of a number of glucose units. It is stored chiefly in the liver, muscle and myocardium and is broken down to its basic glucose units by several enzymes.

The most common form of glycogen storage disease results from the absence of glucose-6-phosphatase. This autosomal recessive condition is known as Von Gierke disease.

Clinical features
Within the first few months of life the infant develops listlessness, vomiting, hypoglycaemia, hepatomegaly and a bleeding tendency.

Diagnosis
Screening test: Urine is positive for reducing substances.

Specific: Glucose-6-phosphatase activity can be determined on a portion of liver obtained from biopsy.

Treatment
Small frequent feeds are recommended, but no specific treatment is available. Most infants die within the first year.

Other types of glycogen storage disease are caused by deficiencies of the following enzymes:

- Acid maltase.
- Debranching enzyme.
- Liver phosphorylase.
- Phosphorylase kinase.

Lactose intolerance

Dietary disaccharides are changed to monosaccharides by enzymes in the gut before absorption. See Table 19.9.

Congenital lactose intolerance is caused by the absence of lactase.

The presence of lactose in the ileocaecal region leads to fermentation of the sugar by intestinal bacteria, with the release of carbon dioxide and lactic acid.

The stools are frothy and sour-smelling and have a low pH.

Clinical features

The infant develops diarrhoea in the first week of life and fails to gain weight.

Diagnosis

Stool liquid tests positive for reducing substances (Clinitest).

Withdrawal of dietary lactose will stop the diarrhoea within 48 hours.

Treatment

Lactose-free diet, such as al 110 milk. At 18 months to 2 years of age, the infant may be able to tolerate small to moderate amounts of lactose in the diet.

Note

Diarrhoea of any origin can produce an acquired lactose intolerance due to a decreased production of lactase. This is more common than the primary type and is treated with a lactose-free milk for several weeks.

Sucrose intolerance is another form of disaccharidase deficiency.

ENDOCRINE SYSTEM
The adrenal gland

The cortex of the adrenal gland originates from coelomic mesoderm during the fifth week of gestation.

Neuroectodermal cells penetrate this structure in the seventh week to form a central medulla. This portion synthesises catecholamines, adrenaline and noradrenaline and remains small until after birth.

The cortex develops into two distinct areas: a fetal zone, which comprises the bulk of the gland in early pregnancy, and a permanent cortex, which emerges during the second trimester.

The fetal cortex produces various metabolites that are converted to oestrogens by the placenta and this zone involutes in the last trimester.

The permanent cortex synthesises gluco- and mineralocorticoids. Cortisol, the main glucocorticoid, plays a major role in maturation of the fetal lungs and the initiation of labour. In addition, glucocorticoids promote gluconeogenesis and the synthesis of liver glycogen. A deficiency will cause hypoglycaemia after birth.

Aldosterone is the predominant mineralocorticoid and it promotes sodium retention and potassium excretion by the kidney. A deficiency is associated with salt loss in a newborn baby.

TABLE 19.9

Enzymes that change disaccharides to monosaccharides		
Disaccharide	Enzyme	Monosaccharide
Lactose	Lactase	Glucose and galactose
Sucrose	Sucrase	Glucose and fructose
Maltose	Maltase	Glucose and glucose

Adrenal haemorrhage

Birth trauma or hypoxaemia may cause bleeding into the adrenal gland. The signs range from pallor to shock and a mass is palpable in the flank.

Features of adrenal insufficiency, such as hypoglycaemia, are unusual and can be delayed.

The clinical presentation may be indistinguishable from renal vein thrombosis and ultrasound, or CAT scanning offers additional assistance.

Calcification usually occurs in the mass within a week and is detected on X-ray examination.

Blood/volume replacement and the correction of shock are the most important aspects of treatment.

Congenital adrenal hyperplasia

This autosomal recessive disorder results from a deficiency of the specific enzymes that are involved in steroid synthesis. Gluco- and mineralocorticoid production is impaired in 90% of cases as a result of 21-hydroxylase deficiency. The CAH gene is situated on the short arm of chromosome 6.

The lack of end-products such as aldosterone, or the overproduction of metabolites such as androgen, cause characteristic physiological derangements.

Androgen excess: In girls this can cause clitoral enlargement and labial fusion.

In boys the penis may be enlarged and progressive virilisation occurs during infancy.

Aldosterone deficiency: A salt-losing state is associated with vomiting, diarrhoea, dehydration and shock.

Diagnosis

An infant with ambiguous genitalia, one who vomits excessively or one with a preceding family history should arouse suspicion.

Appropriate steroid metabolites can be demonstrated in serum and urine.

- 24-hour urine: 17-ketosteroid

excretion is greater than 2,5 mg. Pregnanetriol excretion is greater than 0,5 mg.
- 17-Alpha-hydroxyprogesterone and 11-ketopregnanetriol levels are raised in serum and urine.

In the salt-losing form the serum sodium level may be lowered and renin activity may be increased.

Treatment

Androgen production can be suppressed by lifelong use of cortisone acetate 25 mg/day. The dosage is doubled during stressful situations such as infections or operations.

A mineralocorticoid, fluorohydrocortisone 0,025–0,1 mg/day, will be needed for the salt-losing type, in addition to cortisone acetate.

If dehydration or shock occurs, a volume expander is essential, such as isotonic saline in dextrose 10%. Hydrocortisone and fluorohydrocortisone are used in large doses during the critical stage.

Genitalia: The size of the clitoris may remain static or diminish as the child grows. In this case no surgery is necessary. However, fused labia or a grossly enlarged clitoris will need surgical repair. The prognosis is excellent.

The thyroid gland

The thyroid originates from the primitive pharynx as a thickened layer of endoderm. This invaginates at the base of the tongue, divides into two lobes and descends into the neck. The gland reaches its final site at seven weeks and is attached to the tongue by the thyroglossal duct, which is later obliterated.

At 12 weeks the hormones thyroxine (T4) and triiodothyronine (T3) are synthesised in the gland.

After birth the level of thyroid-stimulating hormone (TSH) from the pituitary rises dramatically, probably in

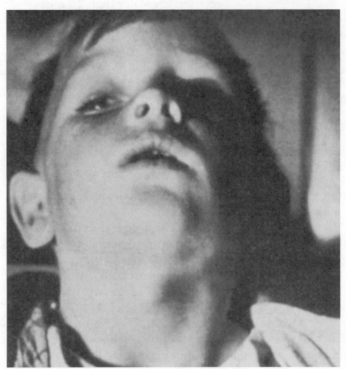

Fig. 19.3 *A thyroglossal cyst. This midline swelling moves up when the tongue is extended*

response to cold stress. This is followed by an increase in T3 and T4. The thyroid plays a critical role in brain development in late pregnancy and infancy. A deficiency of thyroxine can lead to irreversible brain damage, which may occur before or after birth depending on the duration of the inadequacy.

Thyroglossal cyst
The thyroid gland descends from the tongue to the neck in embryonic life and cysts may occur anywhere along this course. They are most likely to be situated in the tongue or the neck (Fig. 19.3). Resection is needed and the outlook is good.

Congenital hypothyroidism
Hypothyroidism occurs in 1 in 4 000 births, probably as a result of aplasia or hypoplasia of the gland.

Affected infants should be identified and treated as soon as possible to prevent adverse effects on the central nervous system.

Clinical features of hypothyroidism are not always obvious at birth and reliance is placed on screening tests.

Thyroid screening
Hypothyroidism can be detected at birth by measuring TSH and thyroid hormones in cord blood.

The normal range for TSH is from 1,5 to 20 μU/ml. T4 levels are estimated on the samples that fall outside this range. Most infants with hypothyroidism will have a TSH level that is greater than 45 μU/ml in cord blood.

Clinical features
At birth the following signs may be noted:
- Excessive length.
- Enlarged fontanelles.
- Depressed nasal bridge.

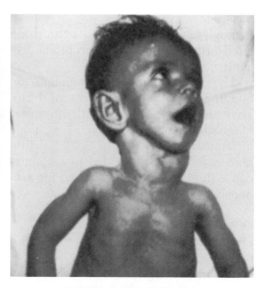

Fig. 19.4 *Infant with a goitre*

After birth other features appear, such as:

- prolonged jaundice
- persistent hypothermia
- abdominal distension and constipation
- lethargy and poor sucking.

Treatment
Thyroxine is the drug of choice. Dose 0,025 mg daily. This is increased to 0,05 mg within a week and a daily dose of 0,15 mg may be required by 18 months of age.

The adequacy of treatment is judged by checking height, bone age and thyroid hormone levels at regular intervals throughout childhood.

Treatment is often lifelong and the outlook for normal growth is good. Mental development depends on the severity of the condition before the commencement of treatment.

Goitrous hypothyroidism (Fig. 19.4)
A hypothyroid infant with a goitre has probably been exposed to drugs such as iodine *in utero*. Goitres rarely result from a deficiency of enzymes needed for thyroxine biosynthesis.

The enlarged gland can compress the trachea to cause asphyxia at birth. It may also interfere with the delivery of the infant.

A partial thyroidectomy may be needed to relieve the obstruction.

Hyperthyroidism
A transient but potentially hazardous form of hyperthyroidism can occur in an infant whose mother has the disorder. This is caused by thyroid-stimulating immunoglobulins, which cross the placenta.

Clinical features include diarrhoea, hyperactivity, tachycardia and cardiac failure. Those with cardiovascular complications may need Lanoxin (p. 199) and Propranolol (p. 307).

Thymus and parathyroids

The thymus is derived from the third pharyngeal pouch in the embryo and continues to develop until puberty. It occupies a considerable portion of the thorax and plays a major role in cellular immunity. This is concerned with the recognition of 'self' and 'non-self' and the prevention of tuberculosis, *Candida*, and protozoal and viral infections.

The cortex of the gland is filled with small T lymphocytes that circulate throughout the body. These lymphocytes become sensitised by antigens, which they then destroy.

The parathyroids originate from the third and fourth pharyngeal pouches and are important regulators of calcium metabolism (p. 263).

Absent thymus and parathyroids
The third and fourth pharyngeal pouches may fail to differentiate into thymus and parathyroid glands. The resultant Di George syndrome is characterised by hypertelorism, cardiac defects, hypocalcaemia, lymphopenia and recurrent *Candida* infections.

The immune defect can be corrected by an implant of fetal thymus, and hypocalcaemia can be controlled by calcium, vitamin D or parathyroid hormone.

Infant of a diabetic mother

The poor control of diabetes during the mother's pregnancy is associated with a significant incidence of fetal overgrowth, intrauterine death, congenital abnormalities and prematurity.

The overgrown infant shows characteristic features at birth:

- The face is puffy and plethoric.
- The skin bruises easily.
- Excessive subcutaneous fat is present, particularly over the shoulders.
- The liver and spleen are enlarged.
- A congenital abnormality may be detected.
- The placenta is large and the umbilical cord is thickened.

The large size of the infant is thought to be owing to a high blood glucose level, which results in pancreatic B-cell hyperplasia, hyperinsulinaemia and the deposition of fat. Occasionally, an infant may be small for gestation. This is likely to occur with severe maternal disease complicated by renal insufficiency.

Complications

Most problems are related to metabolic derangements, prematurity or congenital abnormalities.

Metabolic factors

Hypoglycaemia is likely to occur soon after birth and requires appropriate preventive treatment.

Hypocalcaemia and hypomagnesaemia may occur within days of birth. They are often associated with jitteriness. Magnesium may be given as a single intramuscular injection (p. 307). Calcium gluconate (p. 268) is added to a maintenance fluid (200 ml) and infused intravenously over 24 hours.

Other factors

Hyaline membrane disease, hyperbilirubinaemia and polycythaemia may need specific therapy. Congenital abnormalities may or may not be amenable to correction.

Outcome

The outlook has improved significantly in recent years and babies are rarely overgrown when the maternal blood sugar is maintained within a normal range. The fasting level is kept below 5,5 mmol/l and the postprandial rise should not exceed 6,7 mmol/l. A woman may need hospitalisation to establish these levels. Adequate control of diabetics before and after conception has reduced the risk of intrauterine death, congenital abnormality and excessive fetal growth. Delivery can be planned for 38 or more weeks of gestation, thereby reducing the incidence of prematurity. The chance of developing hypoglycaemia after birth has also been diminished.

CHAPTER 20

Musculoskeletal Disorders

This chapter in outline:

Embryology

Most of the embryo's axial skeleton and musculature evolves from mesodermal somites. These bodies develop on either side of the notochord to form surface elevations on the longitudinal axis of the embryo.

Limbs

Ventrolateral buds appear on the body wall at the end of the fourth week. They are composed of somatic mesoderm and are surrounded by a layer of ectoderm. During the fifth week peripheral nerves grow into these buds from the brachial and lumbosacral plexuses. The limbs partially rotate on their longitudinal axis, the arms revolving laterally and the legs medially.

Bone and cartilage are formed from mesenchyme, a primitive connective tissue derived from mesoderm. The mass of muscle that surrounds the developing bone separates into flexor and extensor groups and limb formation is complete after eight weeks.

Most limb deformities occur as a result of genetic and environmental factors.

SKELETAL MALFORMATIONS

Congenital malformations of the axial skeleton and skull are listed in Table 20.1.

Cleidocranial dysostosis (Fig. 20.1)

This is characterised by:

- total or partial absence of clavicles
- delayed ossification of the bones of the cranial vault.

Aetiology

Cases occur sporadically, but most are due to dominant heredity.

Signs and symptoms

In severe cases the tips of the shoulders can be brought together over the chest.

TABLE 20.1

Important congenital malformations.	
Axial skeleton	*Skull*
Cleidocranial dysostosis	Anencephaly (p. 134)
Klippel–Feil syndrome	Cranium bifidum (p. 135)
Spina bifida	Microcephaly (p. 138)
Pectus excavatum	Craniosynostosis
'Vater' syndrome	

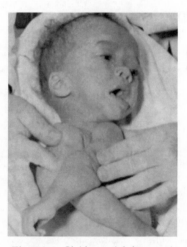

Fig. 20.1 *Cleidocranial dysostosis*

The fontanelles and sutures may remain wide open until adulthood.

Treatment and prognosis
There is no treatment available, but the prognosis for life is good.

Klippel–Feil syndrome
This is characterised by a stiff, short and often twisted neck.

Irregular folds of skin stretch from the ears to the shoulders, thus there is a webbed neck, as in Turner syndrome. It is caused by deformities of the cervical vertebrae, for example aplasia, fusion or maldevelopment.

No treatment is available.

Pectus excavatum
A funnel-shaped deformity of the thorax results from a depressed lower sternum. Surgical correction may be needed in later life for cosmetic reasons or to correct impaired ventilation.

This malformation must be distinguished from the sternal depression that is associated with hyaline membrane disease or chronic lung disease. This resolves within months without treatment.

'Vater' syndrome
Impaired differentiation of mesoderm is thought to cause specific malformations of the vertebrae and other systems.

The acronym 'vater' refers to these malformations, which include vertebra anomalies, anal atresia, tracheo-oesophageal fistula and radial or renal dysplasias.

A mermaid abnormality, which results from a derangement of the caudal axis, may represent the most severe form of this disorder (Fig. 20.2).

Craniosynostosis (Figs. 20.3 and 20.4)
The cranial bones are separated from one another at birth by a layer of fibrous tissue. Growth will be arrested in this region in the event of premature closure of the sutures. The maximum decrease in growth occurs at right angles to an obliterated suture, resulting in various deformities of the skull.

Craniosynostosis is recognisable at

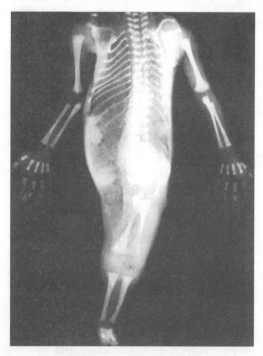

Fig. 20.2 *A 'mermaid' deformity*

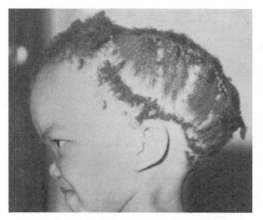

Fig. 20.3 *The elongated narrow head in scaphocephaly*

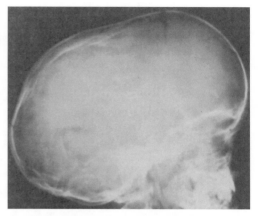

Fig. 20.4 *Scaphocephaly*

birth and occurs four times more frequently in boys than in girls.

Classification
Scaphocephaly (Gr. *skaphé*=boat), i.e. boat-shaped skull: Closure of the sagittal suture results in an elongated narrow head. This is the commonest form of synostosis and may be associated with other abnormalities, like mental retardation.

Brachycephaly (Gr. *brachys*=short), i.e. the breadth of the skull is at least four-fifths its length. Premature closure of the coronal suture gives a high, broad-shaped head with a shortened anteroposterior diameter.

Oxycephaly (Gr. *oxys*=sharp): The coronal and several other sutures are closed and cause the head to be tower-shaped. Serious intracranial complications can occur, such as exophthalmos, papilloedema, optic atrophy.

Plagiocephaly (Gr. *plagio(s)*=oblique), i.e. asymmetrical head: Closure of a suture on one side of the skull, for example lambdoid, can cause this asymmetry. If a single suture is involved then compensatory growth may be adequate to prevent intracranial damage. The condition must be distinguished from other causes of an asymmetrical head, such as positional, moulding, congenital torticollis.

Syndromes associated with craniosynostosis include:

Crouzon syndrome: Characterised by hypoplastic maxillae, beak-shaped nose, hypertelorism, exophthalmos and closure of the coronal and lambdoid sutures.

Apert syndrome: Its features include syndactyly and closure of the coronal suture to produce a tower-shaped head (Fig. 20.5).

Diagnosis
Suspect craniosynostosis if the head has an abnormal shape. A ridge is commonly felt and bones cannot be moved on gentle palpation. The diagnosis is confirmed by radiological examination of the skull.

Treatment
A single, closed suture may not require surgical correction, provided that brain growth is adequate and there are no signs of raised intracranial pressure. Follow-up examinations are essential during the period of skull and brain growth.

Multiple synostosis will need to be corrected to prevent any intracranial complications.

Combined neurosurgical and plastic operations can separate and correct misplaced bones in severe diseases, such as Apert and Crouzon syndromes.

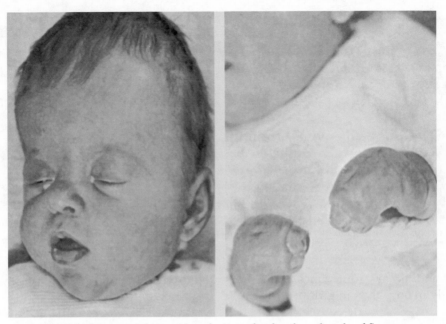

Fig. 20.5 *Apert syndrome. Note the tower head and syndactyly of fingers*

Chondrodystrophies

The longitudinal growth of bone is impaired as a result of defective cartilage function. This leads to dwarfism in which the limb bones are disproportionately smaller than those of the vertebrae or skull. Fibroblast growth-factor genes are defective.

Achondroplasia

This is the commonest form. It may occur spontaneously or be inherited as an autosomal dominant disorder. The circus 'dwarf' is an example of the condition that is characterised by:
- short limbs and small hands
- a relatively normal trunk with lumbar lordosis
- large head, prominent forehead, low nasal bridge
- normal intelligence in most cases.

Rarer forms include the following:
- *Ellis-Van Creveld syndrome:* Features are polydactyly, ectodermal dysplasia and congenital heart defects.

- *Chondrodysplasia punctata:* Features are stippling of epiphyses, for example Conradi syndrome.

Some varieties have a high neonatal mortality rate as a result of respiratory failure. They include the following:
- *Thanatophoric ('death-bringing') syndrome:* Dwarfism is associated with a small thoracic cage.
- *Camptomelic ('bent-limb') syndrome:* The legs are bowed, respiratory tract cartilage is deficient and brain neurons are defective.
- *Asphyxiating thoracic dystrophy:* The thorax is extremely small and respiration may be impaired.

Connective tissue disorders

Marfan syndrome

This is also known as arachnodactyly ('spider fingers') and is inherited as an autosomal dominant disorder. The gene for fibrillin is defective.

Features may not be characteristic at birth.

The following may be observed:

- Long fingers and toes, which are thin and tapering.
- Slender arms and legs.
- High, arched palate.
- Hyper mobile joints.
- Pectus excavatum.

Multiple systems are involved and the outlook depends on the severity of cardiovascular complications such as aortic aneurysm. Beta blocker treatment has been used to retard the growth of the aortic root, thereby diminishing the change of aortic dilitation.

Osteogenesis imperfecta

This is characterised by excessively fragile bones, which fracture with minimal trauma. The sclerae of the eyes may be blue and deafness can develop later.

The skeletal fragility is associated with mutations in genes for type 1 collagen, the major collagen of bone. Four varieties are described: I, II, III, IV. Type II is incompatable with life. In this form, severe fractures occur *in utero* and the infant is often stillborn.

Children with other types develop severe bone deformities as a result of multiple fractures. The incidence of fractures decreases with age. In milder forms, fractures may occur in late childhood.

Treatment

There is no cure and fractures must be treated in the usual way.

Promising advances include the aminobisphosponate drugs and transplants of osteoblastic precursor cells. The former (Pamidronate) blocks osteoclast activity and reduces the turnover rate of bone. The cortex thickens and the number of fractures is reduced.

Limbs

Bow legs (Fig. 20.6)

Outward curving of the tibia is commonly seen at birth. The appearance of bow legs can be exaggerated by the pads of fat on the lateral margin of the legs. This feature is corrected with growth.

Congenital malformations

Various limb malformations are shown in Fig. 20.7. Amelia, the absence of all limbs, is the most severe form. Thalidomide was implicated in an outbreak of these disorders several decades ago.

Digits

Syndactyly (Fig. 20.8)

Digits may be fused by bone or soft tissue. The second and third toes are frequently affected. The feature occurs as an isolated event or may be associated with other anomalies, like Apert syndrome.

Polydactyly (Fig. 20.9)

Extra digits are usually inherited as a dominant trait.

Vestigial ones may occur on the hands and can be tied off if the attachment is a thin band of tissue. Plastic surgery is needed for thicker attachments.

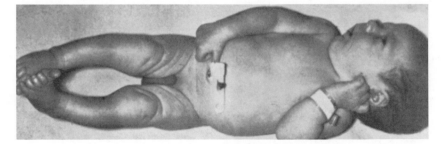

Fig. 20.6 *Normal bowing of the legs at birth. Note asymmetrical thigh folds*

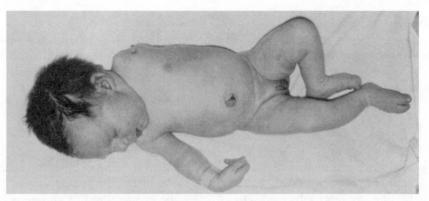

Fig. 20.7 *Limb malformations.* *(a) Extromelia: One whole limb is absent*

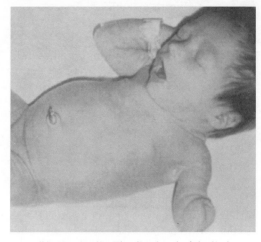

(b) Hemimelia: The distal end of the limb is missing

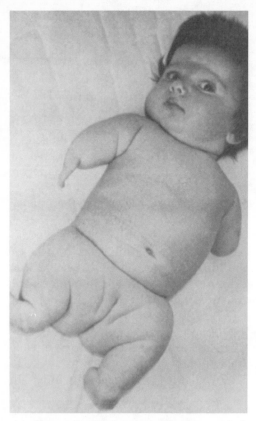

(c) Phocomelia: The hands and feet are attached to the trunk by a short stump

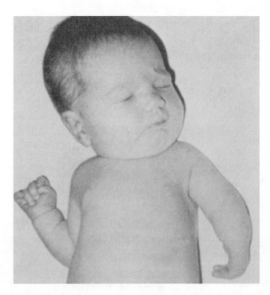

(d) Micromelia: The limb is abnormally short

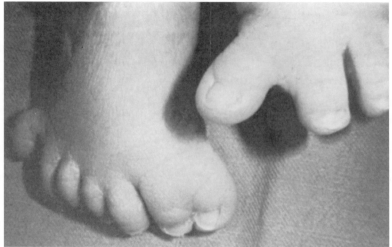

Fig. 20.8 *Poly- and syndactyly of the toes*

Brachydactyly
Abnormally short fingers or toes may be inherited as a dominant trait.

Macrodactyly
An excessively large digit may be linked with other anomalies such as neurofibromatosis.

Foot
Positional abnormalities frequently occur *in utero* and must be distinguished from fixed deformities. A foot that can be manipulated into correct alignment without force will usually adopt a normal position without treatment. A fixed deformity requires orthopaedic attention.

Calcaneovalgus
When the foot is dorsiflexed it can touch the shin with ease. The sole is flat or convex. This positional deformity usually corrects itself, but occasionally needs splintage.

Metatarsus varus (Pigeon toes)
The foot is C-shaped with a convex outer border and concave inner one. This disorder is caused by inward angulation of the forefoot, which may be overcome with gentle manipulation. In this case, spontaneous correction is likely to occur. Fixed angulation requires constant manipulation

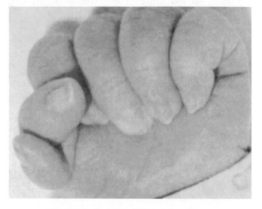

Fig. 20.9 *Polydactyly of the fingers*

and corrective shoes may be needed later.

Inward positioning of the foot can also be caused by torsion of the tibia. Spontaneous correction usually occurs with growth.

Talipes equinovarus (Club foot)
This deformity occurs in 1 of every 1 000 births and affects boys twice as frequently as girls. It is usually isolated, but can be associated with meningomyelocele, dislocated hip or arthrogryposis. The aetiology is unknown.

The foot is plantar flexed (equinus) and medially deviated (varus) and the heel is small (Fig. 20.10). Dorsiflexion beyond 90 degrees is not possible and there are contractures of the medial plantar tissues. Wasting

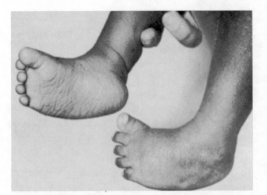

Fig. 20.10 *Talipes equinovarus. The foot is plantar flexed and medially deviated*

of the calf muscles is usually present but may be difficult to detect at birth.

Treatment
Immediate orthopaedic care is essential and involves serial applications of extension strapping to correct the abnormal position. The method is illustrated in Fig. 20.11. Serial plaster casts are also used.

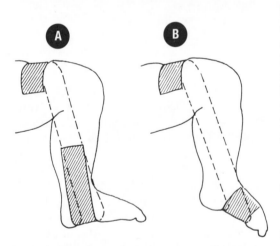

Fig. 20.11 *Immobilisation of a club foot. The leg is sprayed with collodion and then strapped. A. The foot is dorsiflexed as far as possible and extension strapping is applied as illustrated. B. A second length of strapping is applied as shown in order to promote abduction of the foot. (From Davies, P et al. 1972.* Medical Care of Newborn Babies. *London: Heinemann*

Mild cases can be corrected by this treatment. Severe deformities tend to revert to the original position when manipulation is discontinued. Surgical procedures will be needed to release tension in tendons and soft tissues in order to maintain a normal position.

Repeat examinations are essential to assess progress and to detect any deviation from normal. A pleasing functional and cosmetic result can be achieved in most cases.

Joints

Developmental dysplasia of hips
This term is preferred to 'congenital dislocation of hips' because some infants may develop hip dislocation in the first year without abnormal clinical signs at birth (dysplastic hip). Hips should therefore be examined at every opportunity in infancy.

Incidence
True hip dislocation is virtually unknown in black babies. In others it has an incidence of 1,5 per 1 000 births and occurs seven times more frequently in girls than in boys. It may recur in families and is more likely to be found in those born breech with extended legs. The aetiology is unknown. One or both hip joints may be affected, but the dislocation usually occurs on the left side.

Categories
- *Dislocated hip:* The femoral head is not in contact with the acetabulum when the infant is at rest.
- *Dislocatable hip:* The joint is normal at rest, but when subjected to stress (Barlow test), contact is lost between the femoral head and the acetabulum.
- *Subluxatable hip:* Partial contact is maintained between the femoral cartilage and the acetabulum. The hip does not dislocate when subjected to stress.
- *Dysplastic hip:* The femoral head and

acetabulum are abnormally shaped at birth and can dislocate later.

The hip joint may also be dysplastic or dislocated in infants who have gross neuromuscular abnormalities, such as meningomyelocele.

Diagnosis
Signs of a dislocated hip include:
- shortening of a limb
- limitation of abduction (Ortolani test)
- asymmetric thigh creases.

Limb shortening
Dislocation usually occurs posteriorly so that the leg on the affected side appears shortened. When an infant lies supine with the pelvis straightened, legs flexed and feet flat on the surface, the knees should be of equal height. The knee on the affected side is lower than the other.

Limitation of abduction
This feature may be absent shortly after birth when the ligaments and muscles around a hip joint are lax. It is an important, but relatively late sign.

Palpable clunk
The Ortolani and Barlow tests may relocate or dislocate the femoral head with an audible 'clunk'. This characteristic sign of hip dislocation must be distinguished from the innocuous clicks that may be heard in normal hip joints.

Asymmetric skin creases
Thigh creases are asymmetric in 4% of normal babies (Fig. 20.6). This sign may be relatively unimportant on its own, but is significant when associated with other features of a dislocated hip.

Radiology
Normal hip joints show wide variations in radiological features during the early

weeks. Definitive signs of dislocation may not be apparent for six weeks and the value of early investigation is doubtful in the absence of specific clinical signs.

Ultrasound
In the hands of an experienced investigator this non-invasive test is an important advance in the detection of hip dislocation. However, its efficacy as a screening test has yet to be established.

Treatment
Dislocated hip: A truly dislocated hip requires immediate orthopaedic care to avoid the unsatisfactory outcome of late diagnosis and treatment.

The hips are maintained in an abduction splint for several months so that the acetabulum can develop normally. Surgical intervention is often unnecessary following splintage.

Unstable hip: The majority of hips that dislocate only with stressful manipulation (Barlow test) will stabilise later. Repeat gentle examination is important until stability is established. Orthopaedic consultation is mandatory should instability persist beyond a month.

High-risk infant: Ensure orthopaedic consultation for the baby with a family history of hip dysplasia or dislocation as well as a girl who is born breech.

Genu recurvatum
The knee joint can be hyperextended from a breech presentation. This condition occurs more often in girls and also in Ehlers-Danlos, Turner and Klinefelter syndromes. It improves spontaneously. In rare cases the knee dislocates and requires splinting.

Arthrogryposis (Fig. 20.12)
This rare condition occurs mostly in males and is characterised by the fixation of joints in flexion or extension. The cause

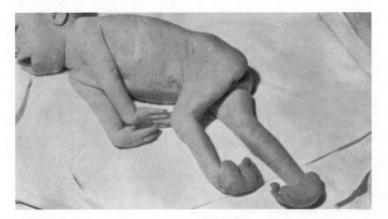

Fig. 20.12
Arthrogryposis multiplex congenita. Note the fixation of all major joints

is unknown. It can occur as an isolated condition or in association with spinal and cerebral disorders that impair fetal movement *in utero*.

Clinical features include:

- immobile joints
- atrophic muscles
- flexion of wrists
- club feet.

Treatment and prognosis
Physiotherapy and surgical repair offer relief, but are not curative. Some improvement occurs with age.

Muscles

Absent abdominal muscles (Fig. 20.13)
Part or all of the musculature of the abdominal wall may be absent at birth. The region resembles a 'prune belly' and the malformation is known as the triad syndrome as it is associated with defects of the urinary system, e.g. hydronephrosis, and genital tract, e.g. undescended testes. It occurs more frequently in males and the cause is unknown.

Most of the infants die from chronic renal failure.

Absent depressor anguli oris (Fig. 20.14)
One side of the lower lip may not move during crying. This is due to hypoplasia of the muscle on that side. It is known as Cayler syndrome and may be associated

with abnormalities such as congenital heart disease. The defect can be distinguished from seventh-nerve palsy in that the eye and cheek muscles are not involved.

Sternomastoid tumour
This unilateral condition is seen mostly with breech deliveries. It probably results from damage to the muscle fibres by bleeding. Signs may be absent during the

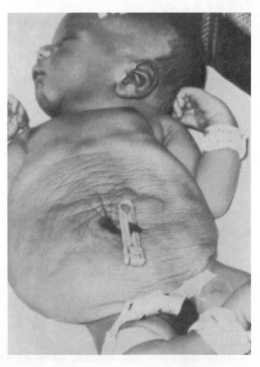

Fig. 20.13 *The 'prune-belly' syndrome*

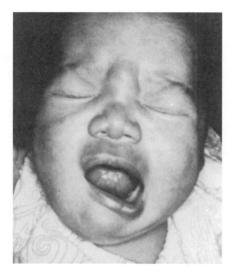

Fig. 20.14 *Cayler syndrome. During crying the eyes can close but the mouth is deviated to one side*

first week of life. Later a firm and painless swelling is noted in the sternomastoid. The muscle shortens and produces torticollis as it pulls the head to one side.

Treatment
Active exercise of the neck. The shortened muscles are stretched by turning the baby's head in the opposite direction and flexing it simultaneously 20–30 times towards the unaffected side. This should be done two or three times a day.

If the condition has not improved by the age of two years, surgical repair should be done.

FRACTURES
Skull
A fracture may present as an isolated finding or it may be associated with intracranial damage.

Causes
Cephalopelvic disproportion. Poorly applied forceps.

Types
Fractures of the cranial bones may be linear, stellate or depressed. They are usually asymptomatic in the absence of intracranial damage and rarely need treatment. Depressed fractures may heal spontaneously or the bones can be elevated with a silastic vacuum cup. Surgical elevation is seldom required if intracranial pressure is normal.

Limbs
The clavicle is the bone most commonly fractured (Fig. 20.15).

Causes
A difficult delivery associated with impacted shoulders or a breech.

The humerus or femur may also be broken as a result of excessive traction on the limbs during delivery (Fig. 20.16).

Ribs can be fractured during vigorous resuscitation.

Diagnosis
The affected limb is not used (pseudo-paralysis). The infant cries when the

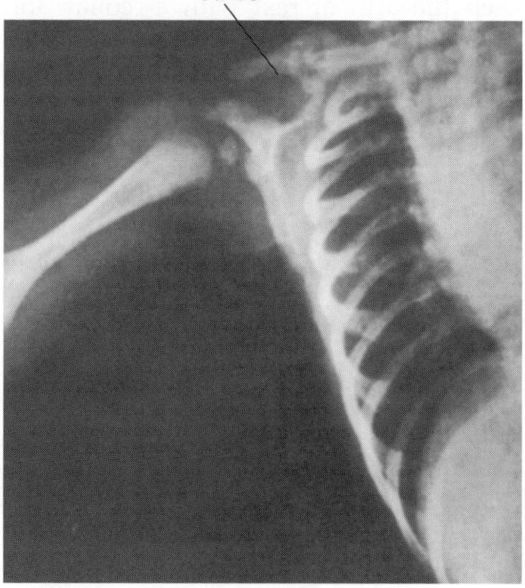

Callus

Fig. 20.15. *Fractured clavicle with callus formation*

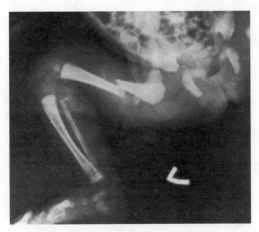

Fig. 20.16 *Fractured shaft of femur*

traumatised area is touched or moved. Swelling may be present over the site of fracture. Crepitus may be felt over the bone. The diagnosis is confirmed on X-ray.

Treatment
Clavicle: No splinting is needed. Do not pull the infant up by the arms. Immobilise the limb on the affected side for a few days by keeping it against the chest under the vest.

Humerus: Flex the elbow to 90° and keep the arm at rest with a 'collar and cuff' sling around the neck and wrist.

Femur: Most fractures require splinting in a Gallow frame.

Prognosis
All fractures have a good prognosis.

Calcification occurs within days to weeks and moulding soon restores the bone to its normal shape.

INFECTIONS

Osteitis and septic arthritis

Bone or joint infections result from septicaemia. Osteitis usually occurs in the metaphysis of long bones, like the femur and humerus, whereas arthritis usually involves the hip joint.

Clinical signs
Local signs of osteitis include:
- pseudoparalysis of a limb
- swelling and tenderness.

Local signs of arthritis include:
- limitation of movement of joint, such as the hip
- swelling and tenderness in that region.

Treatment
- Antibiotics as for septicaemia.

Local therapy includes:
- aspiration of pus from joint
- immobilisation of limb.

Miscellaneous Problems

CRYING
At birth
The only cry eagerly awaited is undoubtedly that which initiates lung expansion at birth. This heralds 'all is well' as air fills the lungs.

A feeble cry at birth must be heeded. It may indicate prematurity, oversedation, hyaline membrane disease, massive aspiration or a generalised abnormality, such as Down's syndrome.

Lack of crying may also be ominous, as it can be associated with respiratory distress, asphyxia or cerebral damage.

After birth
Hunger
This is the most common reason for crying. No healthy baby will keep quiet for more than a few minutes when hungry. The type of cry depends on the infant's personality. It may consist of a few sobs during which the lips are sucked or it may be loud and persistent and accompanied by vigorous sucking of a fist.

Unnecessary crying caused by hunger can be eliminated by feeding the infant on demand.

Loneliness
Illingworth has drawn attention to a problem that occurs more frequently in infants who are kept in nurseries than in those who are kept with their mothers. The nursery infant may cry without any specific reason for up to 2 of the 24 hours.

This is considered to be caused by loneliness and the incidence of crying can be halved by the practice of 'rooming in'.

The only effective way of handling the problem in a nursery is to pick up and cuddle the baby. This does not constitute spoiling, for how can a newborn be considered naughty?

Dissatisfaction
Infants complain vocally if they are too hot, too cold, too tightly wrapped or lying in a damp or soiled nappy.

Babies also resent the switching on of a bright light, being undressed, bathed or placed hastily back into the cot, and will let their feelings be known.

Pain
High-pitched screaming indicates pain, which may be caused by a pin that is pricking the baby's skin, colic or a

fractured bone. In the last condition, the infant usually cries when moved or lifted out of the cot.

Colic

This is one of the most common problems in early life and in some populations affects up to 30% of normal infants. Despite its frequency, no single cause has been identified for all cases.

It is characterised by the rule of three, "crying for more than three hours a day, at least three times a week for more than three weeks".

Early presentation

In the first week of life the baby who is likely to develop colic is excessively alert, unwilling to sleep and restless after feeds.

Clinical features

By the end of the second week the full-blown picture is established.

In a severe case feeding time is interrupted by bouts of high-pitched crying, during which the baby draws up the legs and arches the back. Rocking and patting provide temporary relief, but crying recommences soon after the baby is placed in a cot. Small amounts of milk are sucked and large quantities of air are swallowed.

The mother considers her infant to be excessively hungry and offers more milk, which is eagerly gulped.

Crying can extend from one feed time to the next. The distraught parents consider their baby to be suffering from a serious illness and the tension can be aggravated by neighbours who complain of the noise. A vicious circle ensues as neither mother nor baby are capable of getting sufficient sleep.

In a mild case the spells of restlessness or crying occur after a feed and can last for several hours. This is common after the evening feed. The baby may pass wind, which affords some relief.

Cause

A physical basis has been established. The level of the gut hormone gastrin is raised, but the reason is unclear.

In 60% of cases colic is associated with a sensitivity to cow milk protein. Peptides with antigenic properties can be absorbed from mother's gut into her circulation. They are transported to her breast milk and enter the baby's bowel. Their mode of action is uncertain. Excessive gas fills the large and small intestine and appears to be trapped by spasm of the bowel wall.

Diagnosis

In a healthy baby, a history of recurrent bouts of crying and drawing up of the legs in accoirdance with the rule of three is indicative of colic. The physical examination is normal.

Treatment

Reassurance: Assure parents that their baby is normal and does not have a twisted bowel or ominous disease. Indicate that weight gain is adequate despite crying, and dissuade them from offering extra feeds.

Time off: A colicy baby makes persistent demands on a mother's physical and emotional resources and household members or friends should ensure that she is given frequent breaks. Encourage her to obtain as much sleep as possible, especially at the times when her infant is sleeping.

Antispasmodics: Dicyclamine hydrochloride was used for decades, but since its implication in several cases of apnoea no suitable substitute has been found.

Winding: Excessive air is often swallowed during crying but this does not cause colic.. Remove air by correct winding (p. 49).

Feeds: Colic occurs in both breast- and bottle-fed infants and a change of milk is unlikely to produce relief.

Short-lasting relief: This may be obtained from 2ml. sucrose water 25% sucked from a 'dinky feeder', a car ride, swaddling or carrying baby in a front sling or in a back pouch.

Dietary intervention: Avoidance of cow milk protein by the mother can be dramatically beneficial and a ten-day trial is recommended in severe cases. This implies complete removal and not merely a reduction in the dietary intake. The elimination diet should be supervised by a dietician as a mother may not be aware of occult sources of cow milk protein such as:

- coffee creamers
- packaged soups and cereals
- most margarines
- various sausages, biscuits and chocolates.

The duration of dietary elimination will depend on the infant's response. If colic is cured, introduce one item, such as cheese, after two weeks and note the response. A variable amount of protein may be tolerated before colic recommences. The mother must be provided with adequate calcium if milk products are eliminated for several months.

In bottle-fed babies, a hypoallergenic formula, e.g. NAN HA, can be tried.

Course

Most colicky babies stop crying at about three months – hence 'three-month colic'. "Happy is the physician consulted at the end of a disease", for at this stage most therapies are successful. Those with severe pain improve after three months and are normal by six to nine months.

Earache

Otitis media should be suspected in a baby who cries continuously and cannot be pacified by any means. The eardrums must be examined.

Cerebral cry

Infants who have cerebral damage or meningitis may cry characteristically. They often grunt with each breath in a moaning fashion or cry when the head is touched. When crying is initiated by a stimulus, like a pin-prick, it is often delayed in onset and then persists for longer than normal. Crying may also accompany seizures.

Hoarse or stridulous cry

This may be owing to:
- laryngeal trauma, such as following intubation or vigorous suction
- laryngeal abnormality, for example congenital web
- thyroglossal cyst
- vascular ring
- recurrent laryngeal nerve injury
- goitre.

With experience, it is possible to distinguish the various cries. A mother soon knows whether her infant is hungry or uncomfortable. The cry also serves as a diagnostic sign for specific diseases, e.g. the cry of 'cri-du-chat' syndrome (microcephaly, mental and growth retardation) is cat-like.

PAIN RELIEF

All babies sense pain and the smaller and sicker they are, the more likely are they to experience painful procedures. Quantification of pain is difficult and in hospitals, various scoring systems are used. All have strengths and weaknesses. Scores are based on stress responses such as sleeplessness, crying, grimacing, a raised mean arterial blood pressure, tachycardia and decreased oxygen saturation. If a Score Chart is used, all staff must be familiar with it to ensure validity and reliability.

Nevertheless, certain principles are applicable to all nurseries, none more so than the prevention or limitation of noxious and unpleasant stimuli, so:

- ensure an environment that encourages sleep by avoiding intense light, noise and excessive handling
- offer comforts such as a dummy, soothing talk, gentle stroking, cuddling, nesting, rocking, or kangaroo care and breast-feeding by a mother – this is particularly important following a painful procedure even if analgesia has been used
- change an infant's position frequently and discard soiled or wet napkins
- collect sufficient blood specimens from the minimum number of heel stabs or venesections.

When pain is inevitable, provide appropriate and adequate analgesia prior to a procedure.

- *Sucrose 25% solution:* This is suitable for heel stabs, insertion of catheters, venesections and tracheal suctioning. In premature infants who have a good suck, offer a dummy dipped in the solution about two minutes before the procedure. If sucking is absent instill about 0.1 ml into the mouth with a syringe. For large babies a dose up to 2 ml can be used, followed by a dummy. The effect lasts for up to five minutes and a dose can be repeated if necessary. This does not cause hyperglycaemia.

  Ensure that the solution is renewed daily to prevent bacterial contamination.
- *Paracetamol:* This is suitable for mild to moderate chronic pain such as a headache associated with hypoxic ischaemic encephalopathy. Dose 10 mg/kg. Give this orally up to three times a day for several days.
- *Morphine:* This is reserved for invasive procedures such as tracheal intubation, chest paracentesis, lumbar puncture, restless infants on assisted ventilation and surgical procedures. Dose 0.05 to 0.1 mg/kg,

intravenous or intramuscular about five minutes before the event, when possible.

Example: A 1 kg infant is prescribed 0.05 mg/kg = total 0.05 mg.

Morphine sulphate (5mg/ml). Dilute 0.1ml in 0.9ml of sterile water. This yields a morphine concentration of 0.5 mg/ml. The infant would require 0.1 ml of this solution.

FAILURE TO THRIVE

A baby may fail to gain weight because of an inadequate intake or an excessive loss of food due to vomiting, or diarrhoea. In these cases further investigation and treatment will depend on the underlying cause. Important causes of vomiting are listed on page 203.

Failure to thrive may occur despite a normal intake of food, a normal output of stools and lack of vomiting. In such circumstances the following conditions must be borne in mind:

Late metabolic acidaemia of prematurity

Preterm babies often fail to gain weight after birth. When this continues into the second or third week there is usually an associated metabolic acidaemia, probably as a result of the acidity of cow milk.

But the poor weight gain always precedes acidaemia.

A dramatic gain in weight follows the addition of bicarbonate to the feeds. This substance enhances the absorption of dietary fat.

Dose: Add 3 ml of sodium bicarbonate 4% to each feed for a week.

Idiopathic failure to thrive

A similar failure to gain weight may occur in full-term babies who are fed on cow milk formulae.

These infants usually do not manifest a metabolic acidaemia, but show a rapid gain in weight following the addition of the same amount of bicarbonate to feeds, as indicated above.

Less common, but important, causes of failure to thrive include:

- occult infections, like urinary tract infection and congenital syphilis
- congenital abnormalities, for example a heart defect.

Note

Examine the urine of babies who fail to gain weight, to exclude infection.

Rare cases include:

- inherited metabolic defect (p. 270)
- hypothermia, particularly in the preterm infant
- too little love and attention.

Some babies fail to thrive in an institution but flourish once they are at home in the loving care of their mothers.

FOOD ALLERGY

An infant may produce abnormal amounts of a particular antibody, immunoglobulin E (IgE), to substances called allergens.

These are derived mainly from proteins in food, pollen, mites, animal hairs, etc. The principal allergen in early life is the protein of cow milk.

When an allergen is ingested or inhaled it can stimulate lymphocytes to produce IgE, which is then attached to mast cells in organs such as the skin, respiratory system or gastrointestinal tract.

When the allergen re-enters the body it combines with IgE on the mast cells, which then release vaso-active substances, such as histamine. These act on adjacent smooth muscles, mucous glands and blood vessels to produce a variety of symptoms.

This type of hypersensitivity is known as allergy, but non-IgE mediated sensitivity can also occur in early life from the absorbtion of portions of antigenic proteins like casein or whey through the gut mucosa.

Incidence

The reported incidence varies from 1–4% in infancy and increases to 4–20% in childhood.

The likelihood of allergy depends mostly on a genetic disposition. The infant of an allergic parent has a 40% chance of being affected. The risk increases to 70% if both parents, or one parent and a sibling, are allergic.

Initial sensitisation

Before birth

A raised level of IgE in cord blood is associated with a significant risk of future allergy. The antibody is produced by the fetus and does not cross the placenta. It probably reflects a response to allergens that have been transmitted across the placenta.

After birth

The porous gut of a baby (p. 210) permits large peptides to be absorbed into the circulation. This is the most significant route for sensitisation in infancy and various factors can increase gut permeability. They include:

- prematurity
- necrotising enterocolitis
- gastroenteritis
- IgA deficiency.

Clinical presentation

The signs and symptoms of allergy probably depend on the degree of sensitisation and may not be obvious for weeks, months or years after birth. They cannot be fully discussed in this book.

The involvement of multiple organs in allergy poses a diagnostic dilemma and the widespread features that are compatible with it should be interpreted with caution.

Common manifestations in infants are summarised below.

General: Persistent restlessness, irritability, lack of sleep.

Gastrointestinal: Colic, diarrhoea,

vomiting. Anaemia can result from the loss of red cells in stools.

Respiratory: Persistent blocked nose or nasal discharge. Recurrent colds, cough or wheeziness. Serous otitis media.

Skin: Rough and reddened cheeks. Eczema.

Be suspicious of recurrent or persistent signs like a 'runny nose'. Unless the infant has been in direct contact with an infected person, such a feature is likely to be due to allergy. This and eczema of the cheeks are probably the most frequent early features of allergy and can manifest within weeks of birth.

Treatment
The infant who has been fed cow milk only should respond to a milk formula in which the protein has been extensively hydrolysed (p.56). This is expensive but probably cost effective if hospital, doctor and medication bills are taken into consideration.

The baby on solid food would require a similar milk. In addition, major sensitisers such as wheat, eggs, dairy products, soy and peanuts must be removed. This process must be supervised by a dietician and pursued for several years.

Anaphylactoid reaction
The ingestion of a small quantity of an allergen, such as cow milk, may cause alarming features. This is rare.

Signs include:
- oedema of lips or tongue
- sweating
- tachycardia
- diarrhoea
- vomiting
- cyanosis.

Prevention
Prophylaxis is most important in the newborn. The symptoms of allergy can be delayed or diminished when there is a family history, a high level of IgE in cord blood, or an increase in gut permeability.

- Encourage a lactating woman to avoid foodstuffs that could sensitise her infant, for example cow milk. This advice must be weighed against financial or other difficulties that arise from dieting.
- Ensure exclusive breastfeeding for six months and then introduce single-ingredient foods, one at a time. A suitable weaning cereal is rice, which can be mixed with water or breast milk
- Encourage breast-feeding for 18 months, preferably longer
- Omit wheat, eggs and cow milk for 24 months.
- Avoid peanuts for three years.

A dietary programme should be devised in association with a dietician to ensure adequate nutrition and growth.

The non-breast-fed infant poses a major problem. Soy products have been used as a substitute for cow milk, but sensitisation can occur in up to 40% of infants. This also applies to goat milk.

Nan HA is a partially hydrolysed cow-protein milk that is suitable for prevention but it too can cause sensitisation in about 15 to 20% of cases. If this happens, an extensively hydrolysed product should be considered. A major draw-back is cost.

GRIEF

Parents
The lives of parents can be disrupted by devastating perinatal events, such as the birth of:
- a still birth
- a preterm baby
- a baby who is temporarily or permanently handicapped
- a baby who dies.

The ensuing grief is characterised by stages of shock, disbelief, sadness, guilt and, finally, acceptance. The degree and duration of these is related to the parents' anticipation of the event and their ability to adjust to the situation.

Shock

A mother may experience overwhelming shock when she observes or is informed of her malformed or dying infant.

Pallor, nausea, weakness and confusion occur, and she may be unable to comprehend what has happened or what is being said.

This reaction of shock places great responsibility on the person who has to inform parents of an unpleasant diagnosis, and demands caution, tact and sympathy. The initial comments will always be remembered even though subsequent discussions tend to be forgotten.

Disbelief

The initial blow is cushioned by a denial of the event. The diagnosis may be repeatedly queried and alternative opinions sought or requested. The parents might ignore the seriousness of the situation by referring to their infant in terms that negate any problem.

Sadness and guilt

The reality of the event is eventually perceived and bouts of anger, sadness, frustration, guilt or inadequacy may occur. These are attempts to explain the loss of an infant who was meant to be perfect and to fulfill numerous desires.

Acceptance

The mother's acute physical and emotional disturbances subside as the inevitability of the situation is accepted. Grieving continues for months and is manifested by periods of exhaustion or depression, which are normal features of the process.

Mourning is a painful experience and parents progress through its stages in different ways. Those who have a permanently handicapped child may experience sorrow throughout their lives as persistent demands are made upon their physical and emotional resources. Continual support is essential to enable them to identify and enhance the fruitful aspects of their infant.

They seek help from each other and from close friends, relatives or ministers of religion. They may also need the support of parents who have experienced similar crises and might wish to contact them through relevant organisations, such as Down's Association, preterm infant groups, etc.

For some, solitude is more important than interpersonal relations. Respect this desire to be alone.

Staff

The response of medical and nursing staff to a perinatal crisis can be summarised in a series of questions and answers.

Who should tell?

The doctor in charge of the infant is responsible for imparting relevant information to the parents. This hardship cannot be imposed upon nursing staff committed to a close and constant emotional bond with the parents and infant. Their supportive role will assume greater proportions in the crisis-laden days ahead as they bear the brunt of parental grief, anger and queries.

Whom to tell?

Both parents should be informed of the relevant facts. A mother requires the support of her partner and feels helpless when she is presented with information that is overwhelming. Occasionally this is not possible, for example a father will have to be told of the crisis while the mother is under general anaesthesia.

Where to tell?

Privacy is essential as it allows parents to express their emotions.

What to say?

Caution is of the essence. Devastating details are imparted only when a degree of certainty has been established.

An honest appraisal is essential, yet relevant hope must never be shattered. Always emphasise the normal or correctable aspects of the problem. For example, a baby with a bilateral cleft lip affords an awful spectacle yet has an excellent prognosis. Highlight this by showing the parents pictures of similar lesions that have been successfully corrected.

Why did it happen?

An explanation is constantly sought and questions such as "Do you think that the fall I had during pregnancy could have caused it?" are repeatedly asked. They imply feelings of guilt and parents need the reassurance that their thoughts or actions cannot be implicated.

What can be done?

The anticipated joyful association with a baby is abruptly disrupted and replaced by fears of death or brain damage. Parents may hesitate to name the baby or to make physical contact.

The grief process can be facilitated by encouraging close contact between the parents and baby, regardless of the crisis.

A nurse should prepare the parents for their first encounter by outlining the baby's appearance, such as very immature, always stressing the normal aspects. The actual features, even of a malformed infant, are less alarming to parents than the mental picture they may have formed.

Photographs of the baby may be sent to a mother who is unable to visit.

The nurse may need to allay fears by explaining the functions of an array of equipment that surrounds the baby. She should accompany the parents on their first visit, but subsequently they may wish to be left alone with their infant.

Promote breast-feeding where at all possible and encourage the mother to participate in the daily care of her baby. Kangaroo care is particularly therapeutic and enables the mother to regain self-esteem.

Respect religious affiliations and be ready to summon a minister at the request of parents.

When death is inevitable, urge the parents to hold and cuddle their baby. Monitoring devices are removed, the area is screened and staff withdraw at the moment of death. A mother may wish to caress and dress her dead infant including one who was stillborn before other formalities are completed.

A period of confusion may follow and advice should be offered regarding the necessities of death and registration certificates and a burial or cremation. A doctor may wish to discuss an autopsy, which would aid the diagnosis or outlook of future pregnancies.

Disorders that have long-term implications, such as Down's syndrome or meningomyelocele, are managed with short-term objectives. Encourage parents to master current problems rather than concern themselves with the ultimate outlook. Infancy is not an appropriate time to place a baby in an institution. The matter can be addressed at a later stage.

Will it happen again?

Another baby cannot take the place of the one who is imperfect or dead, and pregnancy should not be contemplated until mourning has been fulfilled. This may take 6 to 12 months and the parents can then prepare for a new infant.

Make every effort to determine the cause of the problem and obtain relevant genetic information in the case of an inherited disease.

Where applicable, adopt an optimistic attitude for future pregnancies and maintain contact so that relevant information can be reviewed from autopsy or other investigations.

ETHICAL AND MORAL ISSUES

The words 'ethics' and 'morals' have similar Greek and Latin roots.

Ethics probes and defines a general doctrine for right and wrong behaviour, such as the Hippocratic oath. Morals refer to the mode of conduct of individuals or communities, like the observation of the Ten Commandments.

These meanings have altered greatly in recent times. The Hippocratic oath, for example, served the medical profession as a code of conduct for over 2 000 years. It is barely recognised at present. The religious convictions that determined an individual's behaviour and served as a conscience have been abandoned in many instances. These changes have influenced attitudes towards ill or learning disabled babies and have prompted many emotive questions, some of which are mentioned below.

Should infants with gross abnormalities be starved?
This has been proposed and promoted in cases where irreparable brain damage has occurred. Treatment has been withheld and sedation has been used to suppress hunger.

Should concern for parents and society equal that for an infant?
Treatment may be withheld for bowel atresia in an infant with Down's syndrome because of the desires and attitudes of the parents.

The legal implications of such actions are uncertain as they have not been subjected to court trial in southern Africa. They could amount to an active promotion of death.

Should infants be treated with all available therapy irrespective of the severity of their handicap or their expectation of life?

A grossly immature baby of 24 weeks' gestation is resuscitated at birth and then kept alive by assisted ventilation and parenteral nutrition. At this age the lungs are barely capable of sustaining life in an air environment, and therapy could be viewed as prolonging the process of death.

At present there are no universal guidelines to these and many other vexing problems.

The following approach reflects the views of the author:

The obligation of medical and nursing staff is primarily towards their patient and then to the parents and society. Consequently, the needs of an infant are considered *before* those of other parties.

Parents are informed of all aspects of a problem and advised that decisions are made in the interest of their infant.

Decisions regarding therapy of a malformed infant, e.g. Down's syndrome, are much the same as those for a normal infant.

Therapy that merely prolongs dying is futile, for example assisted ventilation would not be used for an anencephalic infant. Death should not be induced nor should extraordinary measures be used to extend life.

However, treatment is always provided if doubt exists as to the ultimate outcome of a particular problem.

Infants are entitled to have their basic needs satisfied irrespective of the nature of their problems. This would normally include adequate warmth, food, nursing care and affection.

Ethics committees have been set up in many medical centres. Until recently their main function has been the review and assessment of research programmes. This function has been extended to the problems discussed above and incorporates a wide range of opinions, such as those of clergy, lawyers, social workers, psychiatrists, etc.

CHAPTER 22

Drugs and Dosages

Many drugs are potentially harmful to the developing fetus and newborn infant. Before medication is given to a baby or a pregnant woman, consider the following:

- Is the drug really necessary?
- Is it likely to be effective?
- Is the dosage safe?
- Are side-effects likely to occur?

DRUGS GIVEN TO THE PREGNANT WOMAN

Effect on the fetus

Drugs can impair organ formation, organ function or fetal growth *in utero*.

Organ formation

The period of organogenesis up to 12 weeks is a time of maximum risk for malformations and abortion. No medication can be considered entirely safe during this period and caution must be observed when prescribing for a woman of childbearing age.

Live virus vaccines, such as yellow fever, can severely damage the fetus and should be avoided.

Drugs that may cause malformations are categorised into five groups, depending on risks:

1. No increased risk of abnormalities,

for example folic acid, paracetamol, amoxycillin.
2. Unconfirmed adverse effects, for example amoxycillin with clavulanic acid, ceftriaxone.
3. Inadequate studies to confirm effects; medication requires a prescription, for example rifampicin.
4. Potential risks may be outweighed by beneficial effects; use with caution (Table 22.1).
5. Confirmed risks outweigh beneficial effects; not to be used in pregnancy (Table 22.2).

TABLE 22.1

Drugs to be used with caution in pregnancy	
Name	*Hazard*
ACE inhibitor	Oligohydramnios, growth retardation
Aminoglycoside	Ototoxic, deafness
Aspirin	Gastroschesis, closure *ductus arteriosus*
Benzodiazepine	Cleft lip
Carbamazepine	Spina bifida
Corticosteroid	Cleft lip/palate
Fluconazole	Cranio-facial defects
Lithium	Cardiac abnormalities
Phenytoin	Microcephaly, broad nose
Valproic acid	Spina bifida

TABLE 22.2

Drugs to avoid during pregnancy

Name	Hazard
Alcohol	Microcephaly multiple defects
Androgen	Masculinisation of genitalia
Antimetabolite	Multiple defects
Diethylstilboestrol	Uterine abnormalities, vaginal cancer
Ergotamine	Ototoxic, deafness
Misoprostol	Facial paralysis
Methotrexate	Multiple abnormalities
Retinoic acid	Cranio-facial, heart defects
Tetracycline	Permanent stains of teeth
Thalidomide	Limb defects
Warfarin	Nasal hypoplasia, microcephaly

Organ function (Table 22.3)
The function of fetal organs can be impaired after the stage of organogenesis by a variety of drugs that cross the placenta, for example dicuomarol, which may cause hypoprothrombinaemia and result in severe bleeding and fetal death.

Growth impairment
Maternal addiction to cigarettes or alcohol is associated with impaired fetal growth, particularly during the third trimester.

Effects on the newborn (Table 22.3)
Medication given during pregnancy or in labour can cross the placenta to harm the baby, for example antenatal use of tolbutamide or chloramphenicol may cause fetal thrombocytopenia with resultant purpura after birth. Antiepileptic drugs, for example phenytoin, can cause haemorrhagic disease owing to the depletion of vitamin K_1-dependent clotting factors. Analgesics such as pethidine and morphine can cross the placenta during labour, particularly after intravenous injection, and cause respiratory depression at birth. Anti-inflammatories like indomethacin can cause premature closure of the ductus arteriosus, as well as impaired renal function.

Typical withdrawal effects may be observed in the offspring of mothers who were addicted to so-called 'recreational drugs', such as dagga, heroin and cocaine. Phenobarbitone can also cause these features.

Iodine compounds can produce goitre, and thiouracil may cause hypothyroidism.

Delayed effects
The long-term effects of many drugs are still unknown. Evidence indicates that side-effects can be delayed for many years, for example prolonged oestrogen therapy during pregnancy is associated with an increased risk of genital carcinoma in female offspring 15 to 20 years after birth.

DRUGS EXCRETED IN BREAST MILK

Many drugs ingested by the lactating mother will be excreted in her milk. In the majority of cases, the concentration is insignificant, at less than 1% of maternal dose, and does not contraindicate breast-feeding. In other cases, a drug may be excreted in significant amounts, but either it is not absorbed by the infant's gut, for example streptomycin, or its nature does not warrant discontinuation of feeding, for example penicillin.

Guidelines for breastfeeding mothers:
- Take a medicine only if it is absolutely necessary.
- Use the lowest appropriate dose for the shortest period.
- Take the medicine after a feed to reduce the amount excreted in the milk.
- Observe any reactions in the baby, like rashes, diarrhoea, colic, drowsiness.

TABLE 22.3

Side-effects of drugs given during labour	
Name	*Possible effect on fetus or newborn*
Anaesthetics	
Short-acting barbiturates	Respiratory depression at birth
Volatile anaesthetics	Respiratory depression at birth
Local anaesthetics	Respiratory depression if injected into scalp during labour
Analgesics	
Morphine	Respiratory depression at birth
Pethidine	Respiratory depression at birth
Aspirin	Bleeding tendency
Antibacterials	
Tetracycline	Yellow staining of teeth
Sulphonamide	Increased risk of kernicterus
Antihypertensives	
Reserpine	Stuffy nose
Hexamethonium	Ileus
Induction of labour	
Oxytocin	Hyperbilirubinaemia
Prostaglandin	Hyperbilirubinaemia
Sedative hypnotics	
Diazepam	Poor sucking, lethargy
Midazolam	Poor sucking, lethargy
Magnesium sulphate	Lethargy, hypotonia, respiratory depression

Drugs that have deleterious effects on infants are listed in Table 22.4. They should not be taken during lactation.

TABLE 22.4

Drugs contraindicated in breastfeeding	
Drug	*Side-effect on infant*
Tetracycline	Yellow staining of teeth
Iodine	Thyroid goitre
Ergotamine	Diarrhoea, vomiting
Cytotoxics	Cell damage
Radio-active compounds	Radiation
Phenindione	Bleeding
Lithium	Hypotonia
Bromocriptine	Inadequate milk production

Alternatives can usually be found, for example tetracycline may be replaced by another broad-spectrum antibiotic, while warfarin may be used as a substitute for phenindione.

Pay attention to various creams applied to the nipple, which may be ingested by the infant. A bland preparation such as lanolin is safe, whereas a substance that contains toxic products, for example lead acetate or borax, is not safe.

DRUGS COMMONLY USED

The newborn, particularly if premature, has a limited ability to metabolise and excrete drugs. Consequently, the safe and effective dose of a specific medication is not necessarily based on scaled-down adult values.

Physicians must be familiar with commonly used drugs and their potential side-effects. Nurses must ensure that a prescribed drug is given to the right infant in the correct amount at the precise intervals.

Many drugs used for infants have not been registered for this age group, so avoid new or unfamiliar medications, as the side-effects may be entirely unexpected or unknown.

The following drugs are commonly used for the newborn:

Oxygen
Indication
Hypoxaemia.

Complications
- Retinopathy (retrolental fibroplasias) (p. 155).
- Lung damage (p. 177).

Vitamins
These organic compounds are essential for normal growth.

Vitamin K_1
This product is required for the formation of prothrombin, an essential factor in blood clotting. Hypoprothrombinaemia causes haemorrhagic disease.

Treatment: Give Vitamin K_1 1 mg intramuscularly to all infants at birth to prevent haemorrhagic disease. The initial dose may have to be repeated if a bleeding tendency has been caused by anticoagulants or anticonvulsants.

Vitamin C
The newborn usually has adequate stores of water-soluble vitamin C and does not suffer from scurvy.

Daily requirements: 25–30 mg. Breast milk contains over 4 mg/100 ml and should provide adequate amounts. The vitamin may be lacking in artificial milks as it is destroyed by boiling. Infants on formulae should receive supplementary vitamin C in vitamin drops or fruit juices, for example rose hip syrup.

Vitamin D
Daily requirements:
   Full-term 400 IU.
   (International units.)
   Preterm 800 IU.

Sunlight converts 7-dehydrocholesterol in the skin to vitamin D, but this source cannot be relied upon in winter months and in temperate climates. In such circumstances bottle-fed babies may need supplementary vitamin D as the milk yield is less than 100 IU per day. All preterm babies will require vitamin D supplements. This may be given as vitamin drops.

Toxic effects: Overdosage can cause vomiting, constipation, hypotonia, kidney damage and metastatic calcification.

Note
Human breast milk contains adequate amounts of vitamin D, provided that the mother is well nourished.

Vitamin E
The fat-soluble vitamin E is necessary for muscle development and for erythrocyte stability. Deficiency can cause haemolytic anaemia and is likely to occur in preterm babies.

Daily requirements: 0,5 mg/kg.

Vitamin A
Breast milk is rich in fat-soluble vitamin A. Deficiency can be caused by malabsorption, for example cystic fibrosis, or by a fat-free diet, for example skimmed milk.

Daily requirements: 1 500–3 000 IU.

Toxic effects: Overdosage can cause vomiting, bulging of the fontanelle, papilloedema and thickening of bones.

Vitamin B complex
Breast and cow milk contain adequate amounts of this group and deficiency states are rare in the newborn.
   Daily requirements:
   Thiamine 0,4 mg.
   Riboflavine 0,6 mg.
   Niacin 4,0 mg.

Suitable vitamin preparations
Drops are preferable, as syrups can cause pneumonia if inhaled. Suitable products include Abidec® drops and Vi-daylin® drops.

Note
Overdosage with vitamins can be as harmful as deficiency. Check the vitamin content of milks and cereals before prescribing supplementation.

Iron
Iron is an essential component of haemoglobin. The metal, in the ferrous state, is absorbed from the gut, bound to plasma transferrin and then stored in various organs as ferritin. Red cell breakdown releases iron, which is reused for the formation of haemoglobin in new erythrocytes. The haemoglobin, liver, spleen, kidneys and bone marrow of a newborn are estimated to contain 250 mg of iron.
   Additional iron is required during the growing period as the total red cell mass increases. This must be provided in the diet.
   Daily requirements of elemental iron:
   Full-term 1 mg/kg;
   preterm 1,5–2 mg/kg.

Breast milk contains relatively small quantities of iron, yet absorption is highly efficient and a deficiency is unlikely to occur in the baby who is entirely breast-fed.
   Supplements will be needed in:
- artificially fed full-term babies
- preterm babies.

Iron preparations
Oral products:
   Ferrous sulphate syrup – 25 mg elemental iron per 5 ml.
   Ferrous lactate (Ferro Drops®) – 25 mg elemental iron per 1 ml.
   Ferrous gluconate (Ferlucon®) – 30 mg elemental iron per 5 ml.

Note
Iron supplements are preferably avoided in the first month, as they may saturate transferrin and render an infant more susceptible to bacterial infection, for example *E. coli*.

Antibacterial agents
Indications for antibacterial therapy include:
- a 'contaminated' baby (p. 91)
- established infection, for example pneumonia
- hazardous procedures, for example indwelling arterial catheter.

Discontinue antibiotic therapy within 72 hours if bacterial infection has not been established.
   Severe infections like meningitis, osteomyelitis and septicaemia must be treated for at least 10 to 14 days.

Drugs to avoid
Certain systemic antibacterial drugs can have adverse effects on the newborn and should be avoided. They include the following:
- *Chloramphenicol:* 'Grey syndrome', that is, a shock-like state.
- *Novobiocin:* Increased susceptibility to kernicterus.
- *Sulphonamides:* Increased susceptibility to kernicterus.
- *Streptomycin:* Deafness.
- *Tetracycline:* Yellow staining of teeth.

METHOD OF PRESCRIPTION

A preterm baby could receive more than 20 medications during hospitalisation, for example oxygen, naloxone, bicarbonate, antibiotics, vitamins, iron, theophylline, indomethacin, furosemide, blood, etc.

The risk of dosage errors is ever present, but can be minimised through the use of these guidelines:

- Use only paediatric preparations.
- When prescribing in micrograms, ensure that a conversion from milligrams is correct (Table 22.5) and write 'micrograms' in full. Avoid the abbreviations 'μ' and 'mcg'.
- Two staff members must check the quantity, frequency and duration of a prescribed drug.
- Whenever possible, use the oral route. It is effective and far safer for hazardous drugs like digoxin.
- Determine serum levels of potentially harmful drugs such as oxygen, phenobarbitone, aminophylline, digoxin and aminoglycosides (trough and peak).
- When diluting a drug, draw up some diluent into a 1 ml syringe before introducing the medication. Then add more diluent to the required volume.
- Prescribe potentially hazardous drugs in standard amounts where possible. The frequency of administration will vary with the baby's age after birth and with maturity.

Example
The dose of gentamicin ranges from 3 to 7,5 mg/kg/day, and the quantities ordered for numerous infants in a nursery may vary considerably. The chance of miscalculation can be reduced by prescribing fixed amounts, such as:

- 3 mg to be given 24-hourly – for babies less than 1 500 g
- 3 mg to be given 12-hourly – for larger and older babies.

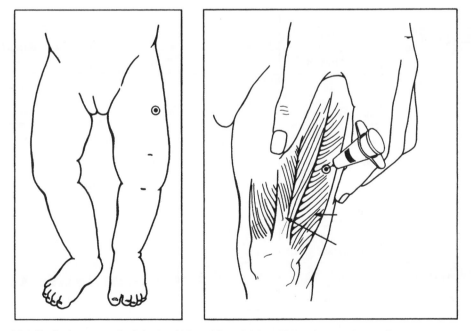

Fig. 22.1 *Site for intramuscular injection (Adapted from Scipien, GM et al. 1979.* Comprehensive Pediatric Nursing. *Place of publication: McGraw-Hill)*

Prescribe each item on a drug chart and fill in dates and times ahead of schedule for the entire course. The dose is entered and initialled in the relevant blocks each time the drug is given.

The initial dose, particularly of antibiotics, should be given immediately and not delayed several hours to fit a customary schedule, for example if gentamicin is prescribed at 07h00, to be given 12-hourly, the first amount is given at 07h00 and not held over until 12 noon.

Potentially harmful drugs are likely to be given intravenously or intramuscularly rather than by mouth because of their composition, for example aminoglycosides, or because of the state of the infant.

For intravenous infusions use a separate infusion pump.

Identify nasogastric and venous tubes with labels of different colours to avoid using the incorrect route.

Intramuscular injection
Use a tuberculin syringe fitted with a 26-gauge needle, and ensure that the total volume to be injected does not exceed 0,5 ml. Squeeze the muscle mass of the antero-lateral thigh between a thumb and forefinger and insert the needle into this site.

Note
NEVER inject into the buttock, as the drug may infiltrate the sciatic nerve and cause permanent damage.

TABLE 22.5

Drug tables

Abbreviations: O = oral; IM = Intramuscular; IV = Intravenous; Top = local, SC = subcutaneous; Prem. = preterm
l = litre; kg = kilogram; mg = milligram; µg = microgram;
ml = millilitre; ppm = parts per million; IU = international units.
Dosages and frequencies are not included for extremely premature infants

Drug	Dose	Frequency	Route	Comment
Analgesics				
Morphine	0.05–0.1 mg/kg/dose	4–6 hours	IM, IV	

Paracetamol
  Term
  Prem
	
	10 mg/kg/dose
	10 mg/kg/dose
		
		6 hours
		12 hours
			
			O
			O	

Anticonvulsants				
Midazolam	20–60 µg/ kg/ hour		IV infusion	Mix 4mg/kg in 20 ml 5% Dextrose water 0.1ml / hour = 20µg/kg/hour
Diazepam	0,2 mg/kg/dose	Once	IV	Can cause apnoea
Phenobarbitone	10–20 mg/kg/dose 3 mg/kg/dose	Once 24 hours	IV O, IM, IV	Loading dose Maintenance
Antimicrobials				
Acyclovir	5–10 mg/kg/dose	24 hours	IV	Herpes simplex
Amikacin	15 mg/kg/dose	24 hours	IM, IV	*Pseudomonas*

Drug	Dose	Frequency	Route	Comment
Amoxycillin	25–50 mg /kg /dose	12 hours	0, IV	
Ceftriaxone	50 mg/kg/dose	24 hours	IM, IV	Avoid calcium
Chloramphenicol ointment	Into eyes	8 hours	Top	Bacterial conjunctivitis
Cloxacillin	25–50 mg/kg/dose	12 hours	0, IM, IV	
Erythromycin Term Prem	 10–20 mg/kg/dose 5–10 mg/kg/dose	 12 hours 12 hours	 0 0	Chlamydia
Flucloxacillin	25–50 mg /kg /dose	Term 8 hours Prem 12 hours	0 0	*Staph. aureus*
Fusidic acid	15 mg/kg/dose	8 hours	0	Enterococcus
Ganciclovir	6 mg/kg/dose	12 hours	IV	Cytomegalovirus (2 weeks)
Gentamicin	3 mg/kg/dose	Term 12 hours Prem 24 hours	IM, IV	serum levels peak 5–8 mg/l trough 1–2 mg/l
Isoniazid	10 mg/kg/dose	24 hours	0	Tuberculosis
Kanamycin Term Prem	 10 mg/dose 5 mg/dose	 2 hours 2 hours	 0 0	Gastroenteritis 3 day course
Nystatin drops	1,0 ml/dose	6 hours	0	*Candida albicans*
Procaine penicillin	50 mg/kg/dose	24 hours	IM	Syphilis (10 days)
Benzyl penicillin	25 mg/kg/dose	12 hours	IM	
Piperacillin	50–100 mg /kg/dose	Term 12 hours Prem 12 hours	IV IV	Infuse over 1 hour Pseudomonas
Vancomycin	15 mg/kg/dose	24 hours	IV	Resistant Staph. organisms
Cardiovascular				
Indomethacin	0,05–0,1 mg/kg/dose	24 hours	IV	Patent ductus arteriosus
Digoxin drops	0.005 mg /kg/dose	Term 12 hours Prem 24 hours	0 0	Heart failure (p. 199)
Propranolol	0,02–0,1 mg/kg/dose	6 hours	IV	Infuse over 10 minutes
Prostaglandin E	125 µg/dose	Hourly	0	Maintain patency of ductus
Furosemide	0,5–1 mg/kg/dose	24 hours	0, IM, IV	

Drug	Dose	Frequency	Route	Comment
Gamma globulins				
Hepatitis B immunoglobulin	200 IU (2 ml)	Once	IM	
Zoster immuno-globulin	0,1 mg/kg/dose	Once	IM	Chickenpox contact within 72 hours
Hormones				
Dexamethasone	0,25 mg/kg/dose	12 hours	O	Three doses for tracheal oedema
reduce to	0,075 mg/kg/dose 0,01 mg/kg/dose	12 hours 12 hours	O O	chronic lung disease (10 days)
Erythropoietin	200 units/kg/dose	Once a week	SC	Prevention of anaemia of prematurity
Fluorohydrocortisone	0,125 mg/kg/dose	12 hours	O	Salt-losing adrenal hyperplasia
Glucagon	50–100 µg/kg/dose	12 hours	IM, IV	Hypoglycaemia
Hydrocortisone	1 mg–3 mg/kg/dose	8 hours	IM, IV	Hypoglycaemia
Prednisone	0,2–1 mg/kg/dose	12 hours	O	
Thyroxine	0,01 mg/kg/dose	24 hours	O	Check T_4 and TSH
Minerals				
Calcium gluconate 10%	100–200 mg/kg/dose (1–2 ml/kg)	Once	IV	Dilute and inject over 10 minutes
Calcium Sandoz syrup	15 mg/kg/dose	8 hours	O	In feeds
Magnesium sulphate 50%	50–100 mg/kg/dose 0,1–0,2 ml/kg	Once	IM	Hypomagnesaemia
Iron drops	1–2 mg/kg/dose	24 hours	O	
Sodium fluoride drops	0,5 mg/dose	24 hours	O	If fluoride in water less than 0,3PPM
Respiratory stimulants				
Theophylline	4–6 mg/kg/dose 1 mg/kg/dose	Once 6 hours	O O	Loading dose Maintenance dose
Naloxone	0,01–0,1 mg/kg/dose	Once	IM, IV	
Sedatives				
Chloral hydrate	15–30 mg/dose	8 hours	O	
Vitamins				
A	1 500 IU/dose	24 hours	O	

Drug	Dose	Frequency	Route	Comment
B				
Thiamine	0,4 mg/dose	24 hours	O	
Riboflavine	0,6 mg/dose	24 hours	O	
Niacin	4,0 mg/dose	24 hours	O	
B6	5,0 mg/dose	24 hours	O	
Folic acid	1,0 mg/dose	24 hours	O, IM	
C	25–30 mg/dose	24 hours	O	
D	400–800 IU/dose	24 hours	O	
E	0,5 mg/kg/dose	24 hours	O	
K_1	1 mg/dose	Once	IM	
Volume expanders				
Normal saline	10–20 ml/kg/dose		IV	
Blood				
Whole	10–20 ml/kg/dose		IV	
Packed cells	5–10 ml/kg/dose		IV	
Stabilised human serum	10–20 ml/kg/dose		IV	

Table 22.6 Conversion Milligrams to Micrograms

Milligram	Microgram	Milligram	Microgram	Milligram	Microgram	Milligram	Microgram
0 ,001	1	0,01	10	0,1	100	1	1 000
0,002	2	0,02	20	0,2	200	2	2 000
0,003	3	0,03	30	0,3	300	3	3 000
0,004	4	0,04	40	0,4	400	4	4 000
0,005	5	0,05	50	0,5	500	5	5 000
0,006	6	0,06	60	0,6	600	6	6 000
0,007	7	0,07	70	0,7	700	7	7 000
0,008	8	0,08	80	0,8	800	8	8 000
0,009	9	0,09	90	0,9	900	9	9 000

Index